Environmental Epidemiology

Principles and Methods

Ray M. Merrill, PhD, MPH
Professor of Biostatistics and Epidemiology
Department of Health Science
Brigham Young University
Provo, Utah

D0162437

JONES AND BARTLETT PUBLISHERS

Sudbury, Massachusetts

BOSTON   TORONTO   LONDON   SINGAPORE

World Headquarters

Jones and Bartlett Publishers
40 Tall Pine Drive
Sudbury, MA 01776
978-443-5000
info@jbpub.com
www.jbpub.com

Jones and Bartlett Publishers
Canada
6339 Ormindale Way
Mississauga, Ontario L5V 1J2
Canada

Jones and Bartlett Publishers
International
Barb House, Barb Mews
London W6 7PA
United Kingdom

Jones and Bartlett's books and products are available through most bookstores and online booksellers. To contact Jones and Bartlett Publishers directly, call 800-832-0034, fax 978-443-8000, or visit our website www.jbpub.com.

Substantial discounts on bulk quantities of Jones and Bartlett's publications are available to corporations, professional associations, and other qualified organizations. For details and specific discount information, contact the special sales department at Jones and Bartlett via the above contact information or send an email to specialsales@jbpub.com.

This publication is designed to provide accurate and authoritative information in regard to the Subject Matter covered. It is sold with the understanding that the publisher is not engaged in rendering legal, accounting, or other professional service. If legal advice or other expert assistance is required, the service of a competent professional person should be sought.

Production Credits

Publisher: Michael Brown
Production Director: Amy Rose
Associate Editor: Katey Birtcher
Production Editor: Tracey Chapman
Production Assistant: Roya Millard
Marketing Manager: Sophie Fleck
Manufacturing Buyer: Therese Connell
Composition: Publishers' Design and Production
   Services, Inc.

Cover Design: Kate Ternullo
Photo Research Manager and Photographer:
   Kimberly Potvin
Photo Researcher: Timothy Renzi
Cover Image: © Lisa Hoang/Shutterstock, Inc.
Printing and Binding: Malloy, Inc.
Cover Printing: Malloy, Inc.

Library of Congress Cataloging-in-Publication Data

Merrill, Ray M.
   Environmental epidemiology : principles and methods / Ray Merrill.
      p. ; cm.
Includes bibliographical references and index.
   ISBN-13: 978-0-7637-4152-5 (pbk.)
   ISBN-10: 0-7637-4152-3 (pbk.)
   1. Environmental health. 2. Environmental monitoring. 3. Environmentally induced diseases—Epidemiology. I. Title.
   [DNLM: 1. Environmental Monitoring—methods. 2. Environmental Health. 3. Epidemiologic Factors. 4. Epidemiologic Methods. WA 670 M571e 2008]
   RA566.M457 2008
   614.5'99—dc22

                                  2007031436
6048

Printed in the United States of America
11 10 09 08 07   10 9 8 7 6 5 4 3 2 1

Contents

About the Author

Ray M. Merrill, PhD, MPH, is a professor of biostatistics and epidemiology at Brigham Young University. He has taught biostatistics and epidemiology classes in the Department of Health Science since coming to BYU in 1998. His graduate training includes an MS in managerial economics from BYU, a PhD in applied statistics from Arizona State University, and an MPH in quantitative methods from Harvard University. In 1995, he became a Cancer Prevention Fellow at the National Cancer Institute, where he worked with leading researchers in the area of cancer epidemiology. Since 1999, he has also held an adjunct faculty position in the Department of Family and Preventive Medicine at the University of Utah. In 2001, he spent a sabbatical working in the Unit of Epidemiology for Cancer Prevention at the International Agency for Research on Cancer in Lyon, France. He is the author of *Introduction to Epidemiology, Fourth Edition*, and more than 150 professional publications in epidemiology and public health journals.

Preface

Environmental epidemiologists study the frequency and pattern of disease and health-related events and attempt to explain the environmental factors that influence these conditions. The study of why and how environmental factors affect peoples' health is the essence of environmental epidemiology. Environmental epidemiology emphasizes the idea that health is largely influenced by environmental factors, and that by identifying these factors and their modes of transmission, the public's health can be better protected.

Originally, environmental epidemiology focused on biological agents (pathogens) and factors such as water supply and sanitation, sewage disposal, housing conditions, and food handling. Regulations and monitoring efforts to improve water, food, and housing quality and sewage treatment and disposal have greatly reduced the burden of diseases associated with biological agents. More recently, environmental epidemiology has expanded its focus by studying the health effects of physical and chemical agents such as radiation, lead, mercury, volatile organic compounds, and pesticides. There has also been some emphasis on studying the health effects of psychosocial factors like family, neighborhood, community, and social groups. Some environmental epidemiologic studies have examined the frequency and patterns of disease and injury in populations struck by natural disasters like flooding, mudslides, fires, earthquakes, and volcanoes. Essentially, the environment studied in environmental epidemiologic studies includes biological, physical, and chemical agents; social settings and factors affecting human contact with these agents; and social environments.

The purpose of this book is to present basic concepts and research methods used in environmental epidemiology and the application of environmental epidemiology to influencing human health and well-being. The first section (Chapters 1–6) covers basic concepts and methods used in environmental epidemiology; the second section (Chapters 7–9) covers approaches for describing disease by person, place, and time; and the third section (Chapters 10–14) involves applications of environmental epidemiology.

In Chapter 1, environmental epidemiology is defined and discussed, a "systems approach" to assessing environmental health problems is presented, and ways in which environmental epidemiology contributes to public health are identified.

In Chapter 2, the research process is presented—from developing a statement of the research problem to identifying appropriate variables, data, and hypotheses—in the context of environmental epidemiology. Methods for assessing exposure and outcome variables are presented.

In Chapter 3, selected types and purposes of environmental monitoring programs are presented, along with indicators commonly used in monitoring programs and some alternative approaches to monitoring in situations where public health indicators are not readily available. Suggested measures of selected environmental health indicators along with potential data sources are presented in Appendices I and II.

In Chapter 4, study designs and factors to consider when selecting a study design are presented. Issues related to internal and external validity are also covered.

In Chapter 5, statistical inference and reliability are discussed, along with a presentation of the statistical models and tests that correspond with the study designs presented in the previous chapter. The Statistical Analysis System (SAS) software programming language is introduced for performing selected analyses. SAS procedure codes and output interpretation are further developed in Appendix III.

In Chapter 6, the important role of causal inference, along with criteria commonly used in causal inference, is presented in the context of environmental epidemiology.

In Chapter 7, concepts and methods of disease clusters are presented, along with the four-stage process for cluster investigation recommended by the Centers for Disease Control and Prevention. The public health role of responding to cluster investigations is discussed, statistical challenges commonly associated with cluster investigations are described, and some alternative approaches for assessment are given for the case where the cluster occurs before the causal hypothesis.

In Chapter 8, mapping and geographic information systems for assessing the relationship between disease clusters and environmental contaminants are presented, with examples and application.

In Chapter 9, the focus is on organizing counts or rates of health-related states or events by time. Time–trend analysis is presented as a useful means for identifying disease outbreaks, for determining incubation or latency periods, and for generating hypotheses about causal relationships.

In Chapter 10, common forms of ambient and indoor air pollution are presented; standards and methods for monitoring ambient and indoor air pollution discussed. Selected health effects from environmental air pollution and monitoring efforts are described.

In Chapter 11, hazardous substances that may contaminate soil and affect the health of animals and humans are identified. Monitoring efforts are described.

In Chapter 12, the role of water in human health is explored. The chapter identifies common waterborne diseases and discusses some of the monitoring efforts used to ensure that safe water standards are met.

In Chapter 13, the electromagnetic spectrum is described, pathways by which people are exposed to radiation are discussed, common health problems associated with radiation exposure are presented, and challenges associated with epidemiologic radiation studies are explored. Radiation monitoring efforts are also considered.

In Chapter 14, the focus is on natural and human sources of global warming, sources and the extent of stratospheric ozone depletion, sources and the extent of deforestation, and policy aimed at curbing human-caused global warming, stratospheric ozone depletion, and deforestation. Epidemiologic evidence of adverse health effects associated with weather changes and ozone depletion are explored.

This book was developed for an introductory course in environmental epidemiology. It is designed for upper-division undergraduate and graduate students in public health, as well as for field public health workers. The chapter topics were selected to represent fundamental concepts, research methods, and application areas in environmental epidemiology. Learning objectives are presented at the beginning of each chapter. The chapters are divided into concise sections with several examples. Tables and figures are used to summarize and clarify important concepts and information. Key words are bolded in the text and defined. Study questions are provided at the end of each chapter.

Introduction to Environmental Epidemiology

LEARNING OBJECTIVES

After completing this chapter, you should be able to:

1. Define environmental epidemiology.

2. Understand the full range of existing environments in environmental epidemiology.

3. Describe the "systems approach" for assessing environmental problems.

4. Describe the four processes of toxicokinetics and how they relate to environmental epidemiology.

5. Describe how human activity has interfered with selected matter cycles and has affected the environment and human health.

6. Identify ways environmental epidemiology contributes to public health.

Introduction

A relation between the environment and human health has been observed for centuries. Hippocrates (460–377 BC), author of *Epidemic I, Epidemic III,* and *On Airs, Waters and Places,* made a connection between disease and environmental conditions, especially in relation to water and seasons.[1] He observed that different diseases occurred in different places and that malaria and yellow fever were most common in swampy areas. Some 2,000 years later, Bernardino Ramazzini (1633–1714), authored the first notable book on occupational health and industrial hygiene, *De morbis artificum diatribe* (*The Diseases of Workers*), published in 1700. In his work he identified several adverse health outcomes associated with chemicals, dust, metals, and other abrasive agents encountered by workers in various occupations.[2–5] For example, he described the dangers of lead poisoning from the glaze used by potters and the dangers of mercury exposure among mirror-makers, goldsmiths, and others. He observed that individuals in these occupations rarely reached old age, but if they did their health was often so bad that they prayed for death. Many of these workers had palsy of the neck and hands, loss of teeth, vertigo, asthma, and paralysis.

In 1775, Percival Pott described an increased risk of scrotal cancer in chimney sweeps, indicating that soot was the causal agent.[6] Later, John Snow (1813–1858) observed and recorded important environmental factors related to the course of cholera.[7] Snow showed that cholera was a waterborne disease that traveled in both surface and groundwater supplies.[8,9] Henry Butlin (1845–1912) observed that scrotal cancer was a more common disease among the English, attributing comparatively low levels in Scotland and America to the protective clothing worn by chimney sweeps in those places.[10] In current times, epidemiologic studies have identified numerous chemical exposures and industrial processes that are causally associated with human cancer.[11] For example, some industrial processes related to human bladder cancer are aluminum production, auramine manufacture, magenta manufacture, and rubber industry. The identified carcinogenic agents produced by these industrial processes include polycyclic aromatic hydrocarbons (PAHs), auramine, magenta, aromatic amine, and solvents.

A large body of research in recent years has greatly added to our understanding of how the environment can protect and sustain human life or contribute to disability and premature death. Some life-promoting features of the environment include

- soil for farming;
- water for drinking;
- air for breathing;

- the stratospheric ozone layer for protection against ultraviolet rays;
- space and facilities for recreation and exercise; and
- standards for food preparation, recycling, and disposal of waste.

On the other hand, some environmental contaminants can be life threatening, such as

- infectious agents (viruses, bacteria, fungi, parasites);
- environmental disruptions (e.g., floods, droughts, earthquakes, fires, tsunamis, mass movements, landslides);
- poor air quality (dusts, pollen, pollution);
- poor water quality (contaminants, inadequate water transport and treatment);
- negative human changes of the environment (global warming, ozone depletion, nuclear accidents, nuclear war, industrial accidents, hazardous material spills, oil spills); and
- social disruptions (ethnic violence, riots, urban fires due to arson, terrorism, bombings, conventional war, chemical/biological weapons).

Many of these environmental exposures are involuntary. For example, exposure to environmental tobacco smoke (also called secondhand smoke or passive smoke) in the home, the workplace, and in public places is often not a conscious choice. Children in particular are often innocent victims who are unable to choose to avoid environmental tobacco smoke. Infants exposed to environmental tobacco smoke are particularly susceptible to bronchitis and pneumonia.[12] In addition, exposed children are at increased risk of middle ear problems and exacerbated and new cases of coughing, wheezing, and asthma.[12,13]

In January 1993, the Environmental Protection Agency (EPA) declared that environmental tobacco smoke was a human carcinogen. Environmental tobacco smoke contains over 250 chemicals that are toxic or cancer causing, such as arsenic, ammonia, benzene, formaldehyde, hydrogen cyanide, and vinyl chloride.[14] The EPA estimates that environmental tobacco smoke contributes to approximately 3,000 lung cancer deaths each year.[12] In addition, a number of studies have linked environmental tobacco smoke with heart disease. A large cohort study involving over 32,000 women showed that constant exposure to environmental tobacco smoke almost doubles the risk of heart attack.[15] Environmental tobacco smoke can have a similar effect in nonsmokers as it does in smokers by causing carotid-wall thickening and compromised endothelial function, which promotes arteriosclerosis (fatty buildup in the arteries) and subsequent heart disease.[16] In the United

States, exposure to environmental tobacco smoke increases the risk of coronary heart disease by approximately 30%, contributing to over 35,000 deaths each year.[17] Recent studies show that much of the cardiovascular system, including platelet and endothelial function, arterial stiffness, atherosclerosis, oxidative stress, inflammation, heart rate variability, energy metabolism, and increased infarct size, is highly sensitive to the toxins in environmental tobacco smoke.[17]

These epidemiologic findings linking environmental tobacco smoke with specific health problems were the impetus for several local, state, and federal authorities to enact public policies designed to protect the public from environmental tobacco smoke. In recent years, clean indoor air laws have been passed in many places. Information detailing smoking restrictions according to state is available elsewhere.[18]

Because many studies have focused on how human health is influenced by environmental factors, the term "environmental epidemiology" has surfaced. The purpose of this chapter is to define environmental epidemiology, identify existing environments in environmental epidemiology, present the "systems approach" to assessing environmental problems, and identify ways environmental epidemiology contributes to public health.

Environmental Epidemiology

To understand the meaning of environmental epidemiology, first consider the meaning of environmental health. The World Health Organization (WHO) defines **environmental health** as those aspects of human health that are determined by physical, chemical, biological, social, and psychological factors in the environment.[19] This includes direct pathologic effects on health by chemicals, radiation, and biological agents as well as indirect effects on health from physical and psychosocial environments such as transportation, housing, socioeconomic status, and social networks. The WHO definition further states that environmental health is the theory and practice of assessing, correcting, controlling, and preventing those environmental factors that have a potentially harmful effect on human populations.[19] Considerable efforts in the United States and elsewhere go into assessment (monitoring and evaluation) of environmental factors associated with health, such as air quality, water quality, noise, solid-waste disposal, housing, occupational conditions, and unsanitary surroundings. On the basis of assessment information, environmental health services can more effectively prevent or reduce the health burden of illness associated with unsafe environmental factors.

In a book compiled by Last, the definition of **epidemiology** provided is "the study of the distribution and determinants of health-related states or events in specified populations, and the application of this study to control for health problems."[20] **Health-related states or events** is used in the definition to capture the fact that epidemiology involves more than just the study of disease states (e.g., respiratory illness), but also includes the study of events (e.g., injury) and behaviors and conditions associated with health (e.g., hand washing). In addition, note that epidemiology is concerned with health-related states or events that occur in populations, not a specific individual. Epidemiologists direct their questions toward a selected population; for example, is there an excess of disease above what is expected in a specified population (**epidemic**) or is the frequency of disease what is normally expected (**endemic**)? When an epidemic is extensive, involving large regions, countries, or continents, it is referred to as a **pandemic** (Figure 1.1).

Outbreak carries the same definition as epidemic but is typically used when the event is confined to a more limited geographic area. In addition, the word "outbreak" may appear less alarming to the public than the word "epidemic." Epidemiologists investigate outbreaks and health disparities in human populations by asking the following:

- Who are the people at greatest risk for disease? Men? Women? Older people? Younger people? People in a given community?
- Why are these people ill and not other people? Physical agent? Biologic agent? Chemical agent? Genetic factor? Lifestyle? Diet? Occupation?
- What is the illness observed? Heart disease? Cancer? Injury?
- How does the disease frequency change over time?
- How does the disease vary from place to place?
- Do disease cases have a given exposure in common?
- What is the strength of the relationship between an exposure and disease?
- How much disease could be avoided by eliminating the exposure?
- Does the totality of evidence provide support for a causal association?
- How can answers to these questions assist in controlling and preventing disease in the future?

It follows that **environmental epidemiology** is the study of distribution and determinants of health-related states or events in specified populations that are influenced by physical, chemical, biological, and psychosocial factors in the environment. It also involves the application of this study to prevent and control health problems. Its population focus and emphasis on identifying causal relations dis-

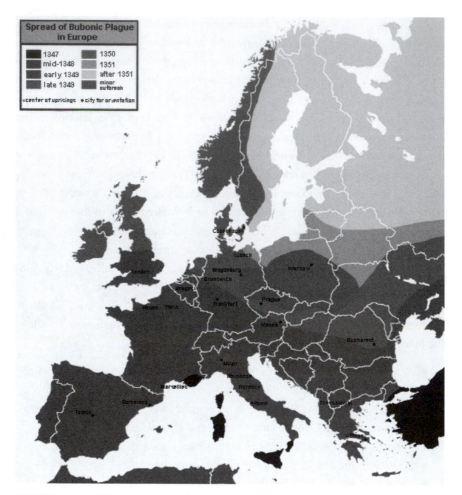

FIGURE 1.1   The spread of the plague throughout Europe from 1346 through 1353. (*Source:* Courtesy of Matich, 2007.)[21]

tinguishes it from environmental health, which is more comprehensive. It seeks to clarify the relation between environmental factors and human health by focusing on specified populations or communities. It is based on the observation that most diseases are not random occurrences, but rather are related to environmental factors that vary according to population subgroups, place, and time. Environmental epidemiologic studies are concerned not only with those who get a disease, but also with those who do not, and in identifying why the two groups differ.

Prior to the second half of the twentieth century, environmental epidemiology focused on disease-causing infectious agents or pathogens and factors such as water quality and supply systems, waste control, and food quality. Supplying safe water, appropriate disposal of waste, and regulation of food handling are environmental measures that have considerably reduced morbidity and mortality levels in many developed parts of the world. Increasing life expectancy and a movement from infectious to chronic disease as the primary cause of disease and death have motivated a change in focus of environmental epidemiology to chemicals and physical agents that have a relatively large impact on chronic illness. These agents include particulate matter, pesticides, radiation, metals, and volatile organic compounds. Epidemiologic studies have shown that particulate matter, especially fine particles, can cause premature death, respiratory-related hospitalization, aggravated asthma, acute respiratory symptoms, chronic bronchitis, decreased lung function, and work and school absences;[22] pesticides can cause birth defects, nerve damage, and cancer;[23] radiation can cause burns and radiation sickness, premature aging, cancer, and death;[24] metals such as lead can cause damage to the nervous system, kidneys, brain, and red blood cells;[25] and volatile organic compounds can cause eye and respiratory tract irritation, headaches, dizziness, visual disorders, memory impairment, and cancer.[26] Environmental epidemiology also examines the effects of social disruptions (e.g., ethnic violence, war, acts of terrorism, and natural disasters) on disease and death.

The Environment

In a medical sense, the **environment** reflects the aggregate of those external conditions and influences affecting the life and development of an organism.[27] John Last defined "environment" for the International Epidemiological Association as "[a]ll that which is external to the human host."[28] The environment may be thought of as physical, biological, social, cultural, and so on, any or all of which can influence health status of populations. Environment has also been presented by how it is associated with human health. Some of the different existing ideas on environments and their perspectives on the interaction with health include:

1. **The inner versus outer environment.** The inner body is protected from outside contaminants by three barriers: the skin, the gastrointestinal tract, and the lungs. When contaminants do penetrate these barriers, the body fortunately has protective mechanisms (e.g., vomiting, diarrhea, detoxification

in the liver, excretion through the kidneys, and coughing). The lungs represent the most susceptible barrier and are considered the most important pathway for environmental contaminants. Consider that the average adult breathes approximately 800 cubic feet (20 cubic meters) or approximately 50 pounds of air each day.[29]

2. **The personal versus ambient environment.** This definition contrasts an environment where a person has control (e.g., diet, smoking, sexual behavior, and alcohol consumption) with the ambient environment where they have little or no control (e.g., food additives, pollution, and industrial products).[29] Many chronic conditions have been largely associated with personal environment. For example, 70% or more of cancer deaths are attributed to diet, smoking, and reproductive and sexual behavior.[30]

3. **The solid, liquid, and gaseous environments.** Routes of human exposure to contaminants are through solid, liquid, and gaseous environments.[29] Soil, food, water, and air are key environments to our existence, and each is subject to contamination. Chemical and biological contaminants can be absorbed in the body through the lungs, gastrointestinal tract, or skin. Common forms of transmission include the air, water, soil, and food. Airborne transmission occurs when droplets or dust particles carry hazardous chemicals (e.g., carbon monoxide, ozone, lead) or biological agents/pathogens (virus, bacteria, fungus) through the air to infect a susceptible host. Waterborne transmission occurs when a harmful chemical or biological agent/pathogen, such as cholera or shigellosis, is carried in drinking water, swimming pools, streams, or lakes. Soilborne contamination occurs when either solid or liquid hazardous substances mix with soil. Soil contaminants may be physically or chemically attached to soil particles or trapped in spaces between soil particles. Soil may become contaminated by hazardous substances that fall out of the air or by contaminated water as it flows over or through it. Foodborne transmission occurs by consuming foods or beverages contaminated by biological agents and poisonous chemicals. The most common foodborne infections are caused by salmonella, listeria, toxoplasma, Norwalk-like viruses, campylobacter, and E. coli O157:H7. It is estimated that foodborne diseases cause approximately 76 million illnesses, 325,000 hospitalizations, and 5,000 deaths each year in the United States.[31,32]

4. **The physical, chemical, biological, and psychosocial environments.** The environment may also be considered according to the avenue or

mechanism by which it affects people. [29] Physical, biological, chemical, and psychosocial aspects of the environment are shown in Table 1.1.

In a broad sense, the study of environmental epidemiology requires consideration of all these definitions of environment and their interrelationship. However, the study of the environment may be restricted by person (e.g., children), place (e.g., workplace, to indoors or outdoors), or time (e.g., summer). It may also be restricted to environments that can be modified.[33] Environmental health interventions typically attempt to modify only the physical, biological, and chemical environments, and corresponding behaviors (e.g., hand washing).

The Systems Approach

A primary goal in environmental epidemiology is to understand how human health problems may arise from environmental factors. An accurate and comprehensive evaluation requires a "systems approach" where the health problem is related to the complexity of environmental exposures. The word "systems" is defined as "a group of interrelated, interacting, or interdependent constituents forming a complex whole."[34] The **systems approach** in environmental epidemiology considers the fact that environmental exposures may derive from multiple sources, they may enter the body through multiple routes, and elements in the environment can change over time because of constant interaction, altering the degree to which

---

TABLE 1.1   Mechanisms by which the environment influences human health

Physical stresses	Excessive heat, cold, and noise; radiation (electromagnetic, ultrasound, microwave, x-irradiation); vehicular collisions; workplace injuries; climate change; ozone depletion; housing; and so on
Chemical	Drugs, acids, alkali, heavy metals (lead and mercury), poisons (arsenic), and some enzymes
Biological	Disease-causing infectious agents or pathogens (viruses, bacteria, fungi, parasites)
Psychosocial milieu	Families and households, socioeconomic status, social networks and social support, neighborhoods and communities, formal institutions, and public policy

Source: Adapted from Moeller, 1992, pp. 6–7. [29]

they are harmful. Understanding the source and nature of environmental contaminants, ways people are exposed, and dose effects often require the combined efforts of epidemiologists, biologists, toxicologists, respiratory physiologists, and public health officials. According to Moeller, viewing a health problem in its entirety through a systems approach involves:

1. Determining the source and nature of each environmental contaminant or stress.
2. Assessing how and in what form it comes into contact with people.
3. Measuring the health effect.
4. Applying controls when and where appropriate.[29]

With the assistance of experts such as air pollution engineers, industrial hygienists, chemists, and quality-control personnel, health standards are then established, monitoring and assessment carried out, and actions taken to reduce contaminants when they exceed specified standards.

Toxicokinetics

Toxicokinetics is an area of study of how a substance enters the body and the course it takes while in the body. The name originates from kinetics, which means movement, and the study of movement of toxic substances. Toxicokinetics involves four processes:

1. Absorption—entrance of the substance into the body. When a substance is ingested or inhaled, it is still considered outside the body until it crosses cellular barriers in the gastrointestinal tract or lungs. Absorption can also be through the skin, implants, conjuctival instillations (eye drops), and suppositories. Hence, there is a distinction between the exposure dose (outside dose) and the absorbed dose (internal dose). For a substance to enter the body, cell membranes (cell walls) must be penetrated. Cell membranes are designed to prevent foreign invaders or substances from entering into bodily tissue.
2. Distribution—movement of the substance from where it enters the body to other sites in the body (e.g., liver, blood and lymph circulation, kidney, lung). After a substance passes the lining of the skin, lung, or gastrointestinal tract, it enters the fluid surrounding the cells of that organ (interstitial fluid) versus fluid inside the cells (intracellular fluid). Interstitial fluid rep-

resents about 15% of body weight and intracellular fluid about 40% of body weight. A toxicant can leave the interstitial fluid in three ways: entering cells of local tissue, entering blood capillaries and the body's blood circulatory system, and entering the lymphatic system. Once in the circulatory system, a chemical can be excreted, stored, biotransformed into metabolites, its metabolites excreted or stored, or it or its metabolites can interact or bind with cellular components.

3. Biotransformation—transformation produced by the body of the substance into new chemicals (metabolites). Biotransformation is essential to survival. It is the process by which absorbed nutrients (food, oxygen, etc.) are transformed into substances required by the body to function normally. While most chemicals undergo biotransformation, the extent to which this is done depends on the storage or excretion of the chemical and its metabolites, the dose level, frequency, and route of exposure. The body is efficient at biotransforming body wastes or chemicals that are not normally produced or expected into water-soluble metabolites excreted into bile and excreted from the body. Biotransformation that metabolizes a substance to lower toxicity is called detoxification. However, it is possible for metabolites to be more toxic (bioactivation). When the metabolite interacts with cellular macromolecules such as DNA, serious health effects (cancer, birth defects) may arise.

4. Excretion—ejection of the substance or metabolites from the body. Toxicants or their metabolites may be ejected from the body through feces, urine, or expired air.

Factors influencing the toxicity severity of a substance that enters the body include route of exposure; duration of exposure; concentration of exposure; rate and amount absorbed; distribution and concentrations within the body; efficiency by which the body changes the substance and the metabolites produced; ability of the substance or metabolites to pass through cell membranes and affect cell components; duration and amount of the substance or metabolites in body tissues; and rate, amount, and site of departure of the substance or metabolites from the body. For example, poor absorption of a highly toxic substance may be less dangerous than a substance with low toxicity but high absorption. Further, two substances of similar toxicity and absorption may pose different hazards, depending on whether biotransformation results in a more toxic metabolite for one versus the other substance.[35]

Polycyclic aromatic hydrocarbons (PAHs) consist of over 100 different chemicals formed during incomplete burning of coal, oil and gas, garbage, tobacco, or charbroiled meat. Some PAHs are manufactured (e.g., coal tar, crude oil, creosote, and roofing tar). Some are used in medicine or used in making pesticides, dyes, and plastics. The Department of Health and Human Services has determined that some PAHs are carcinogenic. People who have breathed or touched mixtures of PAHs over extended periods of time have developed cancer. Points of absorption include the gastrointestinal tract, lungs, and skin by, for example, eating grilled or charred meat; breathing air containing PAHs from cigarette smoke, vehicle exhaust, or asphalt roads; or drinking contaminated water or milk. In the body, PAHs are transformed into chemicals that can attach to substances in body tissues or blood.[36]

The Role of Environmental Epidemiology in Public Health

Environmental epidemiologic research has linked several diseases with environmental factors and has allowed researchers to quantify the public health burden of disease attributed to the environment. Accordingly, environmental factors influence more than 80% of the diseases regularly reported to the WHO. Globally, an estimated 24% of the burden of disease (healthy life years lost) and an estimated 23% of premature deaths have been associated with environmental factors. In children ages 0–14 years, 36% of the disease burden is attributed to environmental factors. Diseases with the strongest absolute burden related to modifiable environmental factors are diarrhea (94%); lower respiratory infections (20%; 42% in developing countries); workplace hazards, radiation, and industrial accidents (44%); and malaria (42%).[33] Diseases with the largest environmental contribution worldwide are presented in Figure 1.2. An estimate of the fraction of cancer deaths occurring in the United States each year that are caused by toxic occupational exposures is 10%.[37] Cigarette smoke is the most common chemical carcinogen, accounting for as many as 40% of all cancer deaths.[38]

Environmental epidemiologic information can provide a means for meeting public health objectives aimed at protecting and improving the health and well-being of human populations. Epidemiologic findings contribute to preventing and controlling health-related states or events by providing useful information for directing public health policy and planning, as well as informing individuals about adverse health behaviors.

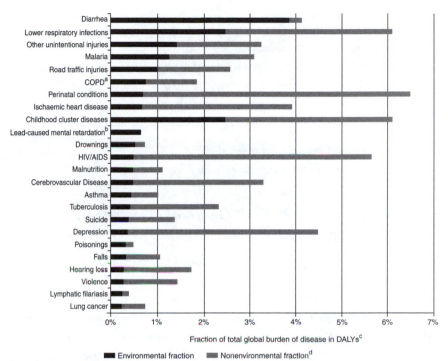

Fraction of total global burden of disease in DALYs[c]

■ Environmental fraction   ■ Nonenvironmental fraction[d]

[a] Abbreviations: COPD = Chronic obstructive pulmonary disease.
[b] Lead-caused mental retardation is defined in the WHO list of diseases for 2002, accessed at: www.who.int/evidence.
[c] DALYs represents a weighted measure of death, illness, and disabillity.
[d] For each disease the fraction attributable to environmental risks is shown in black. Gray plus black represents the total burden of disease.

FIGURE 1.2 Prevalent diseases associated with the environment. (*Source: from Pruss-Ustun & Corvalan, 2006.*)[33]

Public health policy and planning, and individual health decision making should benefit from answers to the following questions:

- What is the extent of the public health problem?
- Who is at greatest risk?
- Where is the health problem greatest?
- When is the health problem greatest?
- What is the likely cause of the health problem?
- What is the natural history of the health problem?
  - susceptibility stage (types of exposure capable of causing disease among susceptible hosts)
  - presymptomatic stage (length of time in the subclinical phase, description of the pathologic changes that occur during this phase)

- symptomatic stage (type of symptoms that characterize the disease)
- outcome stage (probability of recovery, disability, or death associated with different levels of the disease)
- Are prevention and control programs available that are efficacious (i.e., produce desired effect among those who participate in the program)?
- Are prevention and control programs available that are effective (i.e., produce benefits among those who are offered the program; good compliance)?

Some examples of how environmental epidemiologic information influenced public health decisions and policy are provided here.

Example 1: E. Coli O157:H7 Outbreak Associated with Contaminated Alfalfa Sprouts

During the last week of June 1997, the Michigan Department of Community Health observed an increase in laboratory reports of E. coli O157:H7 infection. Over two times the number of infected cases were reported than in the previous month. The increase in cases continued into July. Thirty-eight cases of confirmed O157:H7 infections meeting the case definition from 10 counties in the lower peninsula of Michigan are shown in Figure 1.3. Epidemiologic investigation linked the increased occurrence of illness to consumption of contaminated alfalfa sprouts.[39]

In response, the implicated seed lot discontinued distribution to sprouting companies. Approximately 6,000 pounds of seed were removed from the market-place. The state Division of Food and Drugs held meetings to explain to seed growers the importance of protecting alfalfa and other seeds used in sprouting from possible contamination. Television and radio announcements were made about the risk of contaminated sprouting seeds. In addition, the Center for Food Safety and Quality Enhancement began working with the sprout industry to find ways to make sprouts safer for consumption.[39]

Example 2: E. Coli O157:H7 Outbreak Associated with Contaminated Spinach

In the fall of 2006, an extensive investigation of an E. coli O157:H7 outbreak involving 205 confirmed cases and three deaths found the cause to be contaminated Dole-brand baby spinach grown in California. Some potential environmental risk factors were identified, including contamination near the presence of wild

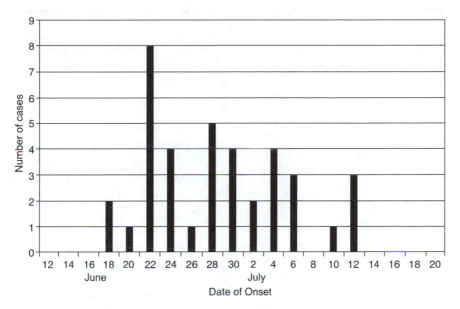

FIGURE 1.3 Number of persons with E. coli O157:H7 infection in Michigan by date, June 15–July 15, 1997. (*Source:* CDC Case Study, 2002.)[39]

pigs and surface waterways exposed to feces from cattle and wildlife. In response to this and other outbreaks, the U.S. Food and Drug Administration (FDA) announced an initiative called "Leafy Greens."[40] This initiative focuses on produce, contamination agents, and related public health concerns. In addition, the FDA has provided recommendations on ways to prevent microbial contamination while processing fresh-cut produce in its publication called "Guide to Minimize Microbial Food Safety Hazards of Fresh-cut Fruits and Vegetables." The FDA also advises consumers to wash all produce thoroughly before eating. Although this would not have prevented the E. coli outbreak involving spinach, it can reduce the risk of contamination from several other sources.

Example 3: Environmental Changes and Health

Changes in the environment caused by human interference in matter cycles has resulted in adverse effects to health. Humans have caused environmental problems by interfering with the **hydrological cycle,** the **nitrogen cycle,** the **phosphorous**

TABLE 1.2   Matter cycles and pollution

Cycles	Human Interference	Environmental Problems
Hydrological cycle	Removal of large quantities of freshwater from rivers, lakes, and groundwater supplies	Depletion of groundwater Vegetation removed
	Because of vegetation removal, rainwater washes away and no longer infiltrates	Groundwater supplies are not restored Groundwater becomes salinated Risk of flooding enhanced Soil erosion increase Landslides increase
	Water quality is compromised because of added nutrients and contaminants	Disruption of ecological processes that usually purify the water
Nitrogen cycle	Fuel combustion releases nitrogen oxides	Nitrous oxide is a greenhouse gas that causes the earth's temperature to increase; can react with ozone to break down the stratospheric ozone layer
	Nitrogen dioxide may react with hydrogen to form nitric acid	Nitric acid causes acid deposition, which damages trees, vegetation, and marine ecosystems
Phosphorous cycle	Removal of phosphates in certain locations to apply to farmland as fertilizers	Because the phosphate supply is mobile, in these locations phosphate levels become too high in surrounding land/soils and groundwater; when crops do not absorb all phosphates, the phosphates end up in water and settle in lakes and reservoirs; the result is eutrophication, which means that water is so rich of nutrients that certain water plants (e.g., green algae) grow extensively; the water then becomes depleted of the oxygen supply causing oxygen-dependent fish and organisms to die and nonoxygen dependent bacteria to thrive

TABLE 1.2 Matter cycles and pollution (continued)

Cycles	Human Interference	Environmental Problems
	Deforestation	The rain washes phosphates away, causing the ground to become unproductive; it takes considerable time for phosphate supplies to be restored because phosphate comes from weathering rocks and oceanic sediments
Sulfur cycle	Humans are responsible for 90% of sulfur salts found on the earth, primarily formed during industrial process (coal combustion, petroleum refining, and melting)	Sulfur compounds (sulfuric acid, sulfur dioxide, and hydrogen sulfide) cause acid deposition on water and soil, influencing life in the soil and water and causing a disturbance to natural processes
Carbon cycle	Deforestation	Removal of trees and plants that absorb carbon dioxide
	Industrial processes (coal and oil combustion)	Carbon emissions to the atmosphere; uptake of excessive carbon dioxide in the atomosphere cannot be taken up by trees, plants, and oceans fast enough; carbon dioxide is a greenhouse gas that causes the earth's temperature to increase
	Extensive burning of fossil fuels, which consist of dead organic matter	Depleting fossil fuel supplies, which take a very long time to restore

Source: Adapted from Lenntech, 2006.[41]

cycle, the **sulfur cycle,** and the **carbon cycle**. A summary of ways humans interfere with these cycles is presented in Table 1.2.

Environmental changes in the climate and stratospheric ozone have prompted investigations of potential health consequences. Good health depends on continued stability and functioning of that part of the earth and its atmosphere that supports life. Climate change may affect human health through increased temperatures and temperature-related illness and death; extreme weather events; air pollution; food and water shortages; and a rise in waterborne, foodborne, vectorborne, and rodentborne diseases. Stratospheric ozone depletion can adversely affect life through increased exposure to ultraviolet radiation. In response, the United Nations Framework Convention on Climate Change (UNFCCC) has taken steps to reduce greenhouse gas emissions and respond to the impacts of climate change.[42] On December 11, 1997, the **Kyoto Protocol** strengthened the UNFCCC by setting standards for greenhouse gas emissions among countries ratifying the protocol.[43] In 1987, the **Montreal Protocol** on Substances That Deplete the Ozone Layer was signed as an international treaty to protect stratospheric ozone by stopping the emission of halocarbon gases and other substances.[44]

Once causal associations are established between environmental factors and human health, public health assessment can be employed to monitor exposure and health-related conditions in the population. Public health surveillance makes possible the identification of individuals and populations at greatest risk for disease and of where the public health problem is greatest.[45] Public health intervention programs can then be developed and effectively evaluated. In addition, people can be warned about the negative effects of certain environmental exposures and alter their conditions and behaviors accordingly.

Key Issues

1. Environmental epidemiology is the study of the distribution and determinants of health-related states or events in specified populations that are influenced by physical, chemical, biological, and psychosocial factors in the environment. It also involves the application of this study to prevent and control health problems.

2. The population focus of environmental epidemiology and emphasis on identifying causal relationships distinguishes it from environmental health, which is more comprehensive.

3. Environmental epidemiology should consider a full range of existing environments: the inner versus outer environment; the personal versus ambient environment; the solid, liquid, and gaseous environments; the chemical, biological, physical, and socioeconomic environments.

4. The systems approach in environmental epidemiology considers the fact that environmental exposures may derive from multiple sources, they may enter the body through multiple routes, and elements in the environment can change over time because of constant interaction, altering the degree to which they are harmful. Viewing a health problem in its entirety through a systems approach involves: (1) determining the source and nature of each

environmental contaminant or stress; (2) assessing how and in what form it comes into contact with people; (3) measuring the health effect; and (4) applying controls when and where appropriate.

5. Toxicokinetics is an area of study of how a substance enters the body and the course it takes while in the body. Toxicokinetics involves four processes: absorption, distribution, biotransformation, and excretion.

6. Changes in the environment caused by human interference in matter cycles (hydrological cycle, the nitrogen cycle, the phosphorous cycle, the sulfur cycle, and the carbon cycle) have resulted in environmental problems and adverse affects to human health.

7. Epidemiologic findings contribute to preventing and controlling health-related states or events by providing useful information for directing public health policy and planning, as well as informing individuals about adverse health behaviors.

Exercises

Key Terms

Define the following terms.

Carbon cycle
Endemic
Environment
Environmental epidemiology
Environmental health
Epidemic
Epidemiology
Health-related states or events
Hydrological cycle
Kyoto Protocol
Montreal Protocol
Nitrogen cycle
Outbreak
Pandemic
Phosphorous cycle
Polycyclic aromatic hydrocarbons
Sulfur cycle

Systems approach
The inner versus outer environment
The personal versus ambient environment
The physical, chemical, biological, and psychosocial environments
The solid, liquid, and gaseous environments
Toxicokinetics

Study Questions

1.1. Define environmental epidemiology.

1.2. Describe the primary purpose of environmental epidemiology.

1.3. What was the original focus of environmental epidemiology, and how has it changed since the mid-twentieth century?

1.4. Compare inner versus outer and personal versus ambient environments.

1.5. Identify and discuss routes of exposure in the environment.

1.6. Identify and give examples of ways that the environment can influence health.

1.7. What is the systems approach for assessing environmental problems?

1.8. How is toxicokinetics related to a systems approach?

1.9. Describe some of the environmental problems related to human interference with the hydrological cycle, the nitrogen cycle, the phosphorous cycle, the sulfur cycle, and the carbon cycle.

1.10. How does environmental epidemiology contribute to public health?

References

1. Jones WHS. (translation). *Hippocrates, Vol. I.* London: William Heinemann; 1923:71–137.

2. Cumston CG. *An Introduction to the History of Medicine.* New York, NY: Alfred A. Knopf; 1926.

3. Garrison FH. *History of Medicine.* Philadelphia, PA: Saunders; 1926.

4. Rosen G. *A History of Public Health.* New York: MD Publications; 1958.

5. Seelig MG. *Medicine: An Historical Outline.* Baltimore: Williams & Wilkins; 1925.

6. Pott P. *Chirurgical Observations.* Vol 3. London: Hawes L, Clark W, Collins R; 1775:177–183.

7. Snow J. *On the Mode of Communication of Cholera.* 2nd ed. 1855. Reproduced by Commonwealth Fund, New York; 1936.

8. Snow on Cholera, Part 1. Available at: http://www.uic.edu/sph/prepare/courses/chsc400/resources/snowcase1.htm. Accessed April 4, 2007.

9. Snow on Cholera, Part 2. Available at: http://www.uic.edu/sph/prepare/courses/chsc400/resources/snowcase2.htm. Accessed April 4, 2007.

10. Waldron HA. A brief history of scrotal cancer. *Br J Ind Med*. 1983;40:390–401.

11. International Agency for Research on Cancer. *Overall evaluations of carcinogenicity: an updating of IARC monographs*. Vols 1–42. IARC Monographs Supplement 7. Geneva IARC; 1987.

12. Environmental Protection Agency. The health effects of exposure to secondhand smoke. Available at: http://www.epa.gov/smokefree/healtheffects.html. Accessed April 5, 2007.

13. Office of Environmental Health Hazard Assessment. Health effects of exposure to environmental tobacco smoke: Final report, approved at the panel's June 24, 2005 meeting. Available at: http://www.oehha.ca.gov/air/environmental_tobacco/2005etsfinal.html. Accessed April 5, 2007.

14. Health and Human Services. The health consequences of involuntary exposure to tobacco smoke: A report of the surgeon general. Available at: http://www.surgeongeneral.gov/library/secondhandsmoke/. Accessed April 5, 2007.

15. Kawachi I, Colditz GA, Speizer FE, et al. A prospective study of passive smoking and coronary heart disease. *Circulation*. 1997;95:2374–2379.

16. Otsuka R, Watanabe H, Kirata K. Acute effects of passive smoking on the coronary circulation in healthy young adults. *JAMA*. 2001;286:436–441.

17. Barnoya J, Glantz SA. Cardiovascular effects of second hand smoke. *Circulation*. 2005;111:2684–2698.

18. American Lung Association. Tobacco control. Available at: http://slati.lungusa.org/. Accessed April 5, 2007.

19. World Health Organization. Protection of the human environment. Available at: http://www.who.int/phe/en/. Accessed September 22, 2006.

20. Last JM, ed. *A Dictionary of Epidemiology*. 3rd ed. New York, NY: Oxford University Press; 1995.

21. Matich J. *The Great Plague*. Available at: http://www.urbanedpartnership.org/target/bridges/greatplague.html. Accessed April 5, 2007.

22. Environmental Protection Agency. Health and environmental effects of particulate matter. Available at: http://www.epa.gov/ttncaaa1/naaqsfin/pmhealth.html. Accessed April 5, 2007.

23. Environmental Protection Agency. Pesticides and food: health problems pesticides may pose. Available at: http://www.epa.gov/pesticides/food/risks.htm. Accessed April 5, 2007.

24. Environmental Protection Agency. Understanding radiation. Health effects. Available at: http://www.epa.gov/radiation/understand/health_effects.htm#whatkind. Accessed April 5, 2007.

25. Environmental Protection Agency. Private drinking water wells. Human health. Available at: http://www.epa.gov/safewater/privatewells/health.html. Accessed April 5, 2007.

26. Environmental Protection Agency. Indoor air quality. An introduction to indoor air quality: organic gases (volatile organic compounds—VOCs). Available at: http://www.epa.gov/iaq/voc.html. Accessed April 5, 2007.

27. *Stedman's Medical Dictionary for the Health Professions and Nursing.* 5th ed. New York: Lippincott, Williams & Wilkins; 2005.

28. Last JM, ed. *A Dictionary of Epidemiology.* 4th ed. New York, NY: Oxford University Press; 2001.

29. Moeller DW. *Environmental Health.* Cambridge, MA: Harvard University Press; 1992.

30. Doll R, Peto R. The causes of cancer; Quantitative estimates of avoidable risks of cancer in the United States today. *J Natl Cancer Inst.* 1981;66(6):1191–1309.

31. Tybor PT, Hurst WC, Reynolds AE, Schuler G. Preventing chemical foodborne illness. Available at: http://pubs.caes.uga.edu/caespubs/pubcd/b1042-w .html. Accessed September 22, 2006.

32. Mead PS, Slutsker L, Dietz V, et al. Food-related illness and death in the United States. 1999. Available at: http://www.cdc.gov/ncidod/eid/vol5no5/ mead.htm. Accessed September 22, 2006.

33. Pruss-Ustun A, Corvalan C. Preventing disease through healthy environments. Towards an estimate of the environmental burden of disease. Geneva, Switzerland: WHO Press. Available at: http://www.who.int/quantifying_ehimpacts/ publications/preventingdisease/en/print.html. Accessed September 22, 2006.

34. *Webster's Ninth New Collegiate Dictionary.* Springfield, MA: Merriam-Webster Inc; 1991.

35. National Library of Science. Toxicology tutor II: toxicokinetics. Available at: http://sis.nlm.nih.gov/enviro/toxtutor/Tox2/amenu.htm. Accessed June 10, 2007.

36. Agency for Toxic Substances and Disease Registry. ToxFAQs: polycyclic aromatic hydrocarbons (PAHs). U.S. Department of Health and Human Services, Public Health Service Agency for Toxic Substances and Disease Registry. Available at: http://www.atsdr.cdc.gov/tfacts69.pdf. Accessed June 10, 2007.

37. Cole P. Cancer and occupation: status and needs of epidemiologic research. *Cancer.* 1977;39:1788–1791.

38. Landrigan PJ, Markowitz SB, Nicholson WJ. Cancer prevention in the workplace. In: Greenwald P, Kramer BS, Weed DL, eds. *Cancer Prevention and Control.* New York, NY: Marcel Dekker Inc; 1995:393–410.

39. Centers for Disease Control and Prevention (CDC) Case Study. A multistate outbreak of E. coli O157:H7 infection. Available at: http://www2a.cdc.gov/ epicasestudies/graphics/ecolii.pdf. Accessed August 23, 2006.

40. Investigation of an Escherichia coli O157:H7 outbreak associated with Dole pre-packaged spinach. Available at: http://www.dhs.ca.gov/ps/fdb/local/PDF/ 2006%20Spinach%20Report%20Final%20redacted%20no%20photosfigures .PDF. Accessed April 4, 2007.

41. Lenntech. Matter cycles and pollution. Available at: http://www.lenntech.com/ matter-cycles-pollution.htm. Accessed June 11, 2007.

42. United Nations Framework Convention on Climate Change. The United Nations Framework Convention on Climate Change: Essential Background.

2006. Available at: http://unfccc.int/essential_background/convention/items/2627.php. Accessed October 17, 2006.

43. United Nations Framework Convention on Climate Change. Kyoto Protocol. Available at: http://unfccc.int/kyoto_protocol/background/items/3145.php. Accessed November 25, 2006.

44. Alternative Fluorocarbons Environmental Acceptability Study. Available at: http://www.afeas.org/montreal_protocol.html. Accessed October 17, 2006.

45. Teutsch SM, Churchill RE. *Principles and Practices of Public Health Surveillance*. 2nd ed. New York: Oxford University Press; 2000.

Basic Elements of Research, Exposure, and Outcome Assessment

LEARNING OBJECTIVES

After completing this chapter, you should be able to:

1. Distinguish between a research problem, a research question, and a hypothesis.

2. Define "variable" and distinguish between dependent and independent variables.

3. Know the primary types of data.

4. Describe direct and indirect methods of exposure and outcome assessment.

5. Define hypothesis.

Introduction

In epidemiologic research, once the health problem has been empirically established, an investigation follows, employing scientific reasoning and methods. The scientific method involves beginning with information or data obtained through observation of the phenomenon of interest. Hypotheses are formed and then tested by further observation or experimentation. Significant results then provide an important piece of evidence used in causal inference. The scientific method is intended to define, classify, or categorize events and their relationships with potential causes; identify causal associations; provide a basis for predicting the effects of certain exposures; and use this information to prevent and control health problems.

Prior to the investigation, the researcher develops a statement of the research problem and identifies appropriate variables, data, and hypotheses. These basic elements of research help transform ideas into concrete research operations. In this chapter these terms are defined and discussed in the context of environmental epidemiology.

Research Problem

The general epidemiology question is how a susceptible host, agent of disease or injury, and permissive environment interact in time and space to produce disease or injury. Formulating this interrelationship is the essence of the **research problem**. The research problem should be clear and specific; otherwise the purpose and methods of the research become meaningless. A good research statement of a health problem is often simple, considering one exposure and one outcome variable such as organic solvents and brain cancer. This does not mean that the economic, social, cultural, and/or political contexts of the problem should not be considered, but these contexts are secondary to the primary problem. The research problem should also be specific with regards to the study subjects and variables to be employed in the analysis. Who is the specified population of interest and what variables will allow us to effectively assess the suspected exposure and health outcome? The research problem should be written prior to the outset of the study in order to focus the research efforts on a specific objective and provide a strong basis for interpreting the results.

Once the research problem is formulated, it is followed by the research question and hypothesis. **Research questions** ask about associations between exposures and health outcomes. A hypothesis is then formulated to predict the result. For example, the research problem may be that there is an elevated rate of hospital admissions for children with respiratory problems in a community that is located near a coke-works site.[1] The research question could be: "Is proximity of the residents to the coke-works site associated with hospital admissions of children for respiratory problems?" The research hypothesis could be that "the risk of hospital admissions for respiratory problems for children increases with proximity to the coke-works site."

Variables

The research process begins by forming concepts to describe health problems in specified populations. A concept is a general idea or understanding derived from specific instances or occurrences.[2] Movement from the conceptual to the empirical involves converting concepts into variables. An empirical approach emphasizes direct observation and experimentation, and variables are used to evaluate hypotheses. A **variable** is a characteristic that differs from one observation to the next and can be measured or categorized. For example, "sex" is a variable because it can be male or female; "severity rating" is a variable because it can take on values like mild, moderate, high; "number of children" is a variable that is limited to integer values (0, 1, 2, etc.); "distance" in meters from one or more hazardous waste sites is a variable because it has different values per individual; micrograms per liter of arsenic in drinking water is a variable because it can take on any value. Consider the variable "temperature," which can take on any value (e.g., $75.3544\ldots^\circ$). On the other hand, "hot" is not a variable, but a description.

Evidence from observation provides knowledge about potential environmental exposures, health risks, and disease occurrence. In environmental health we are often concerned with identifying the change in one variable, called the response or **dependent variable** (e.g., heart disease), as it relates to a given change in another variable (e.g., ground-level ozone), called the explanatory or **independent variable**. The distinction between these two types of variables relates to the research purpose; that is, the researcher chooses how to view the variables, basing the decision on the research problem. Variables may also be included in an analysis to reduce the risk of attributing explanatory power to the suspected exposure variable that in fact may have no association with a disease outcome (i.e., confounding).

An environmental epidemiologic study considers those variables appropriate for addressing the research question. Data are then obtained on those variables under consideration. The compilation of data over all the persons in the study makes up the data set used in the analysis portion of the study. An exception is the ecologic study design where the unit of analysis is on the population level; that is, the unit of analysis represents aggregated data rather than individual level data.

Data

The growth of empirical data collection associated with the environment and health has been astonishing in recent decades. Data about environmental conditions and environmental health risk factors have been widely disseminated in the media and the professional literature. Data motivate and support research hypotheses. **Data** may be thought of as observations or measurements of a phenomenon of interest such as exposure to environmental contaminants or disease information collected about a patient, family, or community. Data are usually established by observation, measurement, or experiment for a select number of variables.

One of the simplest forms of data is **nominal data**, which fall into unordered categories (see Table 2.1). Nominal data are sometimes called qualitative data because they describe the quality of a thing or a person. Distinct levels differ in quality, not quantity. The categories are often represented by numbers. For example, researchers of a study may assign males a value of 1 and females a value of 2. Despite the fact that the sexes are labeled with numbers, both the order and the magnitudes of the numbers are not important. In addition, information that can be captured that is nonnumerical in nature is qualitative data. Examples include text (spoken, written, etc.) and action (video).

When the ordering among categories is important, the data are referred to as **ordinal data**. For example, researchers may assign levels of tension that study par-

TABLE 2.1	Types of data	
	Description	**Examples**
Nominal	Categorical – unordered categories	
	Two levels – dichotomous	Sex, disease (yes, no)
	More than two levels – multichotomous	Race, marital status, education status
Ordinal	Categorical – ordering informative	Preference rating (e.g., agree, neutral, disagree)
Discrete	Quantitative – integers	Number of cases
Continuous	Quantitative – values on a continuum	Dose of ionizing radiation

ticipants experience in their shoulders as 1 never, 2 rarely, 3 occasionally, 4 often, and 5 constantly. A natural ordering exists in the data, with higher numbers representing a higher level of tension. However, as in the case of nominal data, the magnitude of the numbers is not important. We could have reversed the numbers, letting 5 represent never and 1 represent constantly. Consequently, it is not appropriate to apply many arithmetic operations to nominal or ordinal data.

For **discrete data**, both ordering and magnitude are important. Here the data represent quantities (integer values), not just labels. A natural order exists among the data. Because it is meaningful to measure the distance between levels of discrete observations, application of arithmetic computations is appropriate, such as the mean, median, and mode. Unlike discrete data, which is restricted to take on only certain integer values, **continuous data** represent measurable values on a continuum. The difference between two levels of a continuous variable can be arbitrarily small.

If a lesser degree of detail is desired than is available with continuous data, we may transform the data to a discrete, ordinal, or dichotomous form. For example, it is usually not necessary to know a person's exact age (e.g., 18.73 . . .), but to obtain the person's age as an integer value (e.g., 18); some continuous environmental exposures may have a danger threshold (e.g., safe versus dangerous); and it may be adequate to merely identify someone as ill or not ill rather than obtaining the level of the illness (e.g., his or her temperature).

Risk Assessment

Risk assessment is a tool to integrate exposure and health effects in order to identify the potential health hazards in humans. Risk assessment is also used to associate exposure and ecological effects in order to characterize the potential for other hazards in the environment. The definition of risk assessment used by the U.S. Environmental Protection Agency (EPA) is "[r]isk assessment is a process in which information is analyzed to determine if an environmental hazard might cause harm to exposed persons and ecosystems."[3]

Risk assessment involves an array of techniques to measure or estimate whether the exposure poses a threat to health or the ecosystem. Exposure is described more fully in the next section. Later in this chapter, direct and indirect measures of exposure are also discussed. As presented in the previous chapter, factors that influence the toxicity severity of a substance that enters the body include route of exposure, duration of exposure, and concentration of exposure, among other things (see the subsection entitled Toxicokinetics in Chapter 1). Risk assessment is the formal process that is used to establish regulations and standards by the EPA and other organizations. For example, risk assessment has led the Occupational Safety and Health Administration to set a limit of 0.2 milligram of polycyclic aromatic hydrocarbons (PAHs) per cubic meter of air (0.2 mg/m^3). The permissible exposure limit for mineral oil mist containing PAHs is 5 mg/m^3, averaged over 8 hours of exposure. The National Institute for Occupational Safety and Health recommends that coal tar products should not exceed 0.1 mg/m^3, averaged over 10 hours of exposure. Other limits have also been set for workplace exposure to coal, mineral oil, and other things containing PAHs.[4]

Risk assessment is only one step in the **risk management** process. Risk management involves the integration of recognized risk, risk assessment, development of strategies to manage risk, and mitigation of risk through managerial resources.[5] The aim of risk management is to reduce risks to levels deemed acceptable by the community. Risk management includes those types of threats to human health caused by environmental factors. The risk management process is extensive and goes beyond the scope of this book. The interested reader should refer to other sources on this topic, such as the EPA's General Risk Management Program Guidance (http://yosemite.epa.gov/oswer/ceppoweb.nsf/content/EPAguidance.htm# General) or the Risk Management Standard (http://www.theirm.org/publications/ PUstandard.html).

Exposure Data

An **exposure** may represent an actual exposure (e.g., toxic chemical or microorganism), a behavior (e.g., where one works or socializes), or an individual attribute (e.g., age, sex, race). A causal association may be implied in a descriptive study without a direct measure of exposure. However, greater confidence in causal associations between environmental factors and human health requires accurate identification of the primary mechanism (physical, chemical, biological, psychosocial) of the environmental contaminant or stress, and determination of how and in what form the environmental contaminant or stress comes in contact with people. It is necessary to establish whether there is evidence that the environmental contaminant or stress is capable of harming human health. This requires an accurate assessment of exposure.

Measuring the intensity and duration of exposure is often necessary for supporting causal association. Exposure may involve an intense dose over a relatively short period of time, or a low-level prolonged dose over a period from weeks to years. The effects of acute, high-dose environmental exposures may appear within hours or days (e.g., sunburn). On the other hand, the effects of chronic, low-dose exposures may not appear until years later (e.g., cancer).

Identifying an association between dose and an adverse health outcome provides support for causality. The quality of the exposure measurements influences the validity of the study. Validity refers to the "truthfulness" of a measure. A valid measure of a concept measures what it claims to measure. This is often a challenge when the environmental exposure, such as a hazardous chemical or radiation fallout, occurred in the distant past. Reconstructing past exposures may be complicated by limited recall, incomplete measurements, inaccurate records, and variability of exposure from person to person. In this situation, a direct measure of the past exposure may not be possible and can require estimation through modeling.

An exposure may be a specific event and relatively easy to measure, such as exposure to a chemical leak. Other exposures can be subdivided into dose or duration (e.g., number of glasses of water, number of years worked in a coal mine). A disease may require a minimal level of exposure and increase in probability with longer exposure. Such a relationship between exposure and disease may be missed with a dichotomous measure characterizing the presence or absence of the exposure. In many cases it is more appropriate to use ordinal or continuous measures of the exposure, especially when trying to assess a dose–response relationship. It may be useful to restrict the study cohort to those who are most likely exposed or to those with the most years of exposure. This may increase the probability of finding a dose-related effect while increasing the efficiency of the study by requiring fewer numbers of participants.

Although it is often desirable to isolate the association between a given exposure and disease outcome, assessing the combined effects of multiple exposures on human health is a potentially important approach from a public health perspective because public health interventions often target an overall exposure scenario.[6] Combined effects may reflect contaminants where the total effect differs from the sum of the individual effects. For example, automotive exhaust can produce volatile organic compounds and nitrogen oxides that when combined with sunlight produce ground-level ozone.

Measurement of an exposure variable on a continuous scale is the most informative for evaluating associations. Continuous data allow us to measure a dose–response relation between variables. However, in some cases exposure information is available only on a nominal scale—exposed versus unexposed or likely exposed versus unlikely exposed. This may be the only alternative when there are perceived versus documented exposures or the exposure occurred in the past and direct measurement is not feasible. There also exists the basic question as to what to measure; for example, should the peak exposure or the cumulative exposure be measured?[7] When determining what to measure, consider what relates most closely to the incidence and magnitude of a biological response. Is it maximum concentration, average concentration, minimum concentration, or total dose of the biologically active contaminant?[8]

There are both direct and indirect types of data for approximating exposure (see Table 2.2). Data most appropriate for assessing risk factors are those obtained from personal monitoring and use of biological markers. Personal measurement allows for assessment of the contaminant. Biological markers are useful for representing total dose to the body from multiple routes of exposure. These data can provide exposure measures on a continuous scale, which is useful for identifying adverse health outcomes according to dose and whether a threshold exists. Data are also useful that reflect information obtained from quantifying the concentration of toxic contaminants in a specific environment (air, water, soil, and food). These provide direct measures of dose. The remaining types of data listed in the table provide indirect measurements of dose. These data are easier to

---

TABLE 2.2   Direct and indirect measurements of dose

Direct

Quantified personal measurement

Quantified area or ambient measurements in the vicinity of the residence or other sites of activity

Indirect

Estimates of drinking water use, food use, etc.

Distance from site **and** duration of residence

Distance from site **or** duration of residence

Residence or employment in geographic area in reasonable proximity to site where exposure can be assumed

Residence or employment in defined geographical area of the site (e.g., a county)

Source: Modified from National Research Council, 1997, p. 120.[9]

For a list of advantages and disadvantages of various exposure methods see Armstrong, White, and Saracci (1992).[10]

obtain but obviously less precise. Limited time and money may make it necessary to rely on indirect measures of exposure. Although causal inference is strongest when exposure information is directly measured, surrogate measures of exposure can also provide important insights into causality.

Exposure Assessment Methods

Direct Measures

Direct measures of exposure include personal monitoring and use of biologic markers. Personal monitoring involves quantitative measurements of personal exposure to environmental physical stresses, chemical or biological agents, and psychosocial milieu. Personal monitoring devices are worn by individuals while they pursue their normal activities, most often in the workplace. For example, an individual may wear a dosimeter to estimate total exposure to radiation in the workplace through the air, water, and food. A personal air monitor may be worn to measure exposure to air pollutants in the home.

Biologic markers are those specific anatomic, physiologic, biochemical, or molecular characteristics used to measure the presence and severity of a disease or condition. Biological monitoring can involve measurements of concentrations in human tissues (blood lead), metabolic products (dimethylarsinic acid in urine after arsenic exposure), or markers of physiologic effects (e.g., protein adducts induced by beta-naphthylamine in cigarette smoke).[6] Biologic markers can be measured through physical examinations, laboratory assays, and medical imaging. For example, heavy metals and some pesticides can accumulate in the body. Over time the risk of human harm increases. The pollutants, which reflect the amount of pollution in the environment, leave residues in the body that are usually measured in the blood or urine. The approach of measuring pollutant levels in tissue or fluid samples is called **biomonitoring**.[11]

Indirect Measures

Indirect methods for obtaining exposure information include questionnaires, surrogates, existing records, and diaries.

Questionnaires translate the research objectives into specific questions. Answers to these questions provide the data used in data analysis. Questionnaires may be administered through face-to-face interviews, over the telephone, and through the mail or Internet. In a population-based case-control study involving female nonsmokers in Hong Kong, face-to-face interviews were conducted using a standardized questionnaire. There were 200 cases and 285 controls. Cumulative exposure to cooking by various forms of frying increased the risk of lung cancer. The increased risk of lung cancer was greatest when cooking involved deep-frying, followed by frying, and then stir-frying.[12] A telephone-conducted questionnaire of 1,009 American veterans (65% response rate) deployed and not deployed to the Gulf War found that 6% of non–Gulf War veterans reported being exposed to biological or chemical warfare compared with 64% of the Gulf War veterans. Veterans tended to associate exposure with having adverse physical symptoms and receiving an alert from the military.[13] In another questionnaire-based study, data were collected through the mail. This study involved 1,456 Australian Gulf War veterans (80.5% response rate) and a comparison group (56.8% response rate). The study found that the Australian Gulf War veterans had a higher than expected risk of respiratory symptoms and asthma and bronchitis.[14]

Questionnaire data rely on individual recall and knowledge and are thus subject to error. Bias may be introduced by the interviewer's inflections, expressions, gender, and appearance. Telephone interviews are becoming more difficult to conduct because of caller identification, cell phones, and a decreasing tolerance of telemarketing in the population. Historically, many national health surveys in the United States have relied on telephone surveys, yet their response rates have been steadily declining in recent years. For example, the average response rates for the Behavior Risk Factor Surveillance System survey, a national survey conducted every year to monitor health risk-factor behavior, fell consistently between 1997 and 2005, from 68.3% to 51.1%.[15]

Mailed questionnaires avoid interviewer influences but are subject to low response rates. In addition, they exclude individuals who cannot read and do not allow the responder to obtain item clarifications. Electronic mail questionnaires are becoming an increasingly popular way to obtain information because of their relative speed, low cost, and ability to attach pictures and sound files; they often stimulate higher response levels than "snail" mail surveys. However, some challenges to email surveys include obtaining (or purchasing) a list of email addresses, nonresponse to unsolicited email (which may be higher than unsolicited regular mail), and obtaining a representative sample of the general population.

General questions that may be used for characterizing exposure include:

- What is the mechanism (physical, chemical, biological, psychosocial)?
- How potent or intense was the exposure?
- What was the duration of exposure?

- Was there a relation between duration of exposure and disease?
- What is the exposure pathway (air, water, soil, food)?
- How did the pollutant enter the body?
- What clinical signs, if any, are associated with the exposure?

Some exposures may be represented by surrogate measures. Some examples include years of employment, census track, carbon monoxide in indoor air at home, trihalomethanes in water coming out of the tap, self-reported water consumption, and hot shower use. However, such measures are crude and subject to errors. A direct measure would be more accurate, but is often financially prohibitive. Halperin (2002) suggests that cost may be reduced by using an indirect measure of dose, like years of employment in a cohort, and then performing a nested case-control study using a direct measure.[16]

It may also be possible to obtain exposure information from existing records, such as hospital admission or discharge records, pathology records, and crisis assessment prevention intervention services. This approach avoids the problems of interviewer bias, recall bias, and response bias.

Several studies have used diaries to identify exposure. For example, in a prospective cohort of newlywed couples in two districts (Tiexi and Dadong) in Shenyang, China, investigators examined the effects of various environmental and occupational exposures on reproductive outcomes. The study consisted of 165 newlywed, nonsmoking Chinese women with no past history of dysmenorrhea (cramps or painful menstruation) at the time of enrollment. Enrollment began after couples obtained permission to become pregnant. Daily diaries were used to record exposure to environmental tobacco smoke until the occurrence of clinical pregnancy or for up to 1 year. Environmental tobacco smoke was defined as "the mean number of cigarettes smoked per day at home by household members over an entire menstrual cycle before the menstrual period." The adjusted odds ratios of dysmenorrhea associated with tertile groupings of environmental tobacco smoke exposure compared with no exposure were 1.1 (95% CI, 0.5–2.6), 2.5 (CI, 0.9–6.7), and 3.1 (CI, 1.2–8.3), respectively. These data indicate an increased risk of dysmenorrhea among women exposed to environmental tobacco smoke, more so with higher levels of exposure.[17]

Modeling

Pollutants are released from multiple sources (e.g., treatment storage and disposal facilities, industry, government facilities, households, and others). The **fate and transport** of contaminants is an important issue in managing hazardous pollutants. Fate and transport involves groundwater, soil, gas, and atmospheric transport of chemicals. Of primary concern in fate and transport is determination of the transport speed and synergistic effects of chemicals in their environments. Considerable effort has gone into understanding the state and science of the fate and transport of selected substances like mercury in aquatic and terrestrial systems, their transformation processes, and approaches to effectively manage ecological and human exposures to selected substances.[18]

A number of models have been developed to estimate the magnitude of pollutants in the air, water, and soil:

- The Atmospheric Sciences Modeling Division contains information about atmospheric models.
- The Center for Exposure Assessment Modeling provides predictive exposure models for aquatic, terrestrial, and multimedia pathways for organic chemicals and metals.
- The Division of Computational Toxicology applies mathematical and computer models to predict adverse effects and describe the mechanisms through which chemicals may induce harm.
- The Support Center for Regulatory Environmental Model provides model guidance, development, and application.
- The Support Center for Regulatory Air Models is a source of information on atmospheric dispersion (air quality) models.
- ADL Migration Exposure Model was developed to estimate the migration of chemicals from polymeric materials used in the home.
- The Landfill Air Emissions Estimation Model was developed to estimate emissions of methane, carbon dioxide, nonmethane organic compounds, and hazardous air pollutants from municipal solid-waste landfills.
- The Multi-Chamber Concentration and Exposure Model was designed to estimate average peak indoor air concentrations of chemicals from products or materials in homes.
- AQUATOX is a freshwater ecosystem simulation model that predicts the fate of selected pollutants such as organic toxicants and their effects on the ecosystem.
- CHEMFLO is a model for simulating water and chemical movement in unsaturated soils.
- PRESTO-EPA-POP is a computer model for evaluating radiation exposure from contaminated soil layers.[19]

A Physiologically Based Pharmacokinetic (PBPK) model is a physiologically based compartmental (e.g., lung, liver, rapidly perfused tissues, slowly perfused tissues, fat, and kidney) model used to characterize pharmacokinetic behavior (absorption, distribution, metabolism, and excretion) of a chemical. This model has become the tool of choice for predicting the fate of environmental contaminants in humans. Data on blood-flow rates, metabolic, and other processes that the chemical undergoes within each compartment are used to construct a mass-balance framework for the PBPK model.[20] PBPK models have been developed for methylmercury,[21] cadmium,[22] lead,[23] and methyl tert-butyl ether.[24]

Outcome Assessment

The **outcome** refers to the disease state, event, behavior, or condition associated with health that is under investigation. Outcome status refers to the presence or absence of the health-related state or event. Although outcome status is typically measured as a dichotomous variable, it may also be measured as an ordinal variable (e.g., severe, moderate, mild, no disease) or a continuous variable (e.g., concentrations of lead in the blood). The type of data considered is often determined by accessibility.

Accurate assessment of outcome status requires a standard case definition and adequate levels of reporting. A standard set of clinical criteria, or case definition, will ensure that cases are consistently diagnosed, regardless of where or when they were identified and who diagnosed the case. Whatever the criteria, they should be applied consistently and without bias to all those under investigation. A specific case definition will minimize misclassification resulting in bias.

The clinical criteria to be a case, particularly in the setting of an outbreak investigation, may be restricted by person (e.g., to children less than 5 years of age), place (e.g., to employees at a certain work site), and time (e.g., persons with onset of illness within the past 48 hours) variables. The clinical criteria may include laboratory confirmation. Yet acquiring the biological media and having the expertise and resources for assessment may prove difficult. Clinical criteria may also involve a combination of signs, symptoms, and other findings. Clinicians characterize disease status by examining and analyzing the specific symptoms and performing tests on the patient.

The availability of outcome data may also be influenced by the acceptability of the diagnostic test. Diagnostic tests predict the presence of an outcome. Ideally, a diagnostic test will always give the right answer; for example, a positive test in the presence of disease and a negative test in the absence of disease. The test should also be quick, safe, painless, inexpensive, valid, and reliable. The validity of a test is determined by the sensitivity and specificity of the test. **Sensitivity** is the proportion of patients with a given outcome who have a positive test, and **specificity** is the proportion of individuals without a given outcome who have a negative test. Reliability refers to a test's performance over time.

Rarely is a diagnostic test ideal. Validity and reliability of a test typically result in some misclassification. Some occupational and environmental disorders are often difficult to diagnose. In such cases, the outcome of interest is likely to be underestimated. While the best diagnostic tests should be employed, further development of diagnostic procedures is needed, particularly for occupational and environmental disorders that are difficult to diagnose.

The Study (or Research) Hypothesis

A **hypothesis** is a tentative suggestion that certain associations exist in certain activities or a chain of events. The initial hypothesis is generally based on observation, which refers primarily to empirical findings from data systematically collected. Once the hypothesis is in place, it is necessary to determine how to design the study and formulate it in statistical terms. The hypothesis applies to a specified population of interest.

When developing a hypothesis, potential exposures should be described according to their toxicity (including carcinogenicity) and other effects when information is available from experimental studies involving animals and, if available, humans. Health risks associated with potential exposures can be obtained through epidemiologic studies showing the health effects of analogous contaminants in other circumstances. In some instances exposure is not accurately described or a causal factor is not even specified. However, if an excess in disease is observed, based on knowledge about exposure and disease from other sources, it may be possible to hypothesize about the nature of causation.[25]

The methods used in environmental epidemiology are generally observational and not experimental, making it more difficult to make causal inference. In observational studies there is less control over exposure and outcome measures because it is more difficult to control for confounding and there is greater susceptibility to bias. This means that the researcher must rely on inductive methods for making inferences about his or her data. Fundamental to the development of hypothesis testing is inductive reasoning. This is the process leading from a set of specific facts to general statements that explain those facts. Inductive reasoning relies on

1. exact and correct observation;
2. accurate and correct interpretation of the facts in order to understand findings and their relationship to each other and to causality;
3. clear, accurate, and rational explanations of findings, information, and facts in reference to causality;
4. development based on scientific approaches, using facts in the analysis and in a manner that makes sense, based on rational scientific knowledge.[26]

A hypothesis is not necessary in descriptive studies where the distribution of a single variable is being described. On the other hand, a hypothesis is required when an association is being evaluated between exposure and outcome variable.

Key Issues

1. The general epidemiology question is "How do a susceptible host, agent of disease or injury, and permissive environment interact in time and space to produce disease or injury?" Formulating this interrelationship is the essence of a research problem.
2. Movement from the conceptual to the empirical involves converting concepts into variables. Variables are used to evaluate hypotheses.
3. Data may be thought of as observations or measurements of a phenomenon of interest such as exposure to environmental contaminants or disease information collected about a patient, family, or community. Data are usually established by observation, measurement, or experiment for a select number of variables. The four primary types of data are nominal, ordinal, discrete, and continuous.
4. A hypothesis is a tentative suggestion that certain associations exist in certain activities or a chain of events. The initial hypothesis is generally based on observation, which refers primarily to empirical findings from data systematically collected. Once the hypothesis is in place, it is necessary to determine how to design the study and formulate it in statistical terms.

Exercises

Key Terms

Define the following terms.

Biomonitoring
Continuous data
Data
Dependent variable
Discrete data
Exposure
Fate and transport
Hypothesis
Independent variable
Nominal data
Ordinal data
Outcome
Research problem
Research question
Risk assessment
Risk management
Sensitivity
Specificity
Variable

Study Questions

2.1. List some aspects for a good research problem.

2.2. How does a research question differ from a hypothesis?

2.3. What is a variable? How do dependent variables relate to independent variables in a study? Give examples of dependent and independent variables.

2.4. Describe the four types of data presented in the chapter.

2.5. Compare and contrast exposure and outcome data.

2.6. Distinguish between direct and indirect measures of exposure.

2.7. What is the meaning of the term "fate and transport"?

2.8. Explain the stages of hypothesis development.

References

1. Aylin P, Bottle A, Wakefield J, Jarup L, Elliott P. Proximity to coke works and hospital admissions for respiratory and cardiovascular disease in England and Wales. *Thorax.* 2001;56:228–233.

2. *Webster's Ninth New Collegiate Dictionary.* Springfield, MA: Merriam-Webster, Inc; 1991.

3. Environmental Protection Agency. Risk assessment principles & practices. Available at: http://www.epa.gov/OSA/pdfs/ratf-final.pdf. Accessed June 10, 2007.

4. Agency for Toxic Substances and Disease Registry. ToxFAQs: polycyclic aromatic hydrocarbons (PAHs). U.S. Department of Health and Human Services, Public Health Service Agency for Toxic Substances and Disease Registry. Available at: http://www.atsdr.cdc.gov/tfacts69.pdf. Accessed June 10, 2007.

5. Wikipedia: The free encyclopedia. *Risk Management.* Available at: http://en.wikipedia.org/wiki/Risk_management. Accessed June 10, 2007.

6. Hertz-Picciotto I. Environmental epidemiology. In: Rothman K, Greenland S, eds. *Modern Epidemiology.* Philadelphia, PA: Lippincott-Raven; 1998.

7. Bailar JC. Inhalation hazards: The interpretation of epidemiologic evidence. In: Bates DV et al., eds. *Assessment of Inhalation Hazards.* New York, NY: Springer-Verlag; 1989:39–48.

8. Gillette JR. Dose, species, and route extrapolation: general aspects. National Research Council, *Pharmacokinetics in Risk Assessment, Drinking Water and Health.* Vol 8. Washington, DC: National Academy Press; 1989:96–158.

9. National Research Council. *Environmental Epidemiology: Use of the Gray Literature and Other Data in Environmental Epidemiology.* Vol 2. Washington, DC: National Academy Press; 1997.

10. Armstong BK, White E, Saracci R. *Principles of Exposure Measurement in Epidemiology.* New York: Oxford University Press; 1992. Monographs in epidemiology and biostatistics, Vol 21.

11. Environmental Protection Agency. Measuring exposures to environmental pollution. Available at: http://www.epa.gov/indicate/roe/html/roeHealthMe.htm. Accessed April 6, 2007.

12. Yu IT, Chiu YL, Au JS, Wong TW, Tang JL. Dose-response relationship between cooking fumes exposures and lung cancer among Chinese nonsmoking women. *Cancer Res.* 2006;66(9):4961–4967.

13. Brewer NT, Lillie SE, Hallman WK. Why people believe they were exposed to biological or chemical warfare: A survey of Gulf War veterans. *Risk Anal.* 2006;26(2):337–345.

14. Kellsall HL, Sim MR, Forbes AB. Respiratory health status of Australian veterans of the 1991 Gulf War and the effects of exposure to oil fire smoke and dust storms. *Thorax.* 2004;59(1):897–903.

15. Centers for Disease Control and Prevention. Technical information and data: Summary data quality reports. Available at: http://www.cdc.gov/brfss/technical_infodata/quality.htm. Accessed January 22, 2006.

16. Halperin WE. Field investigations of occupational disease and injury. In: Gregg MB, ed. *Field Epidemiology.* 2nd ed. New York, NY: Oxford University Press; 2002:321.

17. Chen C, Cho S, Damokosh AI. Prospective study of exposure to environmental tobacco smoke and dysmenorrhea. *Environ Health Perspect.* 2000;108: 1019–1022.

18. Environmental Protection Agency. Proceedings and summary report: workshop on the fate, transport, and transformation of mercury in aquatic and terrestrial environments. Available at: http://www.epa.gov/nrmrl/pubs/625r 02005/625R02005.pdf. Accessed April 7, 2007.

19. Environmental Protection Agency. *Models.* Available at: http://www.epa.gov/ epahome/models.htm. Accessed April 7, 2007.

20. Environmental Protection Agency. *Glossary archive.* Available at: http://www .epa.gov/iris/gloss8_arch.htm. Accessed April 7, 2007.

21. Shipp AM, Gentry PR, Lawrence G. Determination of a site-specific reference dose for methylmercury for fish-eating populations. *Toxicol Ind Health.* 2000;16(9–10):335–438.

22. Nordbert GF, Kjellstrom T. Metabolic model for cadmium in man. *Environ Health Perspect.* 1979;28:211–217.

23. O'Flaherty EJ. Physiologically based models for bone-seeking elements. IV. Kinetics of lead disposition in humans. *Toxicol Appl Pharmacol.* 1993; 118(1):16–29.

24. Licata AC, Dekant W, Smith CE, Borghoff SJ. A physiologically based pharmacokinetic model for methyl tert-butyl ether in humans: implementing sensitivity and variability analyses. *Toxicol Sci.* 2001;62(2):191–204.

25. National Research Council. *Environmental Epidemiology: Public Health and Hazardous Wastes.* Vol 1. Washington, DC: National Academy Press; 1991.

26. Shindell S, Salloway JC, Oberembt CM. *A Coursebook in Health Care Delivery.* New York: Appleton-Century-Crofts; 1976.

Monitoring Environmental Health

LEARNING OBJECTIVES

After completing this chapter, you should be able to:

1. Identify types and purposes of monitoring programs.
2. Identify several key health indicators and measures.
3. Identify potential data sources of monitoring data.
4. Identify the important role of epidemiology in providing information for environmental monitoring programs.
5. Identify selected challenges and possible solutions to environmental monitoring.

Introduction

Through epidemiologic studies, environmental factors associated with increased risk of human injury, disease, and death have been identified. These studies have also provided a better understanding of exposure pathways of these health indicators. It is upon this basis that environmental standards and monitoring programs are built. Monitoring programs are important because they influence decision making, policy making, and program development in a way that promotes health and well-being.

Monitoring programs attempt to measure and estimate physical conditions and substances in the human environment that influence health. The general aim of monitoring programs is to measure and estimate environmental hazards, to measure adverse health effects and damage to the environment (plants, trees, buildings, air, soil, water), and to evaluate the effectiveness of prevention and control efforts. The purpose of this chapter is to identify types and purposes of environmental monitoring programs, indicators commonly used in monitoring programs, and some alternative approaches to monitoring in situations where public health indicators are not readily available. Later chapters will specifically focus on monitoring programs of air, water, soil and food, radiation, the macro impact of environmental pollution, and disasters.

Types and Purposes of Environmental Monitoring Programs

There are various types of monitoring programs, each with specific purposes. These purposes include assessment of the impact of physical, chemical, and biological stresses; evaluating the local, regional, or global impact of pollutions; assessing contamination levels from industrial facilities, confirming adequacy of pollution controls, and, if necessary, cleanup and restoration efforts; assessing exposure from a single source, multiple sources, and environmental consequences; determining compliance with applicable regulations; and providing relevant information for public relations (see Table 3.1).

Based on Nature of the Stress

Measuring physical stresses involves real-time measurements made in the field. Monitors are put in place near exposure sites. Chemical exposures are evaluated

TABLE 3.1   Types and purposes of environmental monitoring programs

Type of program	Purpose
Based on nature of the stress	
Physical stress	To assess the impact of environmental stresses such as noise and radiation, where the evaluation is based primarily on exposure measurements made in the field, not on samples collected and returned to the laboratory for analysis
Chemical stress	To assess chemical exposures transmitted through solid, liquid, or gaseous environments and interactions with the body through the skin, ingestion, or inhalation
Biological stress	To assess the level of environmental toxins in the body, usually in blood, serum, plasma, or urine
Based on geographic (spatial) coverage	
Local	To evaluate the impact of a single facility on a given area
Regional	To evaluate the combined impact of emissions from several facilities on a larger area
Global	To determine worldwide impacts and trends, such as acidic deposition, depletion of the ozone layer, and the potential for global warming
Based on temporal considerations	
Preoperational	To determine potential contamination levels in the environment prior to operation of a new industrial facility; to train staff; and to confirm the operation of laboratory and field equipment
Operational	To provide data on releases and to confirm adequacy of pollution controls
Postoperational	To ensure proper site cleanup and restoration
Based on monitoring objectives	
Source related	To determine population exposures from a single source
Person related	To determine the total exposure to people from all sources
Environment related	To determine the impacts of several sources on features of the environment such as plants, trees, buildings, statues, soil, and water
Research related	To determine the transfer of specific pollutants from one environmental medium to another and to assess their chemical and biological transformation as they move within the environment; to determine ecological indicators of pollution; and to confirm that the critical population group has been correctly identified and that the models being applied are accurate representations of the environment being monitored

(continued)

TABLE 3.1   Types and purposes of environmental monitoring programs (continued)

Based on administrative and legal requirements	
Compliance related	To determine compliance with applicable regulations
Public information	To provide data and information for purposes of public relations

Source: Adapted from Moeller, 1992, pp. 232–233.[1]

in the air (respirable fraction via air sampling, total particulates via air sampling, and collection of settled particulates), water (nondrinking surface water, groundwater, and drinking water), soil and plants (vegetation and aquatic plants), animals (wildlife, fish, shellfish, and waterfowl), and foodstuffs and milk. Respirable fraction via air sampling, drinking water, wildlife, fish, shellfish, waterfowl, foodstuffs, and milk are direct-dose vectors, which are typically easier to interpret. The appropriate type of sample will be influenced by the relative importance of the medium in contributing to the population exposure. Monitoring biological stresses involves identifying the level of environmental toxins in the body. Ideally this is done by sampling the blood, serum, plasma, or urine.

Monitoring physical stresses is generally simpler than monitoring chemical contaminants. With physical stresses, such as ionizing radiation or workplace injuries, monitoring may involve identifying the source and measuring the magnitude of the problem. For chemical contaminants, monitoring can involve identifying the source, measuring the discharge at the source, determining the exposure pathway (air, water, soil, food), identifying transfer among these media, and determining any chemical or biological transformation within the environment. Air and water are the primary forms of direct transmission through inhalation and ingestion and for transmitting the contaminant from the source to other media such as milk and food. Monitoring devices of the air should be in locations where concentrations and ground deposition of selected contaminants have the greatest likelihood of human exposure. Water samplers should be located above and below the target facility. A sampler should also be located at the first water intake location downstream. Nearby groundwater and other sources of drinking water should also be sampled.[1]

A variety of specific laboratory procedures are now available for measuring biological stresses. These laboratory procedures use biologic markers, also known as biomarkers, to identify and track disease progression prior to or after disease occurrence. **Biomarkers** are defined as anatomic, physiologic, biochemical, or molecular substances that are associated with the presence and severity of specific disease states and are detectable and measurable by a variety of methods including physical examination, laboratory assays, and medical imaging.[2] To illustrate the use of biomarkers in detection of disease occurrence and progression, consider the example of chemical carcinogenesis. As shown in Figure 3.1, the stages of chemical carcinogenesis are environmental exposure, internal dose, biologically effective dose, early biologic effects, and clinical disease. In addition, susceptibility, the inherent or acquired limitation of an organism's ability to respond to a challenge, influences each of the five stages. Although these stages are identified with chemical carcinogenesis in the figure, it is important to note that these stages describe the progression of a number of other health states.

The figure also outlines the types of biomarkers that can be used at each stage. To monitor internal doses, biomarkers are used to measure the actual level of absorption of an agent or the bioaccumulation of metabolite within the body. For

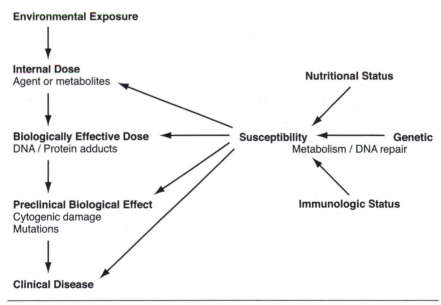

FIGURE 3.1   Stages of chemical carcinogenesis showing the use of biomarkers to identify and track disease. (*Source:* Courtesy of Santella, 2002.)[3]

example, biomarkers are used to measure lead levels in blood, cotinine in serum or urine, urinary phenol levels in benzene exposure, and organochlorines in serum from dietary exposure. To analyze biologically effective doses, biomarkers measure DNA and protein adducts to quantify biochemical, molecular, genetic, immunologic, and physiological mutations in an organism that resulted from the exposure or internal dose. Because biomarkers for biologically effective doses measure initial mutations, they are also useful in identifying or predicting the potential onset of a health impairment or disease. By the stage of preclinical biological effect, biological mutations are beginning to alter not only the structures, but the functions of bodily organs and systems. To measure this early onset of disease, biomarkers are used to further track mutations and to identify the level of cytogenetic damage.[3]

Based on Monitoring Objectives

Monitoring programs also depend on certain objectives. A program may monitor the extent of human exposure resulting from a single source, or the extent of human exposure resulting from multiple sources. Monitoring programs may involve the actual health events, such as the incidence of cardiovascular and respiratory events, or the rates of hospitalization and emergency department visits for acute cardiovascular and respiratory events. Some monitoring programs consider the extent of damage to features of the environment, such as water, soil, buildings, trees, and so on. Monitoring programs may also provide useful information on sources of hazardous pollutants, pathways through the environment, and avenues by which pollutants can result in human exposure.

In the case of environmental uranium, programs monitor human exposure by tracking both environmental damage and health outcomes, and the pathway in between (Figure 3.2). Uranium is a naturally occurring radioactive substance. Uranium is present throughout the earth's crust at a concentration of ~2 mg/kg. As the uranium atoms gradually disintegrate over billions of years, radioactive by-products are formed, consisting of thorium-230, radium-226, radon-222, and "radon daughters," which include lead-210 and polonium-210. Uranium exposure is associated with the nuclear industry, and environmental exposures from mining, food, and buildings. Uranium miners are particularly susceptible to inhalation of uranium through uranium-containing dust particles or aerosols, which can contain large quantities of radioactive radon gas. Uranium-238, which is contained in many

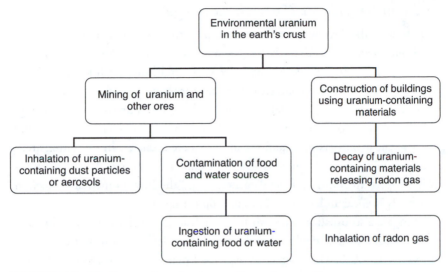

FIGURE 3.2   Pathway of environmental uranium to human exposure

building materials, is also known to decay over time, releasing radon gas into the environment. Because radon is a known carcinogen, uranium can indirectly add to the risk of lung cancer.

In addition to inhalation, environmental uranium can enter the human body through ingestion. Typically, ingestion of uranium occurs indirectly by eating food or drinking water that is contaminated by environmental uranium. Contaminated water and food sources can occur from activities such as mining and the nuclear industry, but are not frequent. Once in the body, uranium is initially absorbed by the lungs or intestines but soon enters the bloodstream. While much of the uranium is quickly excreted from the body through the urinary tract and other pathways, some is deposited in other organs, such as the kidneys, and in bone. Accumulation of uranium in the body can lead to damage of the cardiovascular system, liver, muscle, and nervous system. Because uranium is naturally abundant in the environment and many human activities can enhance the burden of uranium on health, it is important to not only monitor health outcomes from uranium, but environmental changes in uranium.[4]

Based on Geographic (Spatial) Coverage

To understand the distribution of contaminants in the environment, it is important for monitoring programs to track the geographic location of pollutants. On a local level, such environmental monitoring programs for individual facilities are typically handled by each plant or a contractor. On the other hand, regional environmental monitoring programs are generally handled by local and state environmental regulatory agencies. However, in many cases there is overlap between the monitoring efforts of the plant personnel and the local or state agencies. In this latter situation, exchanging samples and cross-checking data may improve the overall monitoring efforts. In addition, federal agencies (e.g., the Environmental Protection Agency) assist local and state facilities in monitoring.

There are also broader efforts to monitor factors that have a global impact, such as global warming, depletion of the ozone layer, deforestation, and acidic deposition. Certain U.S. federal agencies (e.g., the Environmental Protection Agency (EPA), the Agency for Toxic Substances and Disease Registry, and the National Oceanic and Atmospheric Administration) have monitoring programs to assess the level and trends of pollutants in the ambient air, such as carbon monoxide, lead, nitrogen dioxide, ozone, PM_{10}, sulfur dioxide, and tons of criteria pollutants released into the ambient air. In addition, intergovernmental treaties overseen by the organizations such as the United Nations set limits for and monitor the levels of pollutants produced each year in most countries of the world. These treaties include the Kyoto and Montreal protocols, which are discussed in a later chapter. To ensure that monitoring programs are effective in all locations, laws and penalties have been established. These laws and penalties, as well as enforcement agencies, will be further discussed in a later section.

Based on Temporal Considerations

Before a new industrial facility opens, it is important to determine the existing levels of contaminants in the area. Such monitoring efforts include testing soil and nearby water sources for contamination. However, it is also important to determine the amount of contamination the new facility will add to the environment prior to commencing operation. With governmental regulations as guidelines, mathematical models and data from similar facilities can be used to hypothesize the level of contamination the plant will produce. Once the facility is operating, it is crucial that monitoring efforts continue within the plant and surrounding areas to ensure that pollutant levels do not exceed plant projections and federal regulations.

Based on Administrative and Legal Requirements

An important outcome of monitoring programs is to determine compliance with regulations and provide data and information for purposes of public relations. In the United States, there are a number of federal environmental regulations ranging from the Clean Air Act and Clean Water Act to the Noise Control Act and the Occupational Safety and Health Act.[5] Although the EPA oversees federal environmental acts and establishes programs to ensure compliance to regulations, a large amount of responsibility for compliance lies with individual facilities. To prove compliance, individual facilities are required to routinely submit formal reports to state governments and the EPA detailing their monitoring efforts and environmental impacts, including greenhouse gas emissions, radioactive material production, accidents, and so forth. In addition, local governments and the EPA have authority to monitor or inspect facilities regarding environmental issues. If facilities fail to report their environmental impacts or are found to have impacts above regulation limits, penalties are incurred. To inform facilities of pending penalties, a formal notice of noncompliance is first issued. If the notice is ignored and facilities continue to fail regulations, then civil and criminal punishment, including fines or imprisonment, can occur. For example, knowing violators of the Clean Air Act can be criminally prosecuted, resulting in fines up to $25,000 per day of violation or several years of imprisonment.[6] Because noncompliance with federal regulations results in environmental damage and significant penalties, monitoring efforts to ensure compliance is essential.

Environmental Public Health Indicators Project

Several environmental public health indicators have been identified through epidemiologic analytic studies as useful for monitoring environmental contaminants, health effects, and intervention programs. Health indicators should reliably predict the association between human health and the environment. It is recommended that environmental public health indicators be regularly collected, consistently defined, and that standard data collection techniques be used. A measure for a given indicator may change with improved technologies and as epidemiologic studies advance our understanding of sources of disease and injury and their modes of transmission.

The **Environmental Public Health Indicators Project**, sponsored by the Centers for Disease Control and Prevention's Division of Environmental Hazard and Health Effects and the National Center for Environmental Health, has compiled a summary of core indicates. These are listed as follows:

- Air, indoor
- Air, ambient (outdoor)
- Water (ambient, drinking)
- Lead
- Pesticides
- Toxics and waste
- Sun and ultraviolet light
- Sentinel events
- Noise
- Disasters

The Environmental Public Health Indicators Project has provided a comprehensive list of suggested measures for these environmental health indicators along with potential data sources.[7,8] These are presented in Appendices I and II.

The environmental public health indicators also provide a foundation for developing environmental public health surveillance among states. The indicators may provide information for decision making, policy making, and program development. Steps suggested by the Environmental Public Health Indicators Project (2006) are:

1. Select indicator topic(s) relevant to your state.
2. With the selected topic(s), choose relevant indicators.
3. For each indicator selected, identify the measure(s) of interest.
4. For core indicators and measures, use the standard definitions and measurement criteria identified in the technical supplement. If your state uses different standards or criteria, or none are identified in the technical supplement, identify the standards and criteria used or proposed by your state.
5. Identify data sources from which data are used.
   a. Evaluate the usefulness of the identified data sources.
   b. Identify required data elements.
   c. When connecting data for hazards, exposures, health outcomes, and interventions, identify areas in which standards and specifications for automating

differ from those provided by the National Electronic Data Surveillance System (NEDSS). If yours is a new system, develop standards and specifications that are consistent with NEDSS.

   d. Identify data or surveillance systems that need to be stored or made available electronically.

   e. Identify data sources that are useful to public health but restricted from use.

6. Identify additional data collection needs for bridging data gaps for the selected indicators. If the suggested measures are not useful, recommend alternative measures.

7. Summarize data collected for the selected measures to describe the state of environmental public health in your state.

   a. Identify and rank the hazards, exposures, and health effects by level of concern.

   b. Determine whether the data answer questions about the usefulness of public health programs and interventions.

   c. If multiple years of data are available, evaluate trends among selected measures.[7]

Challenges to Monitoring

For many diseases there are no clear environmental etiologies. Difficulty of identifying the at-risk population and limited data are barriers to identifying environmental sources of disease; it remains difficult to identify environmental causes of birth defects, spontaneous abortion, neurological impairment, and cancer, in part because the populations at risk might not have been adequately identified. Further, underpowered studies and indirect sources of data often limit establishment of cause–effect relationships. Yet where potential environmental hazards and exposures harmful to human health are recognized, environmental standards can be set and monitoring programs conducted.

Where the environmental etiologies are in question, environmental epidemiologic studies are needed. Insufficient epidemiologic data limit the setting of appropriate standards. For example, insufficient data exist on the health effects of exposure to magnetic and electric fields to establish sound monitoring standards. In addition, standards may not be specific enough to be meaningful for selected subgroups of the population. Further, basing standards on thresholds may be overly simplistic. It is possible that adverse health events may result from even low dosages, especially after extended periods of exposure.

When risks associated with exposures according to standard limits are not quantified, protection from the standard will not be fully understood across the different standard limits. Unfortunately, contaminant limits in the natural environment are often difficult to establish, although this is less of a difficulty for air and water. Another challenge is that monitoring standards often fail to consider a combination of occupational and environmental pollutants.[9] Small populations affected by environmental contaminants are difficult to apply epidemiologic techniques because of small sample sizes. Some possible solutions may involve meta-analysis, diary records, and disease registries and vital statistics systems. Meta-analysis is useful when a single study is underpowered, diary records are useful because they reduce the problem of recall bias, and disease registries and vital statistics systems may allow us to assess the public health impacts of various sources of exposure.

Meta-analysis

The primary activities and types of meta-analyses will be discussed in Chapter 4: Epidemiologic Study Designs. Briefly, meta-analysis is performed when more than one study has the same conceptual hypothesis. The primary question of interest in a meta-analysis is whether studies with the same conceptual hypothesis produce similar or different results, and what the net result is. Quantitatively synthesizing research requires:

1. Definition of the research question to be summarized.
2. Identification of which research designs will be appropriate.
3. Identification of operational definitions of key constructs allowed, such as treatments, manipulations, and measuring instruments. Exclusion and inclusion criteria should be based on this definition of constructs.

The primary aim of meta-analysis is to summarize and describe existing study results and to compare study results in an effort to provide insights into the exposure and health outcome under investigation and theoretical issues of causation (supported by consistency among studies), reliability, and generalization. Hence, some meta-analyses can make inferences that extend beyond the results of any single study.

Diary Records

In the event of environmental contamination or the occurrence of an environmentally caused disease, diary records may be a useful way to collect information regarding the environmental exposure. By looking at diary records, researchers can find information regarding the time, place, and source of an environmental exposure, in addition to identifying the affected population. For example, the EPA established the Consolidated Human Activity Database (CHAD) to monitor the effects of inhalation of environmental contaminants.[10] Specifically, CHAD analyzes the demographics of participants (age, sex, housing characteristics, and so forth) in relation to their diary records of daily activities. Because diary records are primary accounts written at the time of exposure, diary records avoid the problem of recall bias and can be a valuable source of information relating to environmental exposure.

Disease Registries and Vital Statistics Systems

Disease registries have been around for hundreds of years. In the 1600s in London, John Graunt was one of the first health officials to systematically track the number of deaths per year, including the cause of death and demographics on the deceased, using the "Bills of Mortality."[11] Today there are many disease registries that exist at local and national levels throughout the world. In the United States about half of all physician organizations with 20 physicians or more have a registry for at least one chronic illness.[12] Disease registries provide lists of patients with a given illness, along with clinical information. These disease registries capture information on cancer, renal disease, diabetes, human immunodeficiency virus, acquired immune feficiency syndrome, HIV/AIDS, neurological disorders, diabetes, and so forth. Appendices I and II provide a comprehensive list of health outcomes and data sources or disease registries that contain information regarding risk factors, such as environmental exposures, and demographics of individuals within the registry.

Monitoring Environmental Justice

In recent years, considerable effort has been made to identify and prevent health disparities among racial, ethnic, social, and economic groups in the United States. Disproportionate burdens born by certain groups are showcased by the inequitable distribution of environmental hazards. For example, environmental bias against racial minorities and the impoverished has spawned the term "environmental racism," considered to be a form of neo-racism. Some governmental and organizational actions (or inactions) have targeted these disadvantaged groups so that they are exposed to toxic and hazardous waste more than white, upper-class individuals.[13] Historically, the United States has either been careless in its waste disposal, or communities where racial minorities and impoverished live have suffered from unequal protection against these environmental hazards.[14] Environmental exposures to contaminants have resulted in increased health problems for less affluent sectors of society. These inequities led to the creation of the environmental justice movement, which was formed to ensure equal protection for all against environmental dangers.

The **environmental justice movement** is a grassroots effort to combat the distributional inequities of environmental risks. Although environmental justice had the beginnings of a movement in the early 1960s, it did not take a strong, national hold until 1982, when hundreds of African Americans protested the creation of a hazardous-waste landfill in Warren County, North Carolina.[14] These protests sparked national interest and caused the General Accounting Office and the United Church of Christ Commission for Racial Justice to examine the placement of hazardous-waste landfills. Investigative studies by both groups found a significant relationship between race or socioeconomic status and hazardous-waste sites. The United Church of Christ Commission for Racial Justice found that race was the "most significant factor in close proximity to a hazardous-waste site."[14] Pollution was also strongly linked to racial minorities.

Studies like these led the EPA to form the Office of Environmental Equity in November 1992. Certain regional offices adopted specific policies to address the issue of environmental justice; in 1993 EPA New England issued a policy to ensure "the fair treatment and meaningful involvement of all people, regardless of race, color, national origin, or income, with respect to the development, implementation, and enforcement of environmental laws, regulations and policies."[14] EPA New England has focused on fair treatment of all groups so that no one group suffers a disproportionate burden of environmental hazards.

Environmental justice is primarily concerned with combating current inequalities and preventing future inequalities that lead to disproportionate environmental impacts on the poor and people of color. Because these groups are more likely to be exposed to environmental risks at home and at work, environmental justice is concerned with protecting people where they live, work, and recreate.[13] The movement seeks to influence "cultural norms and values, rules, regulations, behaviors, policies, and decisions" so that racial and poor communities can be confident that their environment will be safe and productive.[14] Frequently, laws have not provided equal protection to minorities or to those without power to challenge extant policies. This movement seeks to guarantee equal protection under all laws. The environmental justice movement utilizes community empowerment to involve citizens in local environmental decisions.[14] Thus, in addition to environmental affairs, this movement concerns itself with social change. Environmental justice activists want more than to simply reduce environmental hazards; they also desire that people reach their greatest potential. Activists realize that people cannot achieve their potential if they are constantly threatened by environmental hazards and the accompanying health problems.

In its fight for equal representation and equal protection, the environmental justice movement has identified several factors that contribute to environmental injustice. The system that so often protects white, wealthy populations is the cause of many injustices to racial and poor minorities. Many of the inequalities stem from "institutional racism in housing, discriminatory zoning and planning practices, the lack of community access to environmental policy making, the absence of many people of color as elected officials, the historically rooted tendency for corporations and governments to follow the path of least resistance in facility siting, market dynamics, and the exclusion of low-income individuals and people of color from the dominant environmental movement."[13] These causes are deeply rooted, which makes it difficult for environmental justice activists to fight against them. However, activists are involving community members to gain legitimacy and power.

Many examples of environmental injustices exist. Historically, African Americans have lived along the banks of the Mississippi River. Oil refineries and petrochemical plants have also congregated in the same area, leaving the African American population unfairly burdened by the health problems associated with proximity to these plants.[14] Polluting industries have typically not been overly accountable to society, and even less so to disadvantaged groups that lack the expertise or political voice to fight the injustices.[13] Another example of environmental injustice is provided by the current push to dispose of nuclear waste on Indian reservations.[15] Even those who have fought with the environmental justice movement for improved quality of life have occasionally harmed disadvantaged groups. Often one set of actions has had negative repercussions on other communities. For example, when some white communities protested against a hazardous-waste site using the slogan "Not in my backyard," they were successful in deterring the companies from creating the site in their community. However, the companies simply moved to another less powerful community, and the unintended consequences became typified by the slogan "Put it in blacks' backyards."[13]

One of the major environmental justice victories occurred in 1994 with Bill Clinton's signing of Executive Order 12989, which obligated all federal agency mandates to speak to environmental justice concerns.[13] This order required those agencies to work for vulnerable populations so that they would not be unfairly burdened with environmental hazards. This focus on vulnerable populations was vital because, although they share an unequal portion of the environmental problems, they rarely possess the resources necessary to make their voices and concerns heard.[14] This order, however, has not been as successful as many had hoped. In 2000, citizens and activists from across the nation came to Washington, DC, to voice their disapproval. Despite the executive order, most agencies had simply paid lip service to environmental justice efforts. The situation had not improved, and racial minorities and the poor were still struggling with the same issues. Poor and racial communities complained that they were under siege, "battling toxic terrorism" by federal agencies, facilities, and chemical industries.[13] Some of the negative environmental consequences cited by the disadvantaged groups include various cancers, respiratory diseases, and nervous system and reproductive disorders.[13] Thus, environmental injustices remain prevalent problems that are not easily solved. The environmental movement continues to fight for disadvantaged communities, providing them with the resources they need to ameliorate the situation. However, fighting these deeply seated problems is never easy.

Key Issues

1. Monitoring programs attempt to measure and estimate physical conditions and substances in the human environment that influence health.

2. The general aim of monitoring programs is to measure and estimate environmental hazards, to measure adverse health effects and damage to the environment (plants, trees, buildings, air, soil, water), and to evaluate the effectiveness of prevention and control efforts.

3. The purposes of monitoring programs include assessment of the impact of physical, chemical, and biological stresses; evaluating the local, regional, or global impact of pollutions; assessing contamination levels from industrial facilities, confirming adequacy of pollution controls and, if necessary, cleanup and restoration efforts; assessing exposure from a single source,

multiple sources, and environmental consequences; determining compliance with applicable regulations; and providing relevant information for public relations.

4. Health indicators should reliably predict the association between human health and the environment. It is recommended that environmental public health indicators be regularly collected and consistently defined, and that standard data collection techniques be used.

5. It is difficult to apply epidemiologic techniques to small populations affected by environmental contaminants because of small sample sizes. Some possible solutions include meta-analysis, diary records, disease registries, and vital statistics systems.

6. Environmental justice is primarily concerned with combating current inequalities and preventing future inequalities that lead to disproportionate environmental impacts on the poor and people of color.

Exercises

Key Terms

Define the following terms.

>Biomarkers
>Environmental justice movement
>Environmental Public Health Indicators Project
>Monitoring programs

Study Questions

3.1. In general, what do monitoring programs attempt to measure?

3.2. List the six specific purposes of monitoring programs.

3.3. With respect to chemical contaminants, monitoring programs may involve what five things?

3.4. What are the five stages of chemical carcinogenesis?

3.5. What are biomarkers typically used to measure?

3.6. List two United Nations treaties directly related to monitor pollutants.

3.7. The Environmental Public Health Indicators Project is sponsored by what federal agency?

3.8. Identify and summarize seven steps provided by the Environmental Public Health Indicators Project to develop environmental public health surveillance among states.

3.9. What are the two barriers to identifying environmental sources of disease?

3.10. What makes it difficult to apply epidemiologic techniques to small populations?

3.11. What is the difference between meta-analysis and a review?

3.12. Who was the first health official to systematically track the number of deaths per year in what he called the "Bills of Mortality"?

3.13. What is environmental injustice? What efforts have been taken to overcome environmental injustice?

References

1. Moeller DW. *Environmental Health.* Cambridge, MA: Harvard University Press; 1992.
2. Center for Biomarkers in Imaging. Imaging biomarkers catalog. 2004. Available at: http://www.biomarkers.org/NewFiles/catalog.html. Accessed November 1, 2006.
3. Santella RM. Mechanisms and biological markers of carcinogenesis. In: Franco EL, Rohan TE, eds. *Cancer Precursors: Epidemiology, Detection, and Prevention.* New York, NY: Springer-Verlag; 2002.
4. Taylor D, Taylor S. Environmental uranium and human health. *Rev Environ Health.* 1997;12:147–157.
5. Goldsteen JB. *The ABCs of Environmental Regulation.* Rockville, MD: ABS Consulting/Government Institutes; 2003.
6. Mackenthun K, Bregman J. *Environmental Regulations.* Boca Raton, FL: Lewis Publishers; 1992.
7. Environmental public health indicators project (indicators); CDC, NCEH, EHHE. Available at: http://www.cdc.gov/nceh/indicators/pdfs/all.pdf. Accessed June 12, 2007.
8. Environmental public health indicators project (sources); CDC, NCEH, EHHE. Available at: http://www.cdc.gov/nceh/indicators/pdfs/sources.pdf. Accessed June 12, 2007.
9. International Commission on Radiological Protection. Recommendations of the International Commission on Radiological Protection. Publication 60. *Annals of the ICRP.* 1991;21:1–3.
10. Environmental Protection Agency. Estimating Inhalation Exposure. Available at: http://www.epa.gov/ttn/fera/data/risk/vol_1/chapter_11.pdf. Accessed November 10, 2006.

11. Merrill RM, Timmreck TC. *Introduction to Epidemiology*. 4th ed. Boston, MA: Jones and Bartlett Publishers; 2006.
12. Schmittdiel J, Bodenheimer T, Solomon NA, Gillies RR, Shortell SM. The prevalence and use of chronic disease registries in physician organizations. *J Gen Intern Med*. 20:855–858.
13. Pellow DN. *Garbage Wars*. Cambridge, MA: MIT Press; 2002.
14. Visgilio G, Whitelaw D. *Our Backyard: A Quest for Environmental Justice*. Lanham, MD: Rowman & Littlefield Publishers; 2003.
15. Mooney L, Bate R. *Environmental Health: Third World Problems—First World Preoccupations*. Woburn, MA: Butterworth-Heinemann; 1999.

Epidemiologic Study Designs

LEARNING OBJECTIVES

After completing this chapter, you should be able to:

1. Define the general meaning of "study design."
2. Distinguish descriptive from analytic study designs.
3. Discuss the rationale, strengths, and weaknesses of the various study designs.
4. Distinguish observational from experimental studies.
5. Define internal and external validity.
6. Identify the six primary activities and three types of meta-analyses.

Introduction

At the heart of an investigation of any environmental health problem is the research or study design. The study design is a scholarly plan that serves as a basis for ultimately obtaining an understanding of the causes of the environmental health problem. With this understanding, appropriate control and prevention efforts may be taken. This chapter will present the study designs commonly used in epidemiology and will discuss factors that should be considered when selecting a study design.

Study Designs

A **study design** is the program that directs the researcher along the path of systematically collecting, analyzing, and interpreting results; it is a formal approach of scientific or scholarly investigation. The methodology may involve observational and experimental assessment. It allows for descriptive assessment of events and for statistical inference concerning relationships between exposure and disease and defines the domain for generalizing the results. The study design can be complex and involve a number of decisions.

There are various study designs in epidemiology used to investigate exposures and health-related states or events, some implicit (descriptive) and others explicit (analytic). For example, a case study involving a single individual may attempt to describe a specific disease condition. A hypothesis is formulated based on an implicit comparison with the usual or "expected" experience of the individual. On the other hand, selection of a comparison group is explicit in analytic study designs where the comparison group is specifically selected to determine if disease cases differ from disease-free cases in terms of exposure. By selecting an appropriate comparison, hypotheses about exposure–disease relationships can be tested.[1]

Descriptive Study Designs

Descriptive study designs focus on assessing a sample without making inferences or causal statements. Descriptive studies are useful for describing the distribution (frequency and pattern) of health-related states or events in specified groups. A descriptive study assists us in (1) providing information about a disease or condition, (2) providing clues to identify a new disease or adverse health effect, (3) identifying the extent of the public health problem, (4) obtaining a description of the public health problem that can be easily communicated, (5) identifying the population at greatest risk, (6) assisting in planning resource allocation, and (7) identifying avenues for future research that can provide insights about an etiologic relationship between an exposure and outcome. Descriptive study designs include the following: case study, cross-sectional studies, and ecologic studies. A brief description of each of these epidemiologic study designs, along with their strengths and weaknesses, is presented in Table 4.1.

TABLE 4.1 Epidemiologic descriptive study designs

	Description	Strengths	Weaknesses
Case study	A snapshot description of a problem or situation for an individual or group; qualitative descriptive research of the facts in chronological order	• In-depth description • Provides clues to identifying a new disease or adverse health effect resulting from an exposure or experience • Identifies potential areas of research	• Conclusions limited to the individual, group, and/or context under study • Cannot be used to establish a cause–effect relationship
Cross-sectional	All the variables are measured at a point in time; there is no distinction between potential risk factors and outcomes	• Control over study population • Control over measurements • Several associations between variables can be studied at same time • Short time period required • Complete data collection	• No data on the time relationship between exposure and injury/disease development • Potential bias from low response rate • Potential measurement bias • Higher proportion of long-term survivors

(continued)

TABLE 4.1   Epidemiologic descriptive study designs (continued)

	Description	Strengths	Weaknesses
Ecological	Aggregate data involved (i.e., no information is available for specific individuals); prevalence of a potential risk factor compared with the rate of an outcome condition	• Exposure and injury/disease data collected from same individuals • Produces prevalence • Takes advantage of preexisting data • Relatively quick and inexpensive • Can be used to evaluate programs, policies, or regulations implemented at the ecologic level • Allows estimation of effects not easily measurable for individuals	• Not feasible with rare exposures or outcomes • Does not yield incidence or relative risk • Susceptible to confounding • Exposures and disease or injury outcomes not measured on the same individuals

Case Study

The aim of a **case study** is to provide a complete understanding of a problem or situation. This type of study includes describing the characteristics of a person or group of people, the setting or community (cultural norms, community values, motives, etc.), the circumstance, and the problem. A case study is useful for obtaining an in-depth understanding of how and why questions. A case study may also provide clues to identifying a new disease or adverse health effect resulting from an exposure or experience.

A case study may involve investigation of an unusual event such as a **cluster**. The Centers for Disease Control and Prevention defines "cluster" as "an unusual aggregation, real or perceived, of health events that are grouped together in time and space and that are reported to a health agency."[2] Epidemiologic evaluations of clusters of cases have resulted in many triumphs in infectious and noninfectious disease control. Some well-known examples include:

- the investigation of cases of pneumonia at the Bellevue-Stratford Hotel in Philadelphia in 1976;[3]
- the 1981 report that seven cases of *Pneumocystis carinii* pneumonia had occurred among young homosexual men in Los Angeles;[4]
- angiosarcoma among vinyl chloride workers;[5]
- neurotoxicity and infertility in kepone workers;[6]
- dermatitis and skin cancer in persons wearing radioactively contaminated gold rings;[7]
- adenocarcinoma of the vagina and maternal consumption of diethylstilbestrol;[8] and
- phocomelia and consumption of thalidomide.[9]

Cross-sectional Study

A **cross-sectional study** involves simultaneous measurement of exposure and outcome factors at a specific point in time for a defined group of individuals. Cross-sectional studies may be thought of as a "snapshot" of the frequency and characteristics of exposure and outcome factors in a group at a particular point in time; in other words, a single examination of a group of individuals takes place. Such data are often obtained through questionnaires or physical examinations (e.g., National Health and Nutrition Examination Survey). Cross-sectional studies provide data that reflect the prevalence of an exposure or outcome in a selected group. However, because cross-sectional data on exposure and outcome factors are collected at the same point in time, the temporal sequence of events cannot be determined. Thus, statements should not be made about causal relationships on the basis of this type of data.

Ecologic Study

An **ecologic study** involves making comparisons between populations or groups of people rather than among individuals. An ecologic investigation of the association between current cigarette smoking and health among adults in the United States is shown in Figure 4.1. Here, as smoking levels increase, the quality of health decreases.

Ecologic studies are often appropriate in environmental settings. For example, injuries are often associated with characteristics in the environment and may best

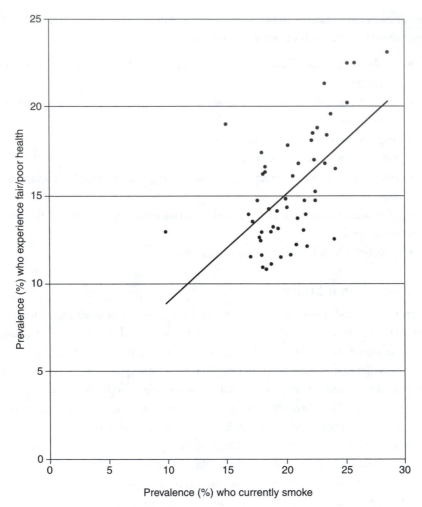

FIGURE 4.1 Ecologic investigation of the association between current cigarette smoking and fair/poor health among U.S. states, ages 18 years and older. (*Source:* Data from CDC, 2006.)[10]

be controlled by group-focused interventions (modifications to physical, social, technological, political, economical, and organizational environments) rather than efforts to change individual behaviors.[11]

In talking about an ecologic study, it is important to have an understanding of the concepts (measurement, analysis, and inference) and rationale underlying this type of study. Morgenstern (1998) classified ecologic measures into three types:

1. **Aggregate measures**—summaries of observations based on individuals within a group (e.g., the proportion of smokers, the incidence rate of lung cancer, or the median household income).

2. **Environmental measures**—physical characteristics of a place such as a home or work site for members of a group (e.g., air-pollution level, water-pollution level, hours of sunlight, or mean temperature). Often individual exposure (or dose) levels remain unmeasured.

3. **Global measures**—attributes of groups for which no analogue at the individual level exists (e.g., population density, number of private medical clinics, laws).[12]

The type of ecologic analysis performed depends on whether the unit of analysis variable(s) in the study is on the individual level or group level. If data are collected on the individual level, a value for each variable is measured for every person in the study. If data are collected on the ecologic level, a value for each variable is measured for the group in the study. Research may involve completely ecologic analysis, partially ecologic analysis, or multilevel analysis.

1. **Completely ecologic analysis**—the units of analysis on all variables are ecologic measures, such as the proportion exposed, the rate of injury, or the rate of disease. The association may be made at the county level.

2. **Partially ecologic analysis**—a combination of individual- and group-level data in the analysis. For example, infant birth weight may be associated with environmental exposure to biogas from a landfill. Individual data could include birth weight, gestational age of the baby, sex, and age of the mother. A surrogate measure of exposure to biogas in the ambient air could be the ecologic measure of "geographic region of residence."

3. **Multilevel analysis**—a modeling technique that combines information at two or more levels. For example, an individual-level analysis within each group could be performed. Then, using the results from the individual-level analysis, ecologic analysis of all groups could be performed.[12]

There are several reasons for the widespread use of ecologic studies, which include:

1. Unavailable data on the individual level. The underlying reason for many ecologic studies is because data are not available on the individual level. It is often not feasible to accurately measure exposure (dose) levels for a large number of people because of resource and time constraints. However,

grouped level data may be easily obtained (e.g., mean radon gas levels from county survey data). Hence, practical constraints require ecologic measurements.[13] This may be especially true in cluster investigations.[14]

2. Design limitations of individual-level studies. If the exposure levels vary little in a given area, it may be of interest to compare exposure levels according to geographic areas. For example, a study that might obtain a wide range of exposure levels could involve an assessment of the association between prostate cancer rates and average daily fat intake for several countries.

3. Low cost and convenient. Ecologic studies often utilize secondary data sources that may be linked to assess given relationships. For example, data obtained from large surveys and cancer registries could be linked on the state level to allow us to associate the proportion of the adult population who smoke and lung cancer rates for each state. Hence, such studies are relatively inexpensive and require little time.

4. Interest in ecologic effects. In some studies the primary interest is in identifying an ecologic effect, such as how a cigarette tax relates to cigarette smoking by state or how a group-focused intervention (modifications to physical, social, technological, political, economical, and organizational environments) relates to injury.[11]

5. Simplicity of analysis and presentation. Large periodic surveys such as the census or national health or risk factor surveys are often assessed ecologically according to combinations of demographic group, year, and region.[12]

For every ecologic study design, the planned unit of analysis is the group and is identified according to place (country, state, city, school, etc.), time, or a combination of place and time. The ecologic study design has been classified as exploratory if no specific exposure of interest exists or is measured, and analytic if a primary exposure variable of interest is measured and considered in the analysis. In an exploratory study, the rate of injury or disease may be compared among many geographic regions during the same time period. The purpose of this comparison is to identify spatial patterns that may indicate an environmental etiology.[12] For example, an investigation of prostate cancer mortality in four U.S. northern plain states found that mortality rates were significantly higher in rural counties than in urban counties.[15] The study suggests that agricultural crop production increases the risk of prostate cancer mortality in these states. Changing patterns of agricultural pesticide use may be responsible for some of the observed association with crop production. The study justifies the need for a subsequent case-control study to assess the relation between prostate cancer and specific agricultural practices.

In an analytic ecologic study, the ecologic association is assessed between the aggregate exposure level and the rate of injury/disease for many groups. This is a common ecologic design where the unit of analysis is typically a geographic region. The steps one usually goes through to conduct an analytic ecologic study follow, along with an example:

1. Develop a hypothesis regarding exposure and outcome. (Is current tobacco smoking associated with fair/poor health compared with very good/good health?)
2. Define and select the ecologic units to be compared. (U.S. states)
3. Obtain summary measures of exposure and outcome. (Prevalence of current smoking and prevalence of experiencing fair/poor health by state)
4. Plot the data for each ecologic unit on a graph. (See Figure 4.1.)
5. Determine if the hypothesized relationship exists. (Do states with higher smoking prevalence have higher prevalence of fair/poor health compared with very good/good health?)

Each point in Figure 4.1's graph represents state-level data. The summary measures are the percentage of the states' adult population who currently smoke and who experience fair/poor health. The scatter plot shows the pattern of points resulting when each point represents the intersection of the values of the two variables. By convention, the explanatory variable is on the horizontal axis and the outcome variable is on the vertical axis. The data are analyzed to determine whether there is an association between the exposure and outcome variables. A least squares regression line was fit to the data, showing a positive association. In the next chapter, the statistical methods for assessing whether the relationship is statistically significant will be presented.

In another example, researchers found an inverse association between the incidence of Crohn's disease and reportable enteric infection at the population level and suggested this may indicate that early exposure to enteric agents yields protection against Crohn's disease.[16] In addition, a positive association between incidence of Crohn's disease and multiple sclerosis may indicate that these two diseases have a common environmental etiology. A good presentation of appropriate statistical methods for assessing such data is presented by Morgenstern (1998).[12]

Time–trend designs can also be classified as exploratory or analytic. In an exploratory time trend (or time series), a comparison of injury/disease rates over time is made for a population in a single geographic area. Age-period-cohort analysis is a special type of **exploratory time–trend analysis**. On the other hand, in an **analytic time–trend analysis**, the ecologic association between average exposure change and disease rate change is made for a population in a single geographic area. When exploratory and analytic time–trend designs include multiple groups, the design is mixed.

To conclude this section on ecologic studies, some mention of their weakness is in order. The primary weakness of this study design is ecologic bias, which occurs when estimates of effect at the ecologic level do not relate to estimates of biologic effect obtained from individual-level analysis.[12] Ecologic studies are also susceptible to confounding. For example, in the example assessing the association between smoking and health, age is a likely confounding factor. In addition, rates and attributable risks cannot be obtained from ecologic data.

Analytic Study Designs

Analytic study designs are distinct from descriptive study designs in that they utilize a comparison group that has been explicitly collected. Analytic study designs are useful for identifying the environmental causes of health-related states or events in specified populations. Descriptive study designs often provide the rationale for conducting an analytic study.

Analytic study designs in environmental epidemiology and epidemiology in general are based on the comparison of individuals who are classified according to exposure and injury/disease status. The unit of analysis is the individual. Analytic study designs fit into two general categories, observational (case-control, cohort) and experimental. In observational studies, researchers evaluate the strength of the relationship between an exposure and health-related state or event. The observed variables are beyond the control or influence of the investigator. On the other hand, in experimental studies some of the participants in the study are deliberately manipulated for the purpose of studying an intervention effect. If the intervention being assessed is an environmental exposure being investigated for its adverse health effects, clearly it would be unethical to assign the intervention. Hence, analytic methods employed in environmental epidemiology are predominantly observational.

In some situations in nature, unplanned events produce a natural experiment. A natural experiment is an unplanned type of experimental study where the levels of exposure to a presumed cause differ among a population in a way that is relatively unaffected by extraneous factors so that the situation resembles a planned experiment.[17] An example of a natural experiment involved John Snow and his investigation of a cholera epidemic in 1854[18]. At the time, the southern districts of London were supplied water by two companies, the Southwark and Vauxhall Company and the Lambeth Company. The districts served by these companies tended to have pipes of both companies going down every street. The Southwark and Vauxhall Company drew its water from the Thames River at a point where it was heavily polluted with human sewage. On the other hand, the Lambeth Company drew its water from the Thames River at a point upstream that was less polluted. Within the southern districts supplied by both companies, Snow determined the water supplier for each household and tracked death due to cholera between July 8 and August 26, 1854. The number and rate of deaths from cholera according to water supplier are shown in Table 4.2.

These results indicate that the rate of death from cholera was 8.4 times higher for those receiving their water supply from the Southwark and Vauxhall Company compared with the Lambeth Company. This example represents a natural experiment because the water supplier used by households was not manipulated by Snow. Instead, Snow took advantage of an unplanned natural situation to investigate his hypothesis that contaminated water was associated with cholera.

Most environmental investigations include both descriptive and analytic studies. The descriptive study describes distributions of health-related states and events in the population. The analytic study examines associations with the ultimate goal to establish cause–effect relationships. Experimental studies typically come last because of their comparatively high cost, difficulty in execution, and narrow focus.

TABLE 4.2 Deaths from cholera in London, July 8 to August 26, 1854, According to water supplier

Water Supplier	Population	Deaths from cholera	Cholera death rate per 1,000
Southwark and Vauxhall Company	98,862	419	4.2
Lambeth Company	154,615	80	0.5

Source: Modified from Snow, 1936.[18]

Of course, no one study design is always better than the others. Various designs have been developed for different circumstances. Each design has its unique strengths and weaknesses. A brief description of each of the epidemiologic study designs, along with their strengths and weaknesses, is presented in Table 4.3.

TABLE 4.3   Epidemiologic analytic study designs

	Description	Strengths	Weaknesses
Experimental	Examines the relation between the intervention and outcome variables in a cohort of people followed over time	• Produces the strongest evidence for causal associations • May produce a faster and less costly answer to the research question than a cohort study • The only appropriate research design for answering certain research questions	• Ethical barriers • Infeasible because the outcome is too rare • Relatively costly and time consuming • Limited generalization to common practice • Potential bias due to loss to follow-up
Cohort	People are followed over time to describe the incidence or the natural history of a condition; assessment can also be made of risk factors for various conditions	• Establishes time sequence of events • Avoids bias in measuring predictors from knowing the outcome • Several outcomes can be assessed • Allows assessment of incidence and the natural history of disease • Yields relative risk	• Large samples often required • May not be feasible in terms of time and money • Not feasible with rare outcomes • Limited to one risk factor • Potential bias due to loss to follow-up

TABLE 4.3   Epidemiologic analytic study designs (continued)

	Description	Strengths	Weaknesses
Case-control	Presence of risk factor(s) for people who have a condition is compared with that for people who do not	• Effective for rare outcomes • Compared with the cohort study, requires less time, money, and size • Yields the odds ratio (when the outcome condition is rare, a good estimate of the relative risk)	• Limited to one outcome condition • Does not provide incidence, relative risk, or natural history • Less effective than a cohort study at establishing time sequence of events • Potential recall and interviewer bias • Potential survival bias • Does not yield incidence or prevalence
Case-crossover	Exposure frequency during a window immediately prior to an outcome event is compared with exposure frequencies during a control time or times at an earlier period	• Controls for fixed individual characteristics that may otherwise confound the association • Effective at studying the effects of short-term exposures on the risk of acute events	• Does not automatically control for confounding from time-related factors

Experimental Study

In a 1747 study of scurvy, James Lind, a Scottish naval surgeon, conducted an experimental study while serving on the HMS *Salisbury*. He took 12 ill patients who had all the classic symptoms of scurvy. He put the sailors in six groups of two and provided different supplements to their diets. One group received a quart of cider each day, and another group consumed an unspecified elixir three times per day; another group drank seawater, while another group received a combination of garlic, mustard, and horseradish; another group had spoonfuls of vinegar, and the last group received two oranges and a lemon. The latter group was the only to make a rapid recovery.[19,20] In the 1870s, Louis Pasteur used the experimental study design to identify the efficacy of a vaccine against anthrax.[19,20] In 1835, Pierre C. A. Louis conducted an experimental study to critique any therapeutic benefit to bloodletting.[21]

The randomized blinded controlled experimental study is considered to be the "gold standard" in epidemiology because it is an effective design for controlling confounding and bias. Randomization of sufficiently large numbers creates a situation where confounding by unmeasured variables is equally likely between groups. Blinding the intervention eliminates unintended interventions (e.g., special attention to treatment group or seeking other treatment for those in the placebo group). Blinding the outcome eliminates ascertainment bias (incorrect conclusions of a study due to the way the data were collected). Variations of the experimental study involving randomization and blinding (i.e., run-in design, factorial design, matched-pair design, and the group randomized design) are described elsewhere.[22]

Methodologically, the strongest design is a between-group design where outcomes are compared between two or more groups of people receiving different levels of the intervention. A within-group design may also be used where the outcome in a single group is compared before and after the assignment of an intervention. An important strength of this design is that individual characteristics that might confound an association (e.g., sex, race, genetic susceptibility) are controlled. However, the within-group design is susceptible to confounding from time-related factors such as climate-related conditions but may be adjusted for in the analysis.

It may be readily apparent that applying the experimental study design for assessing physical, chemical, biological, and psychosocial environments poses ethical challenges. In addition, the outcome of interest may be too rare to feasibly perform an experimental study. Hence, environmental epidemiologic studies tend to rely on descriptive (cross-sectional and ecologic) and analytic (cohort and case-control) observational studies.

Cohort Study

In cohort studies, people are followed over time in order to describe the incidence or the natural history of a health outcome. As time passes, the number of potential health outcomes that may be associated with a specific exposure increases. Cohort studies are characterized by identifying exposure levels and then following over time, with the health outcome of interest assessed in the future. This study design is useful for assessing rare exposures and health outcomes that have a short latency period. For health conditions that have a long latency period, the case–control study design is more efficient. Cohort studies are observational studies that have their unique strengths and weaknesses (see Table 4.3).

Cohort studies can be either prospective or retrospective. In a prospective cohort the study begins by making measurements of exposure at baseline, following the cohort over time, and then measuring selected outcomes according to exposure status. A retrospective cohort is the same as a prospective cohort except assembly of the exposure and outcome variables all happened in the past. In other words, a historical cohort is reconstructed with data on the exposure variable, measured in the past, and data on the outcome variable, measured in the past after some follow-up period. The strength of a prospective cohort design is that it provides better control over exposure and outcome measures than in a retrospective cohort. However, it requires comparatively more time and money to perform than a retrospective cohort study.

In environmental epidemiology it is often convenient to compare cohorts from two separate populations, where the first population reflects people exposed to the potential risk factor and the second population reflects people not exposed or exposed at lower levels of the potential risk factor. For example, two Chilean cities with contrasting drinking water arsenic levels (40 mcg/L vs. < 1 mcg/L) were identified. Higher risk of anemia during pregnancy was found in pregnant women in the exposed city (49% vs. 17%).[23] It may also be convenient to compare the outcomes for people exposed to a potential risk factor at a work site or location with people in the general population. For example, in a cohort study involving British rubber industry workers exposed to beta-naphthylamine, the risk of bladder cancer for these workers was significantly higher than that expected based on national registry data.[24] The study also identified a higher risk of bladder cancer for exposed workers compared with nonexposed workers in the same plant.

Case–Control Study

In a case–control study, the presence of a potential risk factor or factors is compared between those with and those without the health problem of interest. The study begins by identifying cases and controls and then investigating whether the cases were more likely to have been exposed than the controls. Case–control studies are best suited for chronic conditions where the latency period from exposure to disease is years or decades. For example, from a systematic review of 43 case–control studies, a consistent association was identified between benzene exposure (an important industrial chemical and chemical of gasoline) and non-Hodgkin's lymphoma.[25]

A nested case–control study (also called a case–cohort study) is a case–control study "nested" within a cohort study. Levels of the risk factor or factors are compared between cases and a sample of noncases. For example, a recent study conducted a nested case–control study of 362 cases and 1,805 matched controls to assess the association between occupational chemical exposures and prostate cancer incidence. The study found that high levels of trichloroethylene exposure were significantly associated with an increased risk of prostate cancer among workers.[26] In another example, a case–control study nested in a cohort of French uranium miners was conducted. The study identified 100 miners who died of lung cancer and 500 controls matched for age. Information about radon exposure came from the cohort study. Smoking information was obtained retrospectively from a questionnaire and occupational medical records. After adjusting for smoking, the study found a significantly increased risk of lung cancer due to radon exposure.[27]

Nested case–control studies have the scientific benefits of a cohort design. They are also less expensive to conduct than cohort studies. Yet to carry out a nested case–control study, samples or records of interest must be available from before the outcome condition occurred.

Case–Crossover Design

Use of the case–crossover design is becoming increasingly common in environmental epidemiology. It involves comparing the exposure status of a case immediately before its occurrence with that of the same case at a prior time.[28] The argument here is that if precipitating events exist, they should occur more frequently immediately prior to the onset of disease rather than during a period more distant from the disease onset. The **case–crossover study** design is especially appropriate where individual exposures are intermittent, the disease occurs abruptly and the incubation period for detection is short, and the induction period is short.[28,29]

In case–crossover studies, individuals serve as their own controls, with the analytic unit being time—where the time just before the acute event is the "case" time compared with some other time, referred to as the "control" time. Like the within-group design in an experimental study, the case–crossover design assumes that there are no confounding time-related factors, or that they are adjusted for in the analysis. A time-related factor—accumulation of effects—is also assumed not to be present.[30] This simplest case–crossover design is similar to a matched-pair case–control design. Maclure and Mittleman (2000) provide an example illustrated in Figure 4.2.[28] In this illustration, a collision at noon today was the result of exposure to a hazard, such as a puddle, a cell phone call, or a spilled drink (shaded ellipse). How unusual was the exposure? A control group is needed to answer this question, but rather than using a different car, as shown in the bottom of the figure, the same car at noon the day before the accident (top right) can be used as a matched control. Earlier control times could also be used. An advantage of using a traditional control (bottom left) in the study is that their exposures at previous times (bottom right) may serve as an estimate of the magnitude of information bias or possible confounding by factors that vary according to time.

To further illustrate, suppose 200 cardiac events are identified, and you are interested in measuring an association with particulate matter in the air. The "case"

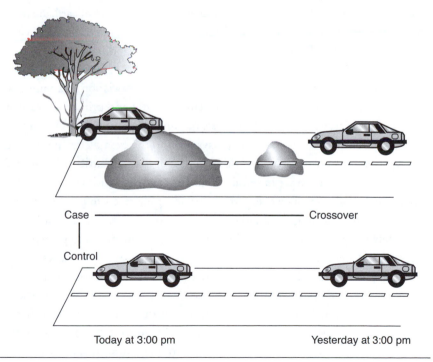

FIGURE 4.2 Case–crossover design

period is designated as the 24 hours preceding the cardiac event, and the "control" period is designated as one week prior to the case period, only one week earlier. Further, let particulate matter be classified as high versus low levels and assume the data are as follows.

	Control	
Case	High	Low
High	60	40
Low	20	80

In other words, among the cardiac patients, 60 experienced high particulate matter during the case and control periods, 40 experienced high particulate matter during the case period but not the control period, 20 experienced low particulate matter during the case period but high particulate matter during the control period, and 80 experienced low particulate matter during both the case and control periods. An odds ratio can be estimated by taking the ratio of discrepant pairs, yielding 2 (40/20). This hypothetical example indicates that a positive association exists between the level of particulate matter and the occurrence of cardiac events. Logistic regression can be used to obtain an adjusted odds ratio in a case–crossover study (see Chapter 5 for matched-paired study, odds ratio, and logistic regression).

In a study by Sullivan and colleagues (2002),[31] an association was found between an increase in exposure to fine particulate matter and primary cardiac arrest among persons with prior heart disease, but limited to current smokers and to increases in fine particulate matter two days prior to the event. This finding suggests that current smokers with preexisting cardiac disease are particularly susceptible to fine particulate matter in the air. It further suggests that it takes a few days rather than being immediate before the heart adversely reacts to particulate matter absorbed into the lungs. In another case–crossover analysis, no association was found between particulate matter with lag of one or more days and primary cardiac arrest.[32] Other studies that have used a case–crossover design to assess the effects of air pollution on health include the following: Barnett and colleagues (2005) found a significantly positive association between air pollutants (NO_2, particles, and SO_2) and hospital admissions for bronchitis, asthma, and respiratory disease in Australia and New Zealand;[33] Forastiere and colleagues (2005) found a positive association between out-of-hospital deaths for coronary heart disease and several air pollutants;[34] and Peel and colleagues (2007) found an increased risk of adverse cardiovascular events with ambient air pollution exposure among individuals suffering from hypertension, diabetes, and chronic obstructive pulmonary disease.[35]

In these examples, information on exposure to particulate matter was obtained objectively. In some case–crossover designs, it may be necessary to rely on a person's recollection of exposure. When individual recall is involved, the threat of recall bias should be considered.

Case–crossover designs may also be used for injury research, but they have three challenges. First, unlike myocardial infarction and other conditions that may occur at any time, occupational injuries often require selected conditions to occur. Hence, identifying the person-time at risk may be a challenge, and only a subset of an individual's person-time may be considered for the study. Second, exposure information may not be available prospectively because most injuries are relatively rare, making prospective data collection inefficient in many settings. Hence, retrospective patient self-reporting of exposure may be necessary, which is prone to recall bias. Third, identifying control periods may be a challenge that is similar to the time when the injury occurs, yet for which the exposure is uncorrelated.[36]

Observational versus Experimental Study

The observational design involves the science and planning of how information will be assembled, described, and related. In an **observational study,** researchers observe events for individuals in the study without altering them. The experimental design involves the science and planning of how an experiment will be conducted in order to obtain valid and reliable results. In an **experimental study**, researchers evaluate the effects of an assigned intervention on an outcome. With the exception of the experimental study, all study designs are observational.

If an observational study design is selected, should the observation be taken at a point in time (cross-sectional study) or should the same subjects be studied over time (**longitudinal study**)? The decision also involves whether to begin with the outcome and then consider past events (**case–control study**) or begin with exposure and follow subjects forward in time to evaluate events that have not yet occurred (**cohort study**).

Observational studies are limited by confounding and bias, and basing causal inference on these studies is more difficult than with experimental studies, especially in environmental epidemiologic studies where the numbers are often small and the exposure is misclassified or poorly measured. In such cases, the strength of the association may be small and not statistically significant. Limited resources may also limit adequate measures of exposure and poorly defined outcomes. Further, cohort studies evaluating long-term exposure may be unethical once a physical, chemical, biological, or psychosocial environment has been identified. When the exposure is identified and people are informed of the environmental contaminant, people will naturally leave the polluted area, if possible, and the study of duration is no longer feasible. Identifying effective ways to meet these limitations is the challenge for modern environmental epidemiology.

Causal inference is strongest when based on experimental studies, followed by cohort studies. Both experimental and cohort studies allow us to establish a time sequence of events. The prospective cohort study is better than the retrospective cohort study, the nested case–control study, or the case–crossover study because there is better control over exposure and outcome measures. Causal inference based on cohort and case–control studies is stronger than when based on cross-sectional or ecological studies because a comparison (control) group is involved. In addition, incidence data obtained from cohort studies are better than prevalence data from cross-sectional studies for making statements about causality. Finally, causal inference is stronger when based on cross-sectional data than when based on ecologic data because ecological data are more prone to confounding.

Study Subjects

The **study subjects** are persons that are the object of scientific investigation. Selecting the study subjects involves two primary decisions. The first decision involves deciding on the selection criteria. Defining the study population essentially involves identifying those individuals best for answering the research question. This will consist of determining clinical criteria and limiting subject selection by geographic area and time boundaries. The second decision involves how to obtain a sample of the population for descriptive and analytic evaluation. For example, in a study of the relationship between occupational exposure to radio frequency/ microwave radiation and brain tumors, selection criteria required that subjects be from one of four neurosurgical clinics, located in Bielefeld, Heidelberg/ Mannheim, and Mainz, Germany. Sampling involved taking all persons at the clinics aged 30–69 diagnosed with brain cancer between October 1, 2000, and October 31, 2003. Controls were frequency matched to the cases by sex, age, and medical center.[37]

Validity

All epidemiologic studies are concerned with validity. The **validity** of an investigation is that component of accuracy reflecting the level of systematic error in the study. There are two types of validity: external validity and internal validity. **External validity** refers to the extent the results of a study are relevant to people who are not part of the study (representativeness). **Internal validity** is the extent the results of a study are not attributable to bias or confounding. For example, results from a hospital based case–control study may not be reflective of the overall population because the controls are hospital patients who, by the mere fact they are in the hospital, likely have poorer health behaviors (e.g., more likely to be smokers, obese, less physically active, heavy drinkers, etc.) than the general population.[38,39] On the other hand, hospital-based case–control studies tend to have a relatively high level of internal validity because controls are (1) easy to identify and available in sufficient numbers, (2) more likely to be aware of antecedent exposures or events, (3) likely to have been subject to the same selection factors that caused the cases to come to this particular hospital, and (4) more likely to cooperate than the general population.[1]

Ensuring a valid study is often determined at the design stage. A high response rate to questionnaires, minimized information bias, and proper control of potential confounders is often determined when designing the study. For example, incentives may ensure an adequate response rate, proper training may minimize interviewer bias, and information gathered on potential confounders at the time of data collection can allow for their adjustment in the analysis. However, there are often unmeasured or unknown potential confounders not considered that cannot be adjusted in the analysis.

Matching or restriction on potential confounders may also be used to improve the internal validity of a study. Matching implies a tailored selection of the study groups in order to make them as comparable as possible. While matching increases internal validity, it decreases external validity.

In environmental epidemiologic studies, samples of people selected for inclusion into the study are restricted by calendar time and geography. Cases have specific clinical manifestations and may be restricted to a narrow range of characteristics (e.g., ages 40–49, men, etc.). Hence, restriction by time, location, and other factors, as commonly done in environmental epidemiologic studies, minimizes the threat of confounding by these factors, thereby improving the internal validity of the study. However, like matching, restriction limits external validity. While there is always a tradeoff between internal and external validity, the primary objective in any environmental epidemiologic study should be on achieving internal validity.

Meta-Analysis

Because environmental studies are not always reliable, causal relationships are hard to establish based on single studies (see Chapter 6: Causal Inference). Therefore, meta-analysis is used to better characterize causal relationships. **Meta-analysis** is "the process or technique of synthesizing research results by using various statistical methods to retrieve, select, and combine results from previous separate but related studies."[40] Meta-analysis is considered a more comprehensive or developed study because it is a systematic comparison of studies that results in the integration of several studies into one analysis. However, it is important to not confuse meta-analysis with a review. While a review summarizes similar studies, meta-analysis combines similar studies to analyze the aggregated information in order to identify consistency of studies, which is important in establishing cause–effect relationships.[41]

Meta-analysis is also used to aggregate subsets of studies, such as information based on age or sex. However, meta-analysis of subsets is less successful in establishing causal relationships because meta-analysis does not allow the selection of subsets to be randomized. Meta-analysis of subsets does provide information on moderator variables.[41] A **moderator variable** can be thought of as a third factor that influences the direction or magnitude of a causal association between an exposure and outcome. For example, cigarette smoking modifies the association between asbestos and lung cancer because those exposed to asbestos who smoke are more likely to develop lung cancer than those exposed to asbestos who do not smoke. Cigarette smoking in this example may also be termed an effect modifier.

For a meta-analysis to establish a causal relationship depends on both the research designs of each primary study and on the methods of meta-analysis employed.

As identified by Cook and colleagues (1992), there are six primary methods or activities within meta-analysis. These six activities are:

1. Assessing evidence that a relationship, or law, exists and that it is relatively nonartificial;
2. Examining the form of a relationship;

3. Analyzing the causal or key conceptual components of the independent variable (treatment) and the key components of the dependent (outcome) variable;

4. Assessing the scope of a relationship;

5. Analyzing the mediating processes that underlie a relationship; and

6. Developing a model that accounts for the variance among study outcomes.[42]

Researchers use one or many of these methods in meta-analysis to accomplish three main outcomes. As identified by Cooper and Hedges (1994), the three outcomes or types of meta-analysis are:

1. Integration of individual studies that all examined a single empirical relation.

2. Assessment of the generability of empirical relationships or associations.

3. Examination of the effect of new theoretical concepts that had not been considered in the primary-level studies.[41]

Of these three variations, assessment the generability of empirical relationships or associations is the most common form of meta-analysis used. Integration of individual studies that all examine a single relation is also commonly used, but in conjunction with assessing generability of empirical relationships. The last type of meta-analysis, examination of the effect of new theoretical concepts that had not been considered in the primary studies, is not commonly used.[41]

Key Issues

1. A study design is a formal approach of scientific or scholarly investigation. It is the program that directs the researcher along the path of systematically collecting, analyzing, and interpreting observations.

2. Descriptive study designs focus on assessing a sample without making inferences or causal statements. Descriptive studies are useful for describing the distribution (frequency and pattern) of health-related states or events in specified groups, and often provide the justification for pursuing an analytic study.

3. Analytic study designs utilize a comparison group that has been explicitly collected. Analytic study designs are useful for identifying the environmental causes of health-related states or events in specified populations.

4. With the exception of the experimental study, all study designs are observational. An observational study involves observing events for individuals in the study without altering them. An experimental study involves evaluating the effects of an assigned intervention on an outcome.
5. Study subjects are persons that are the object of scientific investigation.
6. The validity of an investigation is that component of accuracy reflecting the level of systematic error in the study. External validity is the extent the results of a study are relevant to people who are not part of the study (i.e., generalizable). Internal validity is the extent the results of a study are not attributable to bias or confounding.

Exercises

Key Terms

Define the following terms.

Aggregate measures
Analytic study designs
Analytic time–trend analysis
Case study
Case–control study
Case–crossover study
Cluster
Cohort study
Completely ecologic analysis
Cross-sectional study
Descriptive study designs
Ecologic study
Environmental measures
Experimental study
Exploratory time–trend analysis
External validity
Global measures
Internal validity
Longitudinal study
Meta-analysis
Moderator variable

Multilevel analysis
Observational study
Partially ecologic analysis
Study design
Study subjects
Validity

Study Questions

1.1. Define study design and give three examples of study designs used in environmental epidemiology.

1.2. Compare descriptive and analytic research designs and give examples of each.

1.3. Compare observational studies and experimental studies.

1.4. Discuss the strengths and weaknesses of cohort, case control, and cross-sectional studies.

1.5. What are some of the unique advantages to using a case–crossover design in environmental epidemiology?

1.6. Distinguish between external and internal validity.

1.7. List the six primary methods or activities within meta-analysis.

1.8. List the three types of meta-analysis.

References

1. Hennekens CH, Buring JE. *Epidemiology in Medicine*. Boston, MA: Little, Brown and Company; 1987.
2. Centers for Disease Control and Prevention. Guidelines for investigating clusters of health events. *MMWR*. 1990;39(RR-11):1–23. Available at: http://www.cdc.gov/mmwr/preview/mmwrhtml/00001797.htm. Accessed August 12, 2006.
3. Fraser DW, Tsai TR, Orenstein W, et al. Legionnaires' disease: description of an epidemic of pneumonia. *N Engl J Med*. 1977;297:1189–1197.
4. Centers for Disease Control and Prevention. Pneumocystic pneumonia—Los Angeles. *MMWR*. 1981;30:250–252.
5. Waxweiler RJ, Stringer W, Wagoner JK, Jones J, Falk H, Carter C. Neoplastic risk among workers exposed to vinyl chloride. *Ann N Y Acad Sci*. 1996; 271:40–48.
6. Cannon SB, Veazey JM Jr, Jackson RS, et al. Epidemic kepone poisoning in chemical workers. *Am J Epidemiol*. 1978;107:529–537.

7. Baptiste MS, Rothenberg R, Nasca PC, et al. Health effects associated with exposure to radioactively contaminated gold rings. *J Am Acad Dermatol.* 1984; 10:1019–1023.

8. Herbst AL, Ulfelder H, Poskanzer DC. Adenocarcinoma of the vagina: association of maternal stilbesterol therapy with tumor appearance in young females. *N Engl J Med.* 1987;284:878–881.

9. McBride WG. Thalidomide and congenital abnormalities. *Lancet.* 1961;2: 1388.

10. Centers for Disease Control and Prevention. Behavior Risk Factor Surveillance System Prevalence Data, All States—2006. Available at: http://apps.nccd .cdc.gov/brfss/page.asp?yr=2006&state=All&cat=HS#HS. Accessed June 11, 2007.

11. Stevenson M, McClure R. Use of ecological study designs for injury prevention. *Injury Prevention.* 2005;11:2–4.

12. Morgenstern H. Ecological studies. In: Rothman K, Greenland S, eds. *Modern Epidemiology.* Philadelphia, PA: Lippincott-Raven; 1998:462–480.

13. Morgenstern H, Thomas DC. Principles of study design in environmetal epidemiology. *Environ Health Perspect.* 1993;101(suppl 4):23–38.

14. Walter SD. The ecologic method in the study of environmental health, I: overview of the method. *Environ Health Perspect.* 1991;94:61–65.

15. Rusiecki JA, Kulldorff M, Nuckols JR, Song C, Ward MH. Geographically based investigation of prostate cancer mortality in four U.S. northern plain states. *Am J Prev Med.* 2006;30(2 Suppl):S101–S108.

16. Green C, Elliott L, Beaudoin C, Bernstein CN. A population-based ecologic study of inflammatory bowel disease: searching for etiologic clues. *Am J Epidemiol.* 2006;164(7): 615–623.

17. Oleckno WA. *Essential Epidemiology: Principles and Applications.* Prospect Heights, IL: Waveland Press; 2002.

18. Snow J. *On the Mode of Communication of Cholera.* 2nd ed. 1855. Reproduced by Commonwealth Fund, New York; 1936.

19. Cumston CG. *An Introduction to the History of Medicine.* New York: Alfred A. Knopf; 1926.

20. Garrison FH. *History of Medicine.* Philadelphia, PA: Saunders; 1926.

21. Louis PCA. Recherches sur les effets de la saignée dans quelques maladies inflammatoires, et sur l'action de l'émétique et des vésicatoires dans la pneumonie. Paris: Baillière; 1835.

22. Merrill RM, Timmreck TC. *Introduction to Epidemiology.* 4th ed. Boston, MA: Jones and Bartlett Publishers; 1986.

23. Hopenhayn C, Bush HM, Bingcang A, Hertz-Picciotto I. Association between arsenic exposure from drinking water and anemia during pregnancy. *J Occup Environ Med.* 2006;48(6):635–643.

24. Veys CA. Bladder tumors in rubber workers: a factory study 1946–1995. Occup med 2004;54:322–329.

25. Smith MT, Jones RM, Smith AH. Benzene exposure and risk of non-Hodgkin lymphoma. *Cancer Epidemiol Biomarkers Prev.* 2007;16(3):385–391.

26. Krishnadasan A, Kennedy N, Zhao Y, Morgenstern H, Ritz B. Nested case-control study of occupational chemical exposures and prostate cancer in aerospace and radiation workers. *Am J Ind Med.* 2007;50(5):383–390.

27. Maclure M. The case-crossover design: a method for studying transient effects on the risk of acute events. *Am J Epidemiol.* 1991;133:144–153.

28. Maclure M, Mittleman MA. Should we use a case-crossover design? *Annu Rev Public Health.* 2000;21:193–221.

29. Jaakkola JJK. Case-crossover design in air pollution epidemiology. *Eur Respir J.* 2003;21:81S–85S.

30. Szklo M, Nieto JM. *Epidemiology Beyond the Basics.* Boston, MA: Jones and Bartlett Publishers; 2007.

31. Sullivan J, Ishikawa N, Sheppard L, Siscovick D, Checkoway H, Kaufman J. Exposure to ambient fine particulate matter and primary cardiac arrest among persons with and without clinically recognized heart disease. *Am J Epidemiol.* 2003;157(6):501–509.

32. Levy D, Sheppard L, Checkoway H, et al. A case-crossover analysis of particulate matter air pollution and out-of-hospital primary cardiac arrest. *Epidemiology.* 2001;12(2):193–199.

33. Barnett AG, Williams GM, Schwartz J, et al. Air pollution and child respiratory health: a case-crossover study in Australia and New Zealand. *Am J Respir Crit Care Med.* 2005;171:1272–1278.

34. Forastiere F, Stafoggia M, Picciotto S, et al. A case-crossover analysis of out-of-hospital coronary deaths and air pollution in Rome, Italy. *Am J Respir Crit Care Med.* 2005;172:1549–1555.

35. Peel JL, Metzger KB, Klein M, Flanders WD, Mulholland JA, Tolbert PE. Ambient air pollution and cardiovascular emergency department visits in potentially sensitive groups. *Am J Epidemiol.* 2007;165(6):625–633.

36. Mittleman MA, Sorock GS, Lombardi DA. Overview of case-crossover methods for injury research. Available at: http://www.cdc.gov/Niosh/noirs/abstractsc 3.html. Accessed April 23, 2007.

37. Berg G, Spallek J, Schuz J, et al. Occupational exposure to radio frequency/microwave radiation and the risk of brain tumors: Interphone Study Group, Germany. *Am J Epidemiol.* 2006;164(6):538–548.

38. West W, Schuman KL, Lyon JL, Robison LM, Allred R. Differences in risk estimations from a hospital and population-based case-control study. *Int J Epidemiol.* 1984;13:235.

39. McIntosh ID. Alcohol-related disabilities in general hospital patients: A critical assessment of the evidence. *Int J Addict.* 1982;17:609.

40. *American Heritage Dictionary of the English Language.* 4th ed. Boston, MA: Houghton Mifflin Company; 2000.

41. Cooper H, Hedges L. *The Handbook of Research Synthesis.* New York: Russell Sage Foundation; 1994.

42. Cook TD, Cooper H, Cordray DF, et al. Meta-analysis for explanation: a casebook. New York: Russell Sage Foundation; 1994.

Statistical Modeling and Inference

LEARNING OBJECTIVES

After completing this chapter, you should be able to:

1. Be familiar with types of statistics used in descriptive and analytic studies.

2. Understand basic concepts of hypothesis testing, statistical inference, and reliability.

3. Distinguish between incidence and prevalence measures.

4. Be familiar with common statistical measures of association between exposure and outcome variables.

5. Be familiar with common statistical tests of association between exposure and outcome variables.

6. Be familiar with regression techniques applicable for investigating environmental epidemiologic conditions.

7. Be familiar with basic Statistical Analysis System (SAS) software for assessing environmental epidemiologic data.

Introduction

In the previous chapter, various study designs were discussed. Descriptive study designs are most useful in determining the existence of a health problem and orienting the data in terms of person, place, and time. Descriptive data often provide enough information to provide clues as to the underlying explanation for a given health problem. Summary statistics are employed to evaluate and describe the data. They also assist in formulating the study hypotheses and determining appropriate statistical tests for evaluating those hypotheses. A study hypothesis is developed to explain the presence of a certain pattern or association between elements of a system, such as a chemical exposure and adverse health outcome. Analytic study designs are useful for answering how and why a given health problem occurred.

Statistical models are used to describe patterns in data and to assist in providing evidence to support the study hypothesis. When attempting to identify patterns of association between exposure and outcome variables, obtaining a parsimonious statistical model (simplest model) that adequately describes the data is a primary aim. If the model fits the data reasonably well, appropriate inferences can then be made. Statistical modeling focuses on the shape of the relationship between exposure and outcome variables, as well as whether stratification or regression techniques should be adopted and the choice of variables that will measure those characteristics of the study subjects under investigation.

The current chapter builds on the previous chapter by presenting methods for describing and analyzing data, developing hypotheses, and evaluating associations between variables.

Describing and Analyzing Data

At the heart of any environmental epidemiologic investigation are data that represent numerical information from selected variables. Two important types of statistics that correspond to data from descriptive and analytic studies are presented in Table 5.1. **Descriptive statistics**, also called summary statistics, are used to assess the distribution of data and are used as a final step in editing, characterizing the study participants, supporting hypotheses, and informing choice of analytic statistics. **Analytic statistics** are used to measure and test hypothesized associations.

The type of data involved in an investigation will influence the methods employed for description and analysis. Under the descriptive process, begin by ex-

TABLE 5.1   Steps for describing and analyzing data

Steps	Description	Examples	Purposes
1. Descriptive statistics	Assess distribution of data	Frequency distribution Proportion Mean Median Standard deviation Range, interquartile range	1. Final step of editing 2. Characterize study participants 3. Supporting hypotheses 4. Inform choice of analytic statistic
2. Analytical statistics	Examine and test associations	Contingency table Correlation Regression Analysis of variance	1. Assess the pattern of association between exposure and outcome variables in the sample 2. Compute the appropriate measure of association between variables 3. Estimate the probability that the measured association is due to chance (statistical significance)

Source: Adapted from Feigal et al., 1988.[1]

amining the frequency distribution for each of the variables. A frequency distribution shows the number associated with the levels or categories of each variable. Extreme values in the tails of the distribution can represent data entry errors and should be checked for accuracy. For categorical data, determining the proportion within the levels of each variable is informative. It is often useful to present the data in a bar graph. For continuous data, the frequency distribution shows the shape of the distribution. Continuous data are often grouped into categories and presented in a histogram. With continuous data, the mean, median, and mode (measures of central tendency) and standard deviation and range (measures of dispersion) are often effective for describing the data. The shape of the distribution for the continuous variable influences the measure of central tendency and variability appropriate for describing the data. When the distribution is approximately **normal**, the mean and standard deviation are preferred for describing the data. When the data are highly **skewed**, the median and range are best for describing the data.

After the distribution of the data for each variable has been described, the next step is to assess hypothesized associations between exposure and outcome variables. The hypotheses need to be tested, established, and shown to be consistent or inconsistent with facts. Statistical tests are employed to evaluate hypotheses about associations among variables. If established facts or information are lacking to substantiate a research hypothesis, then more information should be gathered, or we fail to reject the null hypothesis. .

Hypothesis Testing

In Chapter 2, the study (or research) hypothesis was defined as a tentative suggestion of an association and provides focus for the analytic phase of an investigation. The hypothesis represents the research question and serves as the framework for identifying statistical significance. The statistical hypothesis is always formulated in terms of the research question. There are two types of hypotheses considered in hypothesis testing; the **null hypothesis** (H_0) and **study** (also called the alternative or research) **hypothesis** (H_1). The null hypothesis is some postulated value of the population; it is what is currently believed or the status quo. In an assessment of the association between an exposure and outcome variable, it typically states that there is no association. The null hypothesis is a formal basis for a statistical test of association. The alternative hypothesis states that there is an association between the exposure and outcome variables. The test of statistical significance either rejects or fails to reject the null hypothesis.

If the procedure allows the investigator to decide between two hypotheses regarding a population, and is based on sampled data and uses probability to indicate the level of reliability in the conclusion, it is called **statistical inference**. **Relia-**

bility refers to the consistency of the result. Sampled data are evaluated using statistical methods such as regression and correlations, decision theory, and time–series analysis.

Hypothesis testing involves parameters and statistics. A parameter is a measure from the population, and a statistic is a measure from the sample. Statistics are used to characterize data from a sample and measure associations between variables. Parameters are typically unknown and are represented by Greek letters (e.g., α, β, ρ). Statistics are represented by basic Latin letters (e.g., a, b, r). The null and alternative hypotheses are always expressed using parameters that represent the true population values. For example, let's hypothesize that a higher percentage of children immunized against infectious diseases (diphtheria, pertussis, and tetanus) in a given country correlates with a lower under-five mortality rate. Using statistical terminology this means we are testing $H_0 : \rho = 0$ vs. $H_a : \rho < 0$. The sample-based correlation coefficient, denoted by r, is then used to quantify the strength of the relationship between the variables. The correlation coefficient is defined as the quantification of the degree that two random variables are related provided that the relationship is linear. If a plot of the relationship between the data shows that the variables are not linearly related or if outliers (or pairs of data lie considerably outside the range of the other data points), then the Spearman's Rank Correlation Coefficient may be the preferred measure of correlation.

When statistical tests are used to draw conclusions about a population, a corresponding P value is obtained. The ***P*** **value** equals the probability that an effect as large, or larger, than that observed in a particular study could have occurred by chance alone given that there is truly no relationship between the exposure and diseases. The measure of reliability that accompanies every inference distinguishes the science of statistics from fortune-telling. While a fortune-teller can make predictions, there is no level of reliability associated with the prediction as there is with statistics. A basic knowledge of statistics enables people to intelligently evaluate numerical data and statements of reliability. Drawing a conclusion about the presence of a disease and reasons for its existence must be supported by statistical tests.

The P value is directly associated with sample size; that is, as the sample size goes up, the role of chance goes down. If the sample size equals the population size, the P value equals zero. Because statistical significance is directly related to sample size, it is possible for an association to be of practical significance although it is not of statistical significance. This may be particularly true with environmental exposures where studies are often constrained by small sample sizes. For example, in a study assessing the relation between birth weight and mothers' proximity to dump sites during pregnancy, the odds of having a low birth weight child for women living near a high-hazard dump site versus a low-hazard dump site was 1.43 ($p < 0.001$).[2] On the other hand, the odds of a very low birth weight child for women living near a high-hazard dump site versus a low-hazard dump site during pregnancy was 1.49 ($p > 0.05$). Ninety-five percent confidence intervals for these two statistics are 1.12–1.81 and 0.87–2.56, respectively. The larger width of the second interval compared with the first reflects the smaller sample size upon which the 1.49 odds ratio was based.

A primary challenge in drawing inference from sample data to the overall population is that a finding could be entirely due to chance because of random variation from sample to sample. Sample size is directly related to chance. As the sample size increases, the probability that the result is due to chance decreases. Because small numbers of events often characterize environmental studies, limiting significance to the standard criterion that there be a 5% or less likelihood that the results are due to chance may result in overlooking a biologically important association. Researchers have argued, and this may be particularly relevant with environmental studies, that basing significance on P values associated with statistical tests is inadequate.[3] Many favor using the confidence interval over the P value because it shows a range where the true measure of association likely falls, with the width of the interval directly influenced by the sample size.

In some cases a hypothesis may be developed in response to a putative cluster (i.e., post hoc hypothesis). Interpreting the probability of statistical significance in this context is problematic, which will be discussed further in a later chapter. The current discussion on hypothesis testing assumes the hypothesis precedes evaluation of the data for a particular cluster of disease cases.

Incidence versus Prevalence

Categorical dichotomous outcome (or event) variables are most often used in environmental epidemiologic studies to reflect health-related states or events such as injury, primary disease, recurrence of disease, development of side effects, and death. The frequency of the dichotomous outcome variable is defined as the number of people experiencing the outcome. The outcome is defined according to time and characteristics of the event of interest. When the event can be identified by time (e.g., injury, foodborne illness, hospitalization, death), then the number of new events is divided by those people at risk of developing the outcome to obtain a proportion of newly developed cases (**incidence**). On the other hand, if the event is not easily identified by time such as dementia, arthritis, or recovery, then the number of existing events is divided by those people at risk of developing the outcome to obtain a proportion of existing cases (prevalence).

Incidence

Incidence can be derived from cohort studies. There are two types of incidence: (1) **cumulative incidence**, where the denominator in the incidence calculation reflects persons at risk, and (2) **incidence density**, where the denominator in the incidence calculation involves person–time units at risk. The numerator for both types of incidence is constant. Szklo and Neito (2007) provide a good comparison of these two types of incidence, as shown in Table 5.2.

TABLE 5.2   Comparing measures of incidence

	Cumulative Incidence		Incidence Rate	
	If follow-up is complete	If follow-up is incomplete	Individual data (cohort)	Grouped data (area)
Numerator	Number of cases	Classical life table Kaplan-Meier	Number of cases	Number of cases
Denominator	Initial population		Person-time	Average population*
Range	0 to 1		0 to infinity	
Synonyms	Incidence proportion Attack rate		Incidence density†	

Source: Modified from Szklo and Neito, 2007, p. 69.[4]

*Equivalent to person–time when events and losses (or additions) are homogenously distributed over the time interval of interest.

†Rate and density are often used interchangeably.

If follow-up is complete on the individuals in the study cohort, then cumulative incidence is equal to the number of cases occurring over the follow-up period divided by the initial population. Cumulative incidence may also be expressed as incidence proportion or attack rate, and is typically expressed per 100.

$$\text{Attack Rate} = \frac{\text{Number of cases during a short time period}}{\text{Population at risk at the beginning of the time period}} \times 100$$

When follow-up is incomplete such that some cases are lost to follow-up (censored), or no event is experienced by the end of the study (right censored), cumulative incidence (also called cumulative survival) is calculated using the life table or Kaplan-Meier approaches. These approaches have been described by many authors.[4]

When the denominator involves time units contributed by the follow-up period of each individual at risk, rather than individuals, then an incidence rate is derived. Incidence rates are not equivalent to proportions. The time unit used in an incidence rate may be in person-days, person-months, or person-years. Person-years are typically preferred when the outcome of interest is rare.

$$\text{Person - Time Rate} = \frac{\text{Number of cases during observation period}}{\text{Time each person observed; totaled for all persons}} \times 10^m$$

Where 10^m is called the **rate base** and m is typically between 2 and 5. When person-years are used in the rate calculation, a yearly average rate is obtained, such as rates per 100,000 person-years; in other words, a rate per 100,000 persons per year. A time unit is not attached to cumulative incidence and must be specified (e.g., 0.25 cumulative incidence or 25% for 3 weeks of follow-up). A rate and cumulative incidence are only comparable if they are based on the same time unit, such as a rate per person-week and cumulative incidence over a 1-week period.

When the average population is used in the denominator of the incidence calculation, it is equivalent to person-time if the events are evenly distributed over the study time of interest. For example, annual incidence rates of cancer in the United States reported by the National Cancer Institute use the population on July 1 to represent the average population during the year.[5] By assuming the cancer events are homogeneously distributed throughout the year, these rates are expressed as person-years.

Each approach has its advantages and disadvantages. For example, in a cohort study without an internal control group, as may be the case in an occupational epidemiologic investigation, estimation of incidence density rather than cumulative incidence will provide a measure that can be compared with available population rates as control rates. On the other hand, cumulative incidence is often estimated when the focus is on the temporal behavior of an outcome, such as survival assessment after diagnosis of disease.[4]

The incidence rate (density) may be alternatively defined as the **hazard rate**, which is an instantaneous probability of the event at a small time interval (Δt close to zero). It is conditional in the sense that the person was at risk at time t. The hazard rate may be calculated at each specific point in time during the follow-up. Mathematically, the hazard is written as:

$$h(t) = \frac{P(\text{event between } t \text{ and } (t + \Delta t) \,|\, \text{alive at } t)}{\Delta t}.$$

The hazard rate is a useful concept that will be revisited later in this chapter when considering statistical techniques used in time-to-event (or survival) analysis (particularly Cox proportional hazards regression).

Prevalence

Prevalence is the frequency of existing cases of an event among individuals at a point in time (**point prevalence**) or at a certain period of time (**period prevalence**). Point prevalence is conveniently obtained through cross-sectional surveys. Period prevalence is relatively less commonly used and will not be addressed here. Point prevalence is a proportion, typically expressed per 100 people, and is a measure of the magnitude (burden) of the health problem. Prevalence is a measure that combines incidence and duration (survival, recovery). For example, for a disease that has had stable incidence over many years, with 1% incidence per year and duration (survival) of 10 years, the point prevalence proportion is 0.1 (or 10%).

Measures of Association

Categorical Variables

Incidence is an important measure in analytic epidemiology when causal associations are being assessed. For example, if a dichotomous exposure is under investigation, then the event for exposed individuals is compared with the incidence for unexposed individuals. To illustrate, consider the 2 by 2 **contingency table** shown below, where the rows of the table represent exposure status (yes vs. no) and the columns of the table represent disease status (yes vs. no).

	Disease			
Exposed	**Yes**	**No**		
Yes	a	b	$a + b$	
No	c	d	$c + d$	
	$a + c$	$b + d$	$n = a + b + c + d$	

Here a represents the number of observed new cases of disease in the exposed group, c represents the number of observed new cases in the unexposed group, and $a + c$ represents the number of observed new cases of disease overall. The total number of people in the study, n, represents the number of people at risk and disease free at the start of follow-up. For cohort data, cumulative incidence (risk), risk of disease in the exposed group, risk of disease in the unexposed group, and the relative risks are calculated as follows:

$$\text{Overall disease risk} = \frac{(a+c)}{(a+b+c+d)} = r$$

$$\text{Risk for the exposed} = \frac{a}{(a+b)} = r_1$$

$$\text{Risk for the unexposed} = \frac{c}{(c+d)} = r_0$$

$$\textbf{Relative Risk } (RR) = \frac{(a)/(a+b)}{(b)/(c+d)} = \frac{r_1}{r_0}$$

The relative risk is also commonly called the **risk ratio**.

If the follow-up time in person time (in days, months, or years) for the ith person is measured, the 2 by 2 table is modified as follows:

	Disease		
Exposed	**Yes**	**No**	
Yes	a	—	Person Time T_e (t_{ei})
No	c	—	Person Time T_{ue} (t_{uei})
	$a + c$	—	$T \sum (t_{ei} + t_{uei})$

Note that t_{ei} is the follow-up time in person years for the ith person in the exposed group and t_{uei} is the follow-up time in person years for the ith person in the unexposed group. When the denominator in the calculations shown above involves person-time, we use the word "rate," rather than the word "risk." The ratio of incidence density rates is called a **rate ratio**.

The risk (or rate) ratio, denoted by *RR*, allows us to say that those exposed are *x* times as likely to develop the disease as those unexposed. It also may be informative to express the relation of disease risk between exposed and unexposed as a percentage; that is, those who are exposed are *x* percent as likely to develop the disease as those not exposed.

If the $RR > 1$, then the change in percent is $(RR - 1) \times 100$

If the $RR < 1$, then change in percent is $(1 - RR) \times 100$

Some common epidemiologic statistics used to further describe risk (or rate) data are as follows:

Attributable Risk (*AR*) $\qquad\qquad = r_1 - r_0$

Interpretation: Excess risk of disease among the exposed group attributed to the exposure, typically expressed per 100,000.

Attributable Risk Percent (*AR%*) $\qquad = \dfrac{(r_1 - r_0)}{r_1} \times 100$

Interpretation: For disease cases who are exposed, this statistic refers to the percentage of disease cases attributed to their exposure.

Population Attributable Risk (*PAR*) $\qquad = r - r_0$

Interpretation: The excess risk of disease in the population attributed to the exposure, typically expressed per 100,000.

Population Attributable Risk Percent (*PAR%*) $= \dfrac{(r - r_0)}{r} \times 100$

Interpretation: Percentage of the disease in the population that can be attributed to the exposure.

For case–control data involving dichotomous exposure status, the 2 by 2 table can be used to estimate the relative risk using the odds ratio. The relative risk cannot be calculated directly because the exposed group is not necessarily reflective of those exposed. The **odds ratio** is calculated as

$$\text{Odds Ratio (OR): } \frac{a/c}{b/d} = \frac{a \times d}{b \times c}$$

In some case–control studies, controls are pair matched to cases on selected factors (e.g., age, sex, race/ethnicity, smoking status, etc.) to improve the comparability of the cases and controls. Matched case–control studies are analyzed differently than unmatched case–control studies. Although the odds ratio in a matched-paired study is interpreted the same as in an unmatched case–control study, the odds ratio is calculated as

$$\text{Odds Ratio (OR): } b/c$$

This is referred to as a **matched-paired analysis**.

The results of a cross-sectional study can also be analyzed using an n by k contingency table. For simplicity, consider the case where the exposure and outcome variables are dichotomous. On the basis of cross-sectional survey data, the letters a, b, c, and d in the table represent the frequency of exposed persons with the outcome, exposed persons without the outcome, unexposed persons with the outcome, and unexposed persons without the outcome, respectively. The overall prevalence proportion is $(a + c)/n$. If the data represent a probability sample (everyone in the target population has a known chance of selection), this is a point estimate of the prevalence proportion in the population.

The prevalence proportion among the exposed is $PR_1 = a/(a + b)$, and the prevalence proportion among the unexposed is $PR_0 = c/(c + d)$. Thus, the **prevalence ratio** is $PR = PR_1 / PR_0$, which is analogous to the risk ratio.

The risk ratio, rate ratio, odds ratio, and prevalence ratio range from 0 to infinity, where

$RR, OR, PR > 1$ means positive association

$RR, OR, PR = 1$ means no association

$RR, OR, PR < 1$ means negative association

The OR approximates the RR if the probability of disease is rare (affecting 10% or less of the population).

Statistical Tests of Associations Between Categorical Variables

Just as the type of study design used influences the statistical measure of association, it also influences the statistical test used for evaluating an association (see Table 5.3). For the case where both the exposure and outcome variables are dichotomous, the **degrees of freedom** (number of independent pieces of information for basing the precision of a parameter estimate) for the chi-square test are (*rows* − 1)× (*columns* − 1) = 1×1 = 1. The values of chi-square for 1 degree of freedom with cut-off specified proportions in the upper tail of the chi-square distribution are as follows:

	Area in the upper tail					
Degrees of Freedom	0.10	0.05	0.025	0.01	0.005	0.001
1	2.71	3.84	5.02	6.63	7.88	10.83
.	.	.	.	.	.	.
.	.	.	.	.	.	.
.	.	.	.	.	.	.

Note: This is only the top portion of the chi-square table.

To illustrate the relation between the chi-square statistic and the P value in the partial chi-square table above, consider a study exploring whether an occupation requiring a high level of speaking, specifically school teachers, increases the risk of voice disorders. Among 2,531 participants, the percentage who currently had a voice problem was significantly higher for teachers compared with nonteachers [11.0% vs. 6.2%, $\chi^2(1) = 18.2$]. From the table we see that the chi-square value is greater than 10.83, so the corresponding P value is < 0.001. For males, 8.6% of teachers reported a current voice problem as compared with 5.1% of nonteachers, with $\chi^2(1) = 4.4$. The corresponding P value is between 0.05 and 0.01. The exact value is $p = 0.035$. For females, the percentages between teachers and nonteachers were 12.0% compared with 7.0%, with $\chi^2(1) = 11.9$ and $p < 0.001$.[6]

A point estimate, such as the risk ratio, contains no information about the sample size. Although the P value is directly influenced by the sample size, it is also influenced by the level of association between the exposure and health event. Consequently, a small P value may result when there is a strong association between the exposure and event but the sample size is moderate or small. On the other hand, a confidence interval reveals more about the sample size because the width of the

TABLE 5.3 Statistical tests of association for dichotomous exposure and outcome variables according to study design

Study Design	Measure of Association	Test of Association
Cohort	$\text{Risk ratio} = \dfrac{a/(a+b)}{c/(c+d)}$	$\chi^2 = \dfrac{(ad+bc)^2 n}{(a+b)(c+d)(a+c)(b+d)}$
Cumulative incidence	$\text{Rate ratio} = \dfrac{a/T_e}{c/T_{ue}}$	$\chi^2 = \dfrac{\left\{a-\left[T_e(a+c)\right]/T\right\}^2}{\left\{T_e\left[T_{ue}(a+c)\right]/T\right\}^2}$
Incidence density (rate)		
Case-control	$\text{Odds ratio} = \dfrac{a \times d}{c \times b}$	$\chi^2 = \dfrac{(ad-bc)^2 n}{(a+b)(c+d)(a+c)(b+d)}$
Unmatched		$\chi^2 = \dfrac{(b-c)^2}{(b+c)}$
	$\text{Odds ratio} = \dfrac{b}{c}$	
Matched		
Cross-sectional	$\text{Prevalence Ratio} = \dfrac{a/(a+b)}{c/(c+d)}$	$\chi^2 = \dfrac{(ad-bc)^2 n}{(a+b)(c+d)(a+c)(b+d)}$

interval is directly related to the sample size. A **confidence interval** is a range of reasonable values in which a population parameter lies, based on a random sample from the population. A significance level of 0.05 corresponds with a 95% confidence interval.

The confidence interval can also be used to evaluate statistical significance. If the $(1-\alpha) \times 100$ percent confidence interval for the relative risk overlaps 1, this indicates no statistical association. Note that the probability α of a type I error (reject the null hypothesis when it is true) is also called the **level of significance** or the size of the test and is typically selected by the researcher to be 0.05. If a confidence interval overlaps 1, the P value will be greater than α, upon which the confidence interval is based. On the other hand, if the confidence interval does not overlap one, the P value will be less than α.

When assessing measures of association with dichotomous variables (e.g., odds ratio, risk ratio, or rate ratio), if the confidence interval overlaps 1, we fail to reject the null hypothesis, or if the confidence interval does not overlap 1, we reject the null hypothesis. The confidence interval has an advantage over the P value in that the width of the confidence interval is directly related to sample size and says something about the precision of the estimate. As the sample size goes up, the width of the confidence interval goes down. The width of the confidence interval also reflects variability in the data. If the sample size equals the population size, probability no longer plays a role and the confidence interval is not relevant. A summary of the statistical tests and confidence intervals for evaluating selected hypotheses about associations from cohort, case–control, and cross-sectional studies is presented in Table 5.4.

TABLE 5.4   Summary of statistical tests and confidence intervals for evaluating selected hypotheses

- For testing H_0 : *Risk Ratio* = 1 use the chi-square test, Fisher's exact test, or the 95% confidence interval for the risk ratio (ratio of probabilities):[7]

$$95\% \; CI(PR) = \left| \ln PR \pm \left(1.96 \times \sqrt{\left[(b/a)/(a+b) \right] + \left[(d/c)/(c+d) \right]} \right) \right|$$

- For testing H_0 : *Rate Ratio* = 1 use the approximate chi-square test or the confidence interval of a rate ratio (ratio of incidence densities).[8] Definitions for the notations are:

O_1 = observed events in group 1

O_2 = observed events in group 2

L_1 = person-time observed in group 1

L_2 = person-time observed in group 2

$R_1 = O_1/L_1$ = event rate in group 1

$R_2 = O_2/L_2$ = event rate in group 2

$RR = R_1/ R_2$

Step 1: $\hat{P} = \dfrac{O_1}{O_1 + O_2}$

Step 2: $P_L = \hat{P} - \left[1.96 \times \sqrt{\dfrac{\hat{P}(1-\hat{P})}{O_1 + O_2}} \right]; P_U = \hat{P} + \left[1.96 \times \sqrt{\dfrac{\hat{P}(1-\hat{P})}{O_1 + O_2}} \right]$

Step 3: Convert to lower and upper 95% confidence limits on rate ratio.

$$RR_L = \left[\dfrac{P_L}{1-P_L} \right] \times \dfrac{L_2}{L_1}; \; RR_U = \left[\dfrac{P_U}{1-P_U} \right] \times \dfrac{L_2}{L_1}$$

(continued)

TABLE 5.4 Summary of statistical tests and confidence intervals for evaluating selected hypotheses (continued)

An estimate of the 95% confidence interval for the rate ratio can be derived using the following formula:[9]

$$95\%\ CI(Rate\ Ratio) = \exp\left[\ln(Rate\ Ratio) \pm 1.96\sqrt{1/a + 1/c}\right]$$

- For testing $H_0 : PR = 1$ in a cross-sectional study. Use the chi-square test, the Fisher's exact test, or the 95% confidence interval for the prevalence ratio:[7]

$$95\%\ CI(PR) = \exp\left|\ln PR \pm \left(1.96 \times \sqrt{\left[(b/a)/(a+b)\right] + \left[(d/c)/(c+d)\right]}\right)\right|$$

- For testing $H_0 : OR = 1$ in an unmatched case–control study. Use the chi-square test, the Fisher's exact test, or the 95% confidence interval for the odds ratio:[10]

$$95\%\ CI(OR) = \exp\left[\ln OR \pm \left(1.96 \times \sqrt{\frac{1}{a} + \frac{1}{b} + \frac{1}{c} + \frac{1}{d}}\right)\right]$$

- For testing $H_0 : OR = 1$ in a matched case–control study. Use the McNemar's chi-square test or the 95% confidence interval for the odds ratio:[11]

$$95\%\ CI(OR) = \exp\left[\ln OR \pm \left(1.96 \times \sqrt{\frac{1}{b} + \frac{1}{c}}\right)\right]$$

To illustrate the use of confidence intervals with odds ratios, consider a study conducted in Brisbane, Australia, to assess preterm birth in relation to maternal exposure to ambient air pollution. Average maternal exposure estimates for ambient particulate matter (PM_{10}), ozone (O_3), and nitrogen dioxide were associated with preterm birth over the first 3 months after the last menstrual period and over the last 3 months prior to birth. A preterm birth was defined as gestational age of less than 37 weeks. The analysis adjusted for various covariates. A significant positive association between PM_{10} and preterm birth during trimester one was identified, with OR = 1.15, 95% CI 1.06–1.25. A significant positive association was also identified between O_3 and preterm birth during trimester one, with OR = 1.26, 95% CI 1.10– 1.45.[12]

TABLE 5.5   Low birth weight according to proximity to hazardous dump site

| Residence of pregnant women (exposure) | Low birth weight (event) | | Total |
	Yes	No	
Near high-hazard dump site (HH)	181	4268	4449
Near low-hazard dump site (LH)	126	4236	4362
Total	307	8504	8811

Source: Data from Gilbreath & Kass, 2006.[13]

Evaluating Statistical Association Between Categorical Variables

Statistical Analysis System (SAS) software is one of many computer packages useful for assessing measures of association between categorical variables. To illustrate, consider the data that appear in the preceding table, which comes from a study investigating adverse birth outcomes associated with open dump sites in Alaska Native villages (see Table 5.5).

SAS code to generate the 2 by 2 table:

```
DATA DUMP SITES;
   INPUT EXPOSURE $ EVENT $ COUNT;
      DATALINES;
         HH Yes 181
         HH No 4268
         LH Yes 126
         LH No 4236
      ;

PROC FREQ ORDER=DATA;
   TABLE EXPOSURE*EVENT/ CHISQ;
   WEIGHT COUNT;
RUN;
```

The SAS-generated table and other results appear as follows.

Table of EXPOSURE by EVENT

Exposure	Event		
Frequency Percent Row Pct Col Pct	**Yes**	**No**	**Total**
HH	181 2.05 4.07 58.96	4268 48.44 95.93 50.19	4449 50.49
LH	126 1.43 2.89 41.04	4236 48.08 97.11 49.81	4362 49.51
	307 3.48	8504 96.52	8811 100.00

Statistics for Table of EXPOSURE by EVENT

Statistic	DF	Value	Prob
Chi-Square	1	9.1157	0.0025
Likelihood Ratio Chi-Square	1	9.1682	0.0025
Continuity Adj. Chi-Square	1	8.7682	0.0031
Mantel-Haenszel Chi-Square	1	9.1146	0.0025
Phi Coefficient		0.0322	
Contingency Coefficient		0.0321	
Cramer's V		0.0322	

Fisher's Exact Test

Cell (1,1) Frequency (F)	181
Left-sided Pr <= F	0.9990
Right-sided Pr >= F	0.0015
Table Probability (P)	4.808E-04
Two-sided Pr <= P	0.0030
Sample Size = 8811	

The contingency table indicates that the percentage of those women living near high-hazard dump sites during pregnancy who had a low birth weight child was 4.07%. In contrast, women living near low-hazard dump sites during pregnancy had a low birth weight child 2.89% of the time. The chi-square statistic of 9.12 has a corresponding P value of 0.0025, indicating that the risk of low birth weight is significantly higher for children born near high-hazard dump sites compared with low-hazard dump sites.

Had the data been based on a cross-sectional study design, a similar approach could have been taken to evaluate the association between variables.

Note that the **Fisher's exact test**, which appears near the end of the output, is useful when the sample size is small. If any expected cell frequency is less than 2 or if more than 20% of the expected cell frequencies are less than 5, the Fisher's exact test should be used instead of the chi-square test. When the contingency table is 2 by 2, the CHISQ option produces the Fisher's exact test. For a higher dimension table, the EXACT option is required for SAS to produce the Fisher's exact test. Considerable computation time may be required for higher order contingency tables.

To have SAS calculate the odds ratio and risk ratio for the data in the previous example, the SAS code is modified as follows. Now the option CMH replaces CHISQ.

```
PROC FREQ ORDER=DATA;
    TABLE EXPOSURE*EVENT/ NOPRINT CMH;
    WEIGHT COUNT;
RUN;
```

The SAS output generated by this statement is shown in the following table.

Summary Statistics for EXPOSURE by EVENT

Cochran-Mantel-Haenszel Statistics (Based on Table Scores)

Statistic Alternative Hypothesis	DF	Value	Prob
1 Nonzero Correlation	1	9.1146	0.0025
2 Row Mean Scores Differ	1	9.1146	0.0025
3 General Association	1	9.1146	0.0025

Estimates of the Common Relative Risk (Row1/Row2)

Type of Study	Method	Value	95%	Confidence Limits
Case-Control	Mantel-Haenszel	1.4257	1.1313	1.7968
(Odds Ratio)	Logit	1.4257	1.1313	1.7968

Type of Study	Method	Value	95%	Confidence Limits
Cohort	Mantel-Haenszel	1.4084	1.1263	1.7612
(Col 1 Risk)	Logit	1.4084	1.1263	1.7612
Cohort	Mantel-Haenszel	0.9879	0.9801	0.9957
(Col 2 Risk)	Logit	0.9879	0.9801	0.9957
	Total Sample Size 8811			

The **Cochran-Mantel-Haenszel statistic** yields the same P value as the chi-square statistic. This is because we did not adjust for any potential confounding factors. The odds ratio (1.42) and risk ratio (1.41), with their corresponding confidence intervals, both indicate statistical significance. Specifically, these statistics say that those women living near a high-hazard dump site during pregnancy are about 1.4 times as likely as women living near a low-hazard dump site during pregnancy to have a low birth weight child. In general, the odds and risk ratios will not be this close, but they were in this situation because low birth weight is a rare event.

For a matched case–control study involving dichotomous variables, **McNemar's chi-square** test is appropriate. In a study of self-reported pesticide use and breast cancer risk on Long Island, New York, female breast cancer risk was associated with lifetime residential pesticide use. Data from this study appear in Table 5.6.

In this study, controls were age-frequency matched to the cases. The odds ratio is based on the discordant pairs (i.e., OR = 1,243/230 = 5.4). The SAS procedure

TABLE 5.6   Female breast cancer risk associated with lifetime residential pesticide use

	Female breast cancer (event)		
Ever used residential pesticides	Cases	Controls	Total
Yes	1,275	1,243	2,518
No	230	310	540
Total	1,505	1,553	3,058

Source: Data from Teitelbaum et al., 2007.[14]

code used to generate the data and McNemar's chi-square test, which shows statistical significance, is as follows:

```
DATA PESTICIDES;
    INPUT CASES $ CONTROLS $ COUNT;
    DATALINES;
    1 1 1275
    1 2 1243
    2 1 230
    2 2 310
    ;

PROC FREQ DATA=PESTICIDES;
    TABLE CASES*CONTROLS/AGREE;
    WEIGHT COUNT;
RUN;
```

The portion of the SAS output containing the results for the test is as follows.

McNemar's Test	
Statistic (S)	696.6524
DF	1
Pr > S	< .0001

If the exposure variable is categorized into multiple ordinal categories, it may be of interest to evaluate whether increasing levels of exposures are linearly associated with risk of disease. Mantel developed a test statistic called the **Mantel-Haenszel chi-square** (or Mantel's Trend Test) to evaluate whether the observed trend is statistically significant.[15] If it is statistically significant, the null hypothesis of no linear trend is rejected.

To illustrate, consider a study where we surveyed 1962 university students. They were asked to identify from a list of 15 housing problems whether they had experienced any of those problems in the current semester. Students were also asked if they had experienced selected health problems in the prior month (dizziness, headaches, nausea, coughing, breathing problems, or sneezing attacks). There were 51.6% who indicated having experienced one or more of these problems. The number of housing problems from zero to five or more is reported in Table 5.7. For each of these categories, an associated number and percentage of students

TABLE 5.7   Relation between number of housing problems reported and health problems in the past month

Number of housing problems	Health problem[*] No.	Health problem[*] %
0	152	41.4
1	180	42.6
2	233	48.2
3	179	58.5
4	126	65.3
5+	142	74.4

[*]Mantel's trend test = 85.8, p < 0.0001

who reported having had a health problem in the past month are reported. A significant **dose–response relationship** is observed between number of housing problems and having experienced a selected health problem in the past month.

The SAS procedure code used to generate the data in this table and the trend test follows:

```
PROC FREQ;
    TABLE HOUSING_PROBLEM*HEALTH_PROBLEM/CHISQ;
RUN;
```

The portion of the SAS output containing the statistical tests is

Statistics for table of housing problem by health problem			
Statistic	**DF**	**Value**	**Prob**
Chi-Square	5	90.8091	<.0001
Likelihood Ratio Chi-Square	5	93.1244	<.0001
Mantel-Haenszel Chi-Square	1	85.7923	<.0001
Phi Coefficient	0.2151		
Contingency Coefficient	0.2103		
Cramer's V		0.2151	
Sample Size = 1962			

The SAS procedure code used for evaluating a rate ratio can be illustrated using the data found in Table 5.8.

TABLE 5.8   Total cardiovascular disease according to smoking status

	Cases		Person-years
Current smoker	882		220,965
Nonsmoker	673		189,254
Total	1,555		410,219

Source: Data from Iso et al., 2005.[16]

The SAS procedure code used to generate the rate ratio and 95% confidence interval is:

```
DATA SMOKER;
   INPUT SMOKE $ CASES PYEARS;
   LPYEARS=LOG(PYEARS);
   DATALINES;
   1   882   220965
   2   673   189254
   ;

PROC GENMOD;
   CLASS SMOKE;
      MODEL CASES=SMOKE/DIST=POISSON LINK=LOG
      OFFSET=LPYEARS;
      ESTIMATE 'SMOKER' SMOKE 1 -1/EXP;
   RUN;
```

Note that this procedure code involves Poisson regression, which is discussed later in this chapter. A portion of the SAS output generated by this statement is shown in the following table.

Contrast Estimate Results							
Label	Estimate	Standard Error	Alpha	Confidence Limits		Chi-Square	Pr > ChiSq
SMOKER	0.1155	0.0512	0.05	0.0152	0.2158	5.10	0.0240
Exp(SMOKER)	1.1225	0.0575	0.05	1.0153	1.2409		

The rate ratio is 1.12, meaning male current smokers are 1.12 (or 12%) more likely than nonsmokers to develop cardiovascular disease. This increased rate of cardiovascular disease among smokers is statistically significant based on the 95% confidence interval, which does not overlap 1, and the P value that corresponds to the chi-square test, which is less than 0.05.

Evaluating Statistical Association Between Discrete or Continuous Variables with SAS

Bivariate scatter plots or scatter grams are often used to assess the pattern of association between exposure and outcome variables measured on a discrete or continuous scale. For example, ecologic studies aggregate data from secondary sources where the unit of analysis is on a continuous scale such as the percentage of the adult population who smoke cigarettes or the percentage of the adult population who experience fair/poor health (see Figure 4.1). Constructing the scatter plot is important to identify whether the association between discrete or continuous variables is linear or not. For linear associations, **Pearson's correlation** coefficient and linear regression is appropriate. When the relationship between variables is not linear, transformation of the dependent and/or independent variable(s) may be in order or a polynomial regression model may be used to fit the data. Further, graphs of the data are important to identify whether outliers exist in the data or whether the data are normally distributed. When outliers exist in the data, Spearman's rank correlation coefficient is preferred over Pearson's correlation coefficient. When the data are not normally distributed, nonparametric procedures may be used for assessing associations.

The ecologic data in Figure 4.1 are shown in the following SAS data step:

```
DATA ECOLOGIC;
    INPUT STATE $ 1-20 SMOKE 21-24 HEALTH 25-28;
    LABEL SMOKE = 'CURRENT SMOKER';
    LABEL HEALTH= 'FAIR/POOR HEALTH';
DATALINES;
        Alabama              23.2      21.3
        Alaska               24        12.5
        Arizona              18.2      16.3
        Arkansas             23.7      19.6
        California           14.9      19
        Colorado             17.9      11.6
        Connecticut          17        11.5
        Delaware             21.7      12.1
        District of Columbia 17.9      12.9
        Florida              21        16.8
```

Georgia	19.9	14.8
Hawaii	17.5	14.7
Idaho	16.8	13.9
Illinois	20.5	16.1
Indiana	24.1	16.5
Iowa	21.4	13
Kansas	20	14.3
Kentucky	28.5	23.1
Louisiana	23.4	18.4
Maine	20.9	13.7
Maryland	17.7	12.6
Massachusetts	17.8	12.4
Michigan	22.4	15.2
Minnesota	18.3	10.8
Mississippi	25.1	22.5
Missouri	23.2	16.8
Montana	18.9	13.2
Nebraska	18.7	12.9
Nevada	22.2	18.5
New Hampshire	18.7	11.1
New Jersey	18	16.2
New Mexico	20.1	17.8
New York	18.2	16.6
North Carolina	22.1	18.1
North Dakota	19.5	11.5
Ohio	22.4	14.7
Oklahoma	25.1	20.2
Oregon	18.5	14.2
Pennsylvania	21.5	14.7
Rhode Island	19.2	14.1
South Carolina	22.3	17
South Dakota	20.3	11.6
Tennessee	22.6	18.8
Texas	17.9	17.4
Utah	9.8	12.9
Vermont	18	10.9
Virginia	19.3	13.1
Washington	17.1	13.5

```
West Virginia              25.7      22.5
Wisconsin                  20.8      12.2
Wyoming                    21.6      13.9
;
```

The following SAS procedure code produces a scatter plot of the data, similar to that of Figure 4.1:

```
PROC GPLOT DATA=ECOLOGIC;
    TITLE 'Ecologic Scatter Plot';
    PLOT HEALTH*SMOKE;
RUN;
```

To obtain the Pearson and Spearman correlation coefficients, the following SAS procedure code is used:

```
PROC CORR PEARSON SPEARMAN DATA=ECOLOGIC;
    VAR HEALTH SMOKE;
RUN;
```

Corresponding SAS output is as follows:

The CORR Procedure

2 Variables: HEALTH SMOKE
Simple Statistics

Variable	N	Mean	Std Dev	Median	Minimum	Maximum	Label
HEALTH	51	15.29412	3.23638	14.70000	10.80000	23.10000	FAIR/POOR HEALTH
SMOKE	51	20.30392	3.12659	20.10000	9.80000	28.50000	CURRENT SMOKER

Pearson Correlation Coefficients, N = 51
Prob > |r| under H0: Rho=0

	HEALTH	SMOKE
HEALTH	1.00000	0.59213
FAIR/POOR HEALTH		<.0001
SMOKE	0.59213	1.00000
CURRENT SMOKER	<.0001	

Spearman Correlation Coefficients, N = 51
Prob > |r| under H0: Rho=0

	HEALTH	SMOKE
HEALTH	1.00000	0.53815
FAIR/POOR HEALTH		<.0001
SMOKE	0.53815	1.00000
CURRENT SMOKER	<.0001	

The output shows that the average percentage of adults who smoke among U.S. states is 20.3%. The average percentage of adults who experience fair/poor health among U.S. states is 15.3%. The portion of the adult population that currently smokes cigarettes ranges from 9.8% in Utah to 28.5% in Kentucky. The adult population who experience fair/poor health versus very good/good health ranges from 10.8 in Minnesota to 23.1 in Kentucky. In Figure 4.1 a linear line appears to adequately fit the data. The null hypothesis of no linear association between variables can be rejected, based on the Pearson correlation coefficient. The Spearman correlation coefficient also shows a significantly positive association between variables and would be more appropriate to use if considerable outliers occurred in the data.

A summary of selected statistical techniques for testing the association between exposure and outcome variables is presented in Appendix III.

Regression Techniques

Regression is a method for estimating the functional relationship between a dependent variable and one or more independent variables. The regression techniques discussed in this section involve a linear function. The only difference among the models considered is in the outcome variable, related to the explanatory variable or variables in a linear fashion. Such models are collectively referred to as generalized linear models. Four of the most frequently used generalized linear models are (1) **linear regression** (used with a continuous outcome variable), (2) **logistic regression** (used with a categorical outcome variable), (3) **(Cox) proportional hazards** (used with survival analysis), and (4) **Poisson regression** (used with a person-time rate outcome) (see Table 5.9).

The models presented in the table each have multiple independent variables. Hence, they are called **multiple regression** models, as opposed to **simple regression** models where a single independent variable is employed. Multiple regression

TABLE 5.9 Generalized linear models

	Multiple regression model	Interpretation of b_1
Linear	$y = b_0 + b_1x_1 + b_2x_x + \ldots + b_kx_k$	Change in y mean value per unit change in x_1, adjusted for the other variables in the model
Logistic	$\log(odds) = y = b_0 + b_1x_1 + b_2x_x + \ldots + b_kx_k$	Change in the log odds of the outcome per unit change in x_1, adjusted for the other variables in the model
Poisson	$\log(rate) = y = b_0 + b_1x_1 + b_2x_x + \ldots + b_kx_k$	Change in the log rate of the outcome per unit change in x_1, adjusted for the other variables in the model
Cox	$\log(hazard) = y = b_0 + b_1x_1 + b_2x_x + \ldots + b_kx_k$	Change in the log hazard of the outcome per unit change in x_1, adjusted for the other variables in the model

models are useful for adjusting for potential confounding effects of an exposure–disease relationship and are generally more efficient than stratified simple regression models when data in the stratified combinations are sparse.

Linear Regression

In exploring the association between two discrete or continuous variables, such as between ecologic variables, the linear regression technique is often used. It assumes a linear relationship between the outcome and explanatory variables. In other words, the relationship between two variables is thought to follow a straight line, with the scatter of observed points about the line attributed to random error. In this model, the average change in the outcome variable associated with change in the explanatory variable is constant across the range of the explanatory variable. The linear line that fits the data gives the mean expected value of the outcome variable as a function of the explanatory variable. To illustrate, consider again the smoking and health data presented in the previous section. The following SAS procedure code estimates the least-squares regression line:

```
PROC REG;
    MODEL HEALTH=SMOKE;
RUN:
```

Corresponding SAS output appears as follows.

The REG ProcedureModel: MODEL1

Dependent Variable: HEALTH FAIR/POOR HEALTH

Number of Observations Read   51

Number of Observations Used   51

Analysis of Variance

Source	DF	Sum of Squares	Mean Square	F Value	Pr > F
Model	1	183.61845	183.61845	26.46	<.0001
Error	49	340.08979	6.94061		
Corrected Total	50	523.70824			

Root MSE		2.63450	R-Square	0.3506
Dependent Mean		15.29412	Adj R-Sq	0.3374
Coeff Var		17.22560		

Parameter Estimates

Variable	Label	DF	Parameter Estimate	Standard Error	t Value	Pr > |t|
Intercept	Intercept	1	2.84950	2.44744	1.16	0.2500
CURRENT SMOKER		1	0.61292	0.11916	5.14	<.0001

The estimated regression line is

$$Poor\ Health = 2.85 + 0.61 \times Smoke$$

This means that for each percentage increase in smoking, the percentage experiencing fair/poor health increases by 0.61. The slope estimate is statistically significant (i.e., $p < 0.0001$). The intercept is meaningless here because it falls well beyond the range of the data. The coefficient of determination (R-Square) is 0.3506. This indicates that approximately 35% of the variation in fair/poor health status is explained by smoking. A more informative model would adjust for potential confounders such as age, sex, and race by including these variables in the model.

Another example that illustrates a linear dose–response relationship involves cancer. Cancer development has multiple stages that often occur over many years. Multiple exposures to a number of substances may be required before a cancerous growth occurs. A linear dose–response relationship may be appropriate for carcinogens if there is no threshold such that an effect occurs at any dose, and as a dosage of carcinogen increases, so does the risk of cancer. A dose–response curve for a hypothetical carcinogen may look like that shown in Figure 5.1.

In addition to the potency of the dose, assessment should also consider factors that may influence the dose–response relationship, including age and gender. These factors can be adjusted for in the model using multiple-linear regression (see Table 5.9). In this case the estimated regression coefficient for dose represents the estimated average change in the outcome variable associated with a unit change in the dose variable, adjusted for the other variables in the model. The method often used to estimate the regression coefficients in the model is the least-squares method. Several statistics books provide detailed discussion of this method.[17]

In the situation where the explanatory variable is exposure status (yes vs. no), we may arbitrarily assign exposed a value of 1 and not exposed a value of 0, such that the regression coefficient for exposure is dichotomous. In this model, the expected mean value of the outcome variable for those not exposed is b_0, since $x_1 = 0$,

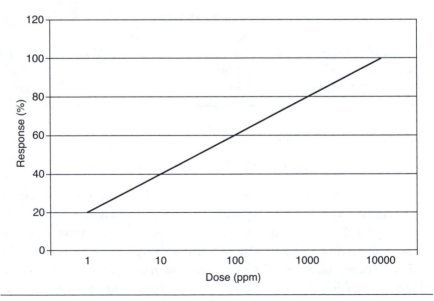

FIGURE 5.1   Dose–response curve for a carcinogen

and b_1 represents the average difference in the outcome variable between exposed and unexposed. As for any multiple regression model, when additional variables are added, b_1 is simultaneously adjusted for the other variables in the model.

When the outcome variable is categorical, such as the occurrence of an event (e.g., injury, disease, or death), a binary multiple-linear regression has been proposed. However, the assumption that the errors are normally distributed is violated. In addition, the estimates of the predicted probability may be less than zero or greater than one. A useful alternative for binary outcome variables is the logistic regression model, which offers a more robust approach to binary multiple-linear regression.

Logistic Regression

The logistic regression model assumes that the probability of a binary outcome variable is related to an explanatory variable as follows:

$$P(y \mid x) = \frac{1}{1 + e^{-(b_0 + b_1 x)}}.$$

The expression $P(y \mid x)$ denotes the probability of the binary outcome (y) for a given value of the explanatory variable. The equation on the right is called the logistic function. The outcome of this probability is constrained to fall within the range 0 to 1, but the relationship between the probability and x is not linear. With some algebra, the equation can be written in the form:

$$\log\left(\frac{P}{1-P}\right) = \log(odds) = b_0 + b_1 x.$$

The expression on the left side of the equality is called the logit (or log odds), and the relationship between the logit and the explanatory variable x is linear. Thus, the logistic model is a linear model in the log odds scale.

The logistic regression coefficient b_1 is the estimated change in the log odds of the outcome per unit change in the value of the explanatory variable. We can also say that it is the odds ratio that corresponds with a one-unit change in x. The odds ratio can be adjusted for potential confounding factors by adding additional variables to the logistic regression model (see Table 5.9).

When the explanatory variable is continuous, the estimated slope coefficient b_1 (and corresponding odds ratio) represents the linear increase in log odds (or exponential increase in odds) per unit change in the explanatory variable over the range of the explanatory variable. If the relationship is not linear over the range of the explanatory variable, then it may be useful to categorize the continuous variable (e.g., dichotomous, tertile, quartile, quintile) or transform the independent variable (e.g., squaring, cubing).

The odds ratio is a biased estimate of the risk ratio (or rate ratio), tending to exaggerate the magnitude of the association. However, when the occurrence of the outcome variable is sufficiently rare (less than 10%), the odds ratio approximates the risk ratio. Several excellent presentations of logistic regression methods using dichotomous response variable are found elsewhere.[18]

Suppose a group of 100 disease cases was identified and a group of 200 controls was randomly selected from the area where the cases originated. The distance of each case and control from their residence to a putative exposure is identified. The mean distance from the exposure for cases and controls can be compared using the two-sample (independent groups) t-test. If the data do not satisfy normality, a nonparametric procedure called the **Wilcoxon rank sum test** is a better choice than the t-test. This is a test of equality of medians rather than of means.

Note that a **parametric test** is based on the assumption that the data are normally distributed on a discrete or continuous scale. Common parametric tests are the z and t tests. On the other hand, a **nonparametric test** does not assume an underlying normal distribution, nor is it required that the data be discrete or continuous. Nonparametric tests are distribution free tests. Common nonparametric tests are the Mann-Whitney test and the chi-square test.

Logistic regression can be used as an alternate to the Wilcoxon rank sum test to estimate the ratio of cases to controls (odds ratio) according to exposure. For example, suppose we are interested in whether the odds of disease change according to distance from a putative exposure. Bands of distance from the exposure must be selected prior to analysis. Suppose these are divided into 5 bands, from 1 to 5 kilometers. Now consider the following hypothetical case–control data:

Distance from Plant (Kilometers)	Cases	Controls	Odds Ratio	95% CI
1	40	100	3.33	1.65, 6.73
2	35	100	2.92	1.43, 5.94
3	30	100	2.50	1.21, 5.16
4	15	100	1.25	0.56, 2.80
5	12	100	1.00	—

A dose–response relationship is evident. Specifically, the odds of disease increase with closer proximity to the exposure. With a dichotomous outcome variable (case vs. control), logistic regression can be used to estimate the odds ratios and corresponding confidence intervals. SAS code for generating the odds ratios and 95% confidence intervals in the above table is:

```
DATA LOGISTIC;
INPUT DISTANCE CASE $ COUNT;
DATALINES;
    1 YES 40
    1 NO 100
    2 YES 35
    2 NO 100
    3 YES 30
    3 NO 100
    4 YES 15
    4 NO 100
    5 YES 12
    5 NO 100
    ;

PROC LOGISTIC DATA=LOGISTIC DESC;
    CLASS DISTANCE/DESC;
    MODEL CASE=DISTANCE;
    WEIGHT COUNT;
RUN;
```

A portion of the SAS output that corresponds to this procedure code is:

Odds Ratio Estimates			
Effect	Point Estimate	95% Wald Confidence	Limits
DISTANCE 5 vs 1	0.300	0.149	0.605
DISTANCE 4 vs 1	0.375	0.195	0.722
DISTANCE 3 vs 1	0.750	0.433	1.298
DISTANCE 2 vs 1	0.875	0.514	1.489

Here we can see that the odds of being a case significantly decreases with greater distance away from the site.

We can also treat distance as a discrete variable and calculate the odds of disease according to distance from the exposure. The odds of disease significantly decrease with distance from the exposure (OR = 0.74, 95% CI: 0.64, 0.85). The SAS code to generate this estimate and corresponding confidence interval is:

```
PROC LOGISTIC DATA=LOGISTIC DESC;
   MODEL CASE=DISTANCE;
   WEIGHT COUNT;
RUN;
```

Another example is based on the study of Doll and Hill (1966) where they examined among male British doctors the association between death from coronary disease and smoking status according to age.[19] The SAS data step is as follows:

```
DATA CORONARY;
INPUT AGE $ SMOKE $ DEATHS PYEARS;
LPYEARS=LOG(PYEARS);
DATALINES;
35-44      YES    32     52407
45-54      YES    104    43248
55-64      YES    206    28612
65-74      YES    186    12663
75-84      YES    102    5317
35-44      NO     2      18790
45-54      NO     12     10673
55-64      NO     28     5710
65-74      NO     28     2585
75-84      NO     31     1462
;
```

The SAS procedure code for estimating the rate ratio of death by smoking status for smokers and according to age groups is as follows:

```
PROC GENMOD;
   CLASS AGE SMOKE/DESC;
```

```
MODEL DEATHS=AGE SMOKE/DIST=POISSON LINK=LOG
OFFSET=LPYEARS;
    ESTIMATE 'SMOKER' SMOKE 1 -1/EXP;
RUN;
```

A portion of the resulting SAS output is as follows:

Contrast Estimate Results							
Label	Standard Estimate	Error	Alpha	Confidence	Limits	Chi-Square	Pr > ChiSq
SMOKER	0.3545	0.1074	0.05	0.1441	0.5650	10.90	0.0010
Exp(SMOKER)	1.4255	0.1531	0.05	1.1550	1.7594		

Hence, after adjusting for age, smokers have 1.43 times the mortality rate of nonsmokers.

Cox Proportional Hazards Model (Cox Model)

Many environmental health outcomes are related to time. The Cox model, also called the proportional hazards model, is a useful model for analyzing time-to-event (or survival) data.[20,21] The model indicates the probability that a person will experience an event (e.g., death) in the next interval of time, given that he or she has survived until the beginning of the interval. The model assumes an underlying hazard function $h_0(t) \times B$, which describes how hazard (or risk) changes over time for a baseline or reference group (e.g., risk among the unexposed). Exposure to a certain risk factor, such as a biologic pathogen or chemical agent, is associated with a fixed relative increase in an instantaneous risk of the associated outcome compared with. Mathematically we can say:

$$h_1(t) = h_0(t) \times B.$$

B denotes a constant multiplication factor. Letting $B = e^{b_0 + b_1 x_1 + \ldots + b_k x_k}$ implies that the risk of an event in a short interval of time will follow an exponential model. The equation can be reformatted as

$$h_1(t) = h_0(t) \times e^{b_0 + b_1 x_1 + \ldots + b_k x_k}, \text{ or } HR = \frac{h_1(t)}{h_0(t)} = e^{b_0 + b_1 x_1 + \ldots + b_k x_k}.$$

Taking the logarithm of both sides gives:

$$\log(HR) = b_0 + b_1 x_1 + \ldots + b_k x_k$$

The regression coefficients obtained from the Cox proportional hazards model take into account the time to occurrence for each event. They also take into account the time of censoring for the individuals not observed for the entire follow-up period. The hazards are assumed to be proportional over time such that one hazard ratio is estimated for the entire follow-up period. If the hazard ratio changes during the follow-up time (i.e., a time by exposure interaction exists), the model should be stratified according to follow-up time. A variable is time dependent if the difference in its values between two individuals changes with time (e.g., cumulative exposures such as smoking) compared with fixed variables such as sex or race. By convention, cumulative exposures are often put into less precise dichotomy scales such as exposed versus not exposed instead of more meaningful time to exposure. Several texts provide detailed descriptions of the Cox proportional hazards model and the incorporation of time-dependent exposures (e.g., Kleinbaum, 1996).[22] The hazard ratios obtained from the Cox proportional hazards regression are analogous to relative risks.

In one study, researchers explored whether adults with asthma could have symptomatic exacerbation after exposure to secondhand smoke. Exposure to secondhand smoke during the previous 7 days was measured using a nicotine badge that 189 patients each wore. The hazard ratio (relative risk) of asthma severity for those in the highest tertile of nicotine versus the lowest level was 1.56 (95% CI 0.18–2.95), adjusted for sociodemographic covariates and previous smoking history. Estimates of exposure to secondhand smoke in the previous 3 months were estimated using hair nicotine and cotinine levels. The second and third tertiles of hair nicotine exposure during the previous month were associated with a greater baseline prospective risk of hospital admission for asthma (adjusted HR 3.73; 95% CI 1.04–13.30 and adjusted HR 3.61; 95% CI 1.0–12.9, respectively).[23]

An important strength of Cox proportional hazards regression is that adjusted relative risk estimates can be generated. In the previous example, relative risk estimates were adjusted for sociodemographic covariates and previous smoking history. In a nested case–control study within the European prospective investigation involving cancer and nutrition, daily exposure (many hours) to environmental tobacco smoke during childhood was significantly associated with lung cancer in adulthood. Using a Cox proportional hazards model, the hazard ratio (relative risk) was 3.6, with 95% CI 1.2–11.1.[24] The relative risk was adjusted by sex, smoking status, country, education level, energy intake, fruit and vegetable consumption, and physical activity.

In SAS, the procedure for performing Cox proportional hazards regression is PHREG. To illustrate the use of PHREG, consider the following hypothetical data, which represent time to event for people exposed versus not exposed.

```
>   DATA COX;
INPUT TIME CENSORED EXPOSURE;
DATALINES;
43  0  0
28  1  0
72  0  0
3   1  1
7   1  1
12  1  0
15  1  0
33  0  0
6   1  1
31  1  0
28  1  1
32  1  1
8   1  1
5   1  1
25  1  1
5   1  0
17  0  1
2   1  1
;

PROC PHREG DATA=COX;
    MODEL TIME*STATUS(0)=EXPOSED/RL;
  RUN;
```

In this example TIME is the time-to-event variable, STATUS is the censoring indicator (0 for no event and 1 for event), and EXPOSED, in this example, represents exposure status (yes vs. no). The RL option provides confidence intervals in the SAS output. Suppose the study population involves asthmatic never smokers and TIME is in days until an asthma attack and EXPOSED reflects living with someone who smokes (yes vs. no). Perhaps the censored individuals had not experienced an asthma attack when the study ended. The SAS output that results from this data set and SAS code is as follows.

The PHREG Procedure								
Analysis of Maximum Likelihood Estimates								
Variable	DF	Parameter Estimate	Standard Error	Chi-Square	Pr > ChiSq	Hazard Ratio	95% Hazard Confidence	Limits
EXPOSURE	1	1.13650	0.56163	4.0948	0.0430	3.116	1.036	9.368

The estimate 3.1 (95% CI 1.0, 9.4) indicates that for asthmatics who have never smoked, the relative risk of an asthma attack is greater if they live with a smoker than if they do not live with a smoker.

There are several issues related to Cox proportional hazards regression that go beyond the scope of this book (e.g., adjustment for ties, the need for interaction or stratification, model checking, etc.). Before applying Cox proportional hazards regression, it is recommended that you refer to a more in-depth coverage of this topic (e.g., Kleinbaum, 1996).[22]

Poisson Regression

Poisson regression is appropriate when the dependent events occur infrequently, the events occur independently, and the events occur over some continuous medium such as time or area. The probability of a single event occurring is influenced by the length of the time interval. Counts or rates of rare diseases are well suited for modeling with Poisson regression.[25]

Poisson regression assumes that the data follow a Poisson distribution, which is frequently encountered when a rate exists at which events occur, for example, 6 injuries per hour, 18 cases per 1,000 person-years, 44 cases per 100 people. The rate can be multiplied by exposure to obtain expected number of health-related states or events; that is, 6 injuries per hour over 5 hours means 30 injuries; 18 cases per 1,000 person-years multiplied by 2,000 person-years means 36 cases; and 44 cases per 100 people multiplied by 150 people means 66 cases. Traditional regression assumes a symmetric distribution of errors. However, the Poisson distribution is skewed. Traditional regression can produce negative predicted values. However, the Poisson distribution is nonnegative. Finally, traditional regression assumes constant variance. However, for the Poisson distribution the variance increases as the mean increases. Poisson regression uses a log-transformation that adjusts for the skewness and prevents model predictions of negative values. In addition, Poisson regression models the variance as a function of the mean.

Poisson regression can analyze both count and rate data. Above we showed the relation between rates and counts. Fitting a model using rates requires that we have the number of health-related states or events (i.e., the numerator of the rate) and the measure of time, area, or people (i.e., the denominator of the rate). The Poisson model is fit to the counts using the log of the denominator as an offset variable.[26]

When counts and rates of disease are not rare, logistic regression or survival analysis should be considered. In addition, Poisson regression is appropriate when we have observed and expected counts by exposure status (cohort data), whereas logistic regression is appropriate when we have cases and controls by exposure status (case–control data).

Suppose we are interested in estimating a rate or counts of disease and identifying the relationship the rate has or counts have with a set of explanatory variables. It may also be of interest to know how a ratio of observed to expected rates or counts varies over the levels of an explanatory variable. In the following example, we present observed and expected counts of disease X in relation to the distance from a chemical plant suspected of being the source of an environmental pollutant linked with the disease. Consider the following hypothetical data:

Distance from Plant (Kilometers)	Observed	Expected	Rate Ratio	Observed to Expected (% Higher)
1	8	4	2.00	100%
2	5	3	1.67	67%
3	10	6	1.67	67%
4	14	8	1.75	75%
5	20	13	1.54	54%
6	21	16	1.31	31%
7	22	16	1.38	38%
8	18	16	1.13	13%
9	20	17	1.18	18%
10	17	17	1.00	0%

The SAS command for employing Poisson regression to estimate the trend in the ratio of observed and expected counts with distance from the plant is presented as follows.

```
DATA X;
    INPUT DISTANCE O E;
    LE=LOG(E);
    DATALINES;
    1    8    4
    2    5    3
    3    10   6
    4    14   8
    5    20   13
    6    21   16
    7    22   16
    8    18   16
    9    20   17
    10   17   17
    ;

PROC GENMOD DATA=X;
    MODEL O=DISTANCE/DIST=POISSON LINK=LOG OFFSET=LE;
RUN;
```

The PROC GENMOD statement in SAS allows us to employ Poisson regression. The number of observed cases in the putative cluster is the dependent variable and the distance from the plant is the independent variable. The option DIST=POISSON specifies the Poisson distribution and the option LINK= LOG specific that the link function is the log function. The variable LE is the natural log of the expected counts. Hence, the model fits a loglinear model to the ratio of observed to expected counts. A portion of the SAS output is as follows:

Parameter	DF	Standard Estimate	Wald Error	95% CI		Chi-Square	P Value
Intercept 0.0004	1	0.7666	0.2161	0.3431	1.1901	12.59	
Distance 0.0218	1	-0.0729	0.0318	-0.1352	-0.0106	5.26	
Scale	0	1.0000	0.0000	1.0000	1.0000		

Note: The scale parameter was held fixed.

Label	Estimate	Standard Estimate	95% CI		Chi-Square	P Value
Beta	-0.0729	0.0318	-0.1352	-0.0106	5.26	
Exp(Beta)	0.9297	0.0296	0.8735	0.9894		0.0218

The ratio of observed to expected counts changes by a factor of 0.9297 for each kilometer increase in distance from the plant. For 10 kilometers the decrease in the ratio of observed to expected counts is 48% (= $0.9297^{10} \times 100$). The *P* value is 0.0218, so the ratio significantly decreases over the 10 kilometers from the plant. A good comparison of Poisson regression results with ordinary least squares, and negative binomial regression is presented elsewhere by Hutchinson and Holtman (2005).[27]

Selecting the Correct Statistical Model

The appropriate statistical model is influenced by the type of the study and the type of the exposure and outcome variables. Multivariate techniques are used to assess the influence of multiple factor on the outcome variables as well as to adjust for potential confounders. Table 5.10 provides summaries of statistical models and adjusted measures of association related to the study design and variable type.

Conducting statistical analyses has been greatly facilitated in recent years because of the computer and powerful computer software. A word of caution, however, is that when selecting a statistical technique for assessment, it is often important to evaluate model assumptions. The need for careful examination of the raw data by means of frequency distributions, bivariate scatter plots, normal probability plots, and so on is critical. It is recommended that when applying an analytic regression

TABLE 5.10 Summary of statistical models and adjusted measures of association related to selected study designs and variable types

Type of study	Outcome variable (type)	Statistical technique	Adjusted measures of association
Any	Continuous	Linear regression Analysis of variance	Linear regression coefficient Difference in means
Cross-sectional	Dichotomous	Direct adjustment*	Prevalence ratio
		Indirect adjustment†	Standardized prevalence ratio
		Mantel-Haenszel	Odds ratio
		Logistic regression	Odds ratio
Case-control	Dichotomous	Mantel-Haenszel	Odds ratio
		Logistic regression	Odds ratio
Cohort	Cumulative incidence (by the end of follow-up)	Direct adjustment	Relative risk
		Indirect adjustment	Standardized incidence ratio
	Cumulative incidence (Time-to-event data)	Cox model	Hazard ratio
	Incidence rate (per person-time)	Poisson regression	Rate ratio
Nested case-control	Time-dependent disease status	Conditional logistic regression	Hazard ratio
	(Time-to-event data)	Cox model with staggered entries	

Source: Modified from Szklo and Nieto, 2007, p. 290.[4]

*A method of rate adjustment used when the specific rates (e.g., age-specific rates) in each population being compared are available and stable.

†A method of rate adjustment used when one or more of the specific rates (e.g., age-specific rates) in one of the populations being compared is either unavailable or unstable. The direct and indirect methods are presented in most principles books in epidemiology (e.g., Merrill and Timmreck, 2006).[28]

technique, consultation be made with a statistician. It is often best to involve a statistician early in the research process, preferably at the study design stage of the investigation.

Key Issues

1. Data represents numerical information from selected variables. The type of data involved in an investigation will influence the methods employed for description and analysis.
2. Data analysis is statistical examination of the pattern of relationship between the variables under investigation.
3. Statistical tests are employed to evaluate hypotheses about associations between exposure and outcome variables.
4. Statistical inference involves a procedure that allows the researcher to decide between two hypotheses about a population based on sampled data and uses probability to indicate the level of reliability in the conclusion.
5. When assessing measures of association with dichotomous variables the confidence interval can be used to indicate statistical interaction. A confidence interval is preferred over the *P* value because the width of the interval also reflects the level of precision in the estimate.
6. Linear regression is used when the outcome variable is continuous, logistic regression is used when the outcome variable is categorical, Cox proportional hazards model is used with time-to-event (survival) data, and Poisson regression is used with a person-time rate outcome variable.

Exercises

Key Terms

Define the following terms.

Analytic statistics
Attributable risk
Attributable risk percent
Cochran-Mantel-Haenszel statistic
Confidence interval
Contingency table

Cumulative incidence
Degrees of freedom
Descriptive statistics
Dose–response relationship
Fisher's exact test
Hazard rate
Incidence
Incidence density
Level of significance
Linear regression
Logistic regression
Mantel-Haenszel chi-square
Matched-paired analysis
McNemar's chi-square
Multiple regression
Nonparametric test
Normal distribution
Null hypothesis
Odds ratio
P value
Parametric test
Pearson's correlation
Period prevalence
Point prevalence
Poisson regression
Population attributable risk
Population attributable risk percent
Prevalence
Prevalence ratio
Proportional hazards
Rate base
Rate ratio
Regression
Relative risk
Reliability
Risk ratio
Simple regression

Skewed distribution
Statistical Analysis System
Statistical inference
Study hypothesis
Wilcoxon rank sum test

Study Questions

5.1. List four purposes for assessing data using descriptive statistics.

5.2. List three purposes for performing analytic statistics.

5.3. How does statistical inference relate to hypothesis testing?

5.4. What is the primary distinction between incidence and prevalence?

5.5. What is the primary distinction in cumulative incidence and incidence density (also called incidence rate)?

5.6. List two advantages of using a confidence interval over a P value in statistical inference.

5.7. Match the following:

____ Cumulative incidence	a. Risk ratio (involving person time)
____ Incidence density (rate)	b. Odds ratio (b/c)
____ Unmatched case-control	c. Odds ratio ($a \times d/c \times B$))
____ Matched case-control	d. Prevalence ratio
____ Cross-sectional	e. Risk ratio

5.8. Match the following:

____ For testing $H_0 : Risk\ Ratio = 1$

a. $\chi^2 = \dfrac{(ad - bc)^2\, n}{(a+b)(c+d)(a+c)(b+d)}$

____ For testing $H_0 : Rate\ Ratio = 1$

b. $\chi^2 = \dfrac{(b-c)^2}{(b+c)}$

____ For testing $H_0 : PR = 1$

c. $\chi^2 = \dfrac{\left\{a - \left[T_e(a-c)\right]\big/T\right\}^2}{\left\{T_e\left[T_{ue}(a+c)\right]\big/T\right\}^2}$

____ For testing $H_0 : OR = 1$ (unmatched C-C)

____ For testing $H_0 : OR = 1$ (matched C-C)

5.9. What are two statistical measures useful for identifying whether an association exists between discrete or continuous variables? Discuss.

5.10. Match the following:

Model	Outcome variable
___ Linear regression	a. Person-time rate
___ Logistic regression	b. Continuous
___ Proportional hazards	c. Categorical
___ Poisson regression	d. Time-to-event

5.11. Describe the general features of nonparametric methods.

5.12. List three advantages that Poisson regression has over traditional regression when dealing with modeling the number of cases of a health-related state event as a function of exposure and other variables.

References

1. Feigal D, Black D, Grady D, et al. Planning for data management and analysis. In: Hulley S, Cummings S, Browner W, et al. *Designing Clinical Research: An Epidemiologic Approach*. Baltimore, MD: Williams & Wilkins; 1988.

2. Gilbreath S, Kass PH. Adverse birth outcomes associated with open dump sites in Alaska Native villages. *Am J Epidemiol*. 2006;164:518–528.

3. Rothman K. *Modern Epidemiology*. Boston, MA: Little, Brown and Company; 1986.

4. Szklo M, Nieto FJ. *Epidemiology Beyond the Basics*. 2nd ed. Boston, MA: Jones and Bartlett Publishers; 2007.

5. Ries LAG, Melbert D, Krapcho M, et al. SEER Cancer Statistics Review, 1975–2004, National Cancer Institute. Bethesda, MD. 2007. Available at: http://seer.cancer.gov/csr/1975_2004/. Accessed June 12, 2007.

6. Roy N, Merrill RM, Thibeault S, Parsa RA, Gray SD, Smith EM. Prevalence of voice disorders in teachers and the general population. *J Speech Hear Res*. 2004;47(2):281–293.

7. Katz D, Baptista J, Azen SP, Pike MC. Obtaining confidence intervals for the risk ratio in cohort studies. *Biometrics*. 1978;34:469–474.

8. Ederer F, Mantel N. Confidence limits on the ratio for two Poisson variables. *Am J Epidemiol*. 1974;100:165–167.

9. Ahlbom A. *Biostatistics for Epidemiologists*. Boca Raton, FL: Lewis Publishers; 1993.

10. Woolf B. On estimating the relation between blood group and disease. *Ann Hum Genet*. 1955;19:251–253.

11. Schlesselman JJ. *Case-Control Studies: Design, Conduct, Analysis*. New York: Oxford University Press; 1982.

12. Hansen C, Neller A, Williams G, Simpson R. Maternal exposure to low levels of ambient air pollution and preterm birth in Brisbane, Australia. *BJOG, An International Journal of Obstetrics and Gynaecology*. 2006;113(8):935–941.

13. Gilbreath S, Kass PH. Adverse birth outcomes associated with open dump sites in Alaska Native villages. *Am J Epidemiol.* 2006;164:518–528.

14. Teitelbaum SL, Gammon MD, Britton JA, Neugut AI, Levin B, Stellman SD. Reported residential pesticide use and breast cancer risk on Long Island, New York. *Am J Epidemiol.* 2007;165(6):643–651.

15. Mantel N. Chi-square tests with one degree of freedom: extensions of the Mantel-Haenszel procedure. *J Am Stat Assoc.* 1963;58:690–700.

16. Iso H, Date C, Yamamoto A, et al. Smoking cessation and mortality from cardiovascular disease among Japanese men and women. The JACC study. *Am J Epidemiol.* 2005;161(2):170–179.

17. Pagano M, Gauvreau K. *Principles of Biostatistics.* 2nd ed. Pacific Grove, CA: Duxbury; 2000.

18. Stokes ME, Davis CS, Koch GG. *Categorical Data Analysis Using the SAS System.* Cary, NC: SAS Institute Inc; 1995.

19. Doll R, Hill AB. Mortality of British doctors in relation to smoking; observations on coronary thrombosis. In: Epidemiological Approaches to the Study of Cancer and Other Chronic Diseases. Haenszel W, ed. *Natl Cancer Inst Monogr.* 1966;19:204–268.

20. Cox DR. Regression models and life-tables (with discussion). *J R Stat Soc, Ser B.* 1972;34:187–220.

21. Cox DR., Oaks D. *Analysis of Survival Data.* London: Chapman and Hall; 1984.

22. Kleinbaum DG. *Survival Analysis: A Self-Learning Text.* New York: Springer-Verlag; 1996.

23. Eisner MD, Klein J, Hammond SK, Koren G, Lactao G, Irbarren C. Directly measured second hand smoke exposure and asthma health outcomes. *Thorax.* 2005;60:814–821.

24. Vineis P, Airoldi L, Veglia P, et al. Environmental tobacco smoke and risk of respiratory cancer and chronic obstructive pulmonary disease in former smokers and never smokers in the EPIC prospective study. *BMJ.* 2005;330(7486): 277.

25. Frome EL, Checkoway H. Use of Poisson regression models in estimating incidence rates and ratios. *Am J Epidemiol.* 1985;212:309–323.

26. McCullagh P, Nelder JA. *Generalized Linear Models.* London: Chapman and Hall; 1983.

27. Hutchinson MK, Holtman MC. Analysis of count data using Poisson regression. *Res Nurs Health.* 2005;28:408–418.

28. Merrill RM, Timmreck TC. *Introduction to Epidemiology.* 4th ed. Boston, MA: Jones and Bartlett Publishers; 2006.

Causal Inference

LEARNING OBJECTIVES

After completing this chapter, you should be able to:

1. Define causal inference.
2. Know selected criteria for establishing a cause–effect relationship.
3. Formulate and test hypotheses in the search for causal associations.
4. Define risk factor.
5. Understand how webs of causation can be used as tools in environmental epidemiology.

Introduction

In the previous chapter focus was on measuring and testing associations between exposure and outcome variables. Suppose we establish that an exposure is statistically associated with an outcome variable. The next step is to determine whether the statistical association reflects a causal association. At the heart of all scientific investigation is the notion of causality. Causality plays a vital role in injury and disease investigations in environmental epidemiology. Concluding that there is a valid statistical association is only one of the criteria used in establishing a causal association. A valid statistical association, although required for there to be a causal association, is not sufficient to determine a causal association. Other criteria should be considered before drawing conclusions about causality, including temporality of events and dose–response relationships. The study design influences whether temporal sequence of events and dose–response relationships can be established.

Once causal association is established and important risk factors made clear, a protection attitude can arise rather than a mere reaction to environmental crises, such as having a supply of food and water in case of natural disasters. Education of risk factors can be achieved through schools, churches, business and industry, trade associations and professional organizations, advertising and news media, and government agencies.[1]

The purpose of this chapter is to define the term "causal inference" and present those criteria commonly used in causal inference.

Causal Inference

Whereas associations between and among variables are observed, causation is inferred. A **causal inference** is a conclusion about the presence of a disease and the reasons for its existence. The connection between human health and physical, chemical, biological, social, and psychosocial factors in the environment is based on causal inference. To better understand this term, consider that in our daily lives each of us infers that something is true or highly probable based on our expectations and experiences. We may practice the piano expecting that it will improve our performance skills or lock our doors believing that it will prevent crime. Inference in environmental epidemiology is similar to inference in daily life in that it is also based on expectations and experience. Only in science, expectations are referred to as hypotheses, theories, or predictions, and experiences are called results, observations, or data. Inference in everyday life serves as a basis for action.[2] Similarly, causal inferences provide a scientific basis for medical and public health action.

We make inferences in our daily lives in a different manner than scientists do. The inferences we make are informal and are based on our expectations about the given event, reasons for its occurrence, and experience with similar situations. On the other hand, in science inference is typically made after the application of formal methods. For instance, **statistical inference** draws a conclusion about a population based on sampled data and uses probability to indicate the level of reliability in the conclusion. Sampled data are evaluated using statistical methods such as regression and correlations, decision theory, and time-series analysis. Causal inferences are made with methods comprising lists of criteria or conditions applied to the results of scientific studies. Inferences are then made based on "judgment" and "logic" and are generally considered to follow an acceptable mode of scientific reasoning.[2]

The methods of causal inference were initially developed by Jacob Henle (1809–1885) and his student Robert Koch (1843–1910), both German physicians. Three postulates or guidelines were developed called **Koch's postulates** (or Henle-Koch postulates), published in 1880.[3] These postulates were applied by Koch to establish the etiology of anthrax and tuberculosis, although they can be generalized to other diseases. The postulates state:

1. The parasite occurs in every case of the disease in question and under circumstances that can account for the pathologic changes and clinical courses of the disease.
2. It occurs in no other disease as a fortuitous and nonpathogenic parasite.
3. After being fully isolated from the body and repeatedly grown in pure culture, it can induce the disease anew.

These postulates remain a benchmark for judging whether a causal relationship exists between an organism and a disease. However, they have been found to be inadequate for most diseases, especially noninfectious chronic diseases.[4] A number of individuals have since contributed to the development of causal inference. Table 6.1, previously presented by Weed (1995), summarizes criteria thought to be important in causal inference. A few conditions were added over the time period covered in the table, but for the most part, the evolutionary

TABLE 6.1   Criteria used in causal inference

Lilienfeld (1959)[5]	Sartwell (1960)[6]	Surgeon General (1964)[7] and Susser (1973)[8]	Hill (1965)[9]	MacMahan and Pugh (1970)[10]
• Consistency	• Replication	• Consistency	• Consistency	• Strength of association (including magnitude of association and dose–response)
• Magnitude of effect	• Strength of association	• Strength of association (including magnitude of effect and dose–response)	• Strength of association	• Temporality
• Dose-response	• Dose-response	• Temporality	• Biological gradient	• Experimentation
• Biological mechanism	• Temporality	• Biological coherence	• Temporality	• Consonance with existing knowledge
	• Biological reasonableness	• Specificity	• Experimental evidence	• Biological mechanisms
			• Biological plausibility	• Consistency
			• Biological coherence	• Exclusion of alternative explanations
			• Specificity	
			• Analogy	

Source: From Weed, 1995, p. 292.2

changes between 1959 and 1973 were minor. Causal methods used since are essentially the same.

The general **causal criteria** used in the 1964 Surgeon General's report to assess the extent that available information supports causal inference are consistency, strength of association, temporality, biologic coherence, and specificity. These are presented and described as follows:

1. **Consistency.** Consistency occurs when associations are replicated by different investigators in different settings and populations with different methods. It is unlikely that similar relations will occur in studies involving different settings and populations by chance alone, unless each study is biased in a similar manner. For example, cigarette smoking has been shown to be the principal cause of lung cancer in hundreds of studies and over 27 reports by the U.S. Surgeon General. On the other hand, a lack of consistency may be due to methodological differences and/or systematic changes in effect over time. Meta-analysis may be an effective way to combine relations found across several studies but requires that the studies employ similar study designs and assumes the studies apply sound methods that minimize bias.

2. **Strength of association.** A strong direct association between an exposure and disease outcome increases the likelihood of there being a causal association. In general, weak associations provide little support of causal association. Stronger associations are less likely explained by chance, bias, or confounding.

   A causal relation implies that a valid statistical association exists, which is not due to chance, bias, or confounding. When sampled data are used to assess the effect of an exposure on a disease outcome, the findings could be due to **chance**. **Bias** involves the deviation of the results from the truth and is controlled for by carefully designing and carrying out the study. Because there is usually very little that can be done once bias has occurred, avoiding bias at the design level of a study is critical.[11] **Confounding** occurs when the relationship between an exposure and outcome is influenced by a third factor, where the factor is related to the exposure and, independent of this relationship, is also a risk factor for the disease or outcome. Given that the observational study designs used in environmental epidemiology do not allow us to balance out the effect of confounding factors through randomization, considerable care is required to deal with this potential problem. Approaches such as matching and restriction have been used at the design level of study, while stratification and multiple-regression have been used at the analysis level of study to control for confounding.

After ruling out chance, bias, and confounding as possible explanations for association, statistical associations provide grounds for a clear causal relationship. For example, large statistical associations between smoking and lung cancer were found this way. The risk of dying from lung cancer is 22 times higher among men who smoke and 12 times higher among women who smoke compared with nonsmokers.[12]

A **dose–response relationship** means the risk of disease changes in direct proportion to the level of the exposure. For example, incidence rates of skin melanoma, a cancer of pigment producing cells residing in skin epidermis, is generally inversely correlated with latitude of residence, with higher rates closer to the equator.[13] Removal of the exposure should reduce or eliminate the disease risk, unless irreversible damage has occurred. Where multiple types of exposure contribute to a given disease, removal of one type of exposure may reduce but not eliminate the disease risk.

For diseases and conditions where causal relationships are indirect, such as when a mediating variable is involved, evaluating the strength of an association is more complex. Multiple-regression, structural equation modeling, or other statistical methods may be required for assessing statistical associations. Keep in mind that such statistical modeling must be supported by theoretical relationships.

3. **Temporality.** For an exposure to cause a disease it must temporally precede the disease at a reasonable interval. Incubation periods from exposure to the onset of clinical symptoms can be a few hours, days, weeks, or years. Although **incubation period** is a term used with acute conditions, **latency period** is typically used to represent the time from exposure to clinical symptoms for chronic conditions. The best study design for establishing a time sequence of events is the cohort study. In cohort studies exposure status is first identified, and persons with the disease of interest are excluded from the study. Exposed and unexposed groups are then followed to see if there is a difference in disease risk. For example, Richard Doll published results from a cohort study in 1955 showing that men exposed to asbestos in their work for 20 or more years were almost 14 times more likely to develop lung cancer than expected.[14] Establishing a temporal sequence of events is typically more difficult with diseases having longer latency periods.

4. **Biological coherence.** Biological coherence is the association between an exposure and disease outcome supported in terms of basic human biology. With respect to cancer, the International Agency for Research on Cancer has classified 150 chemicals or biological agents as known or probable carcinogens based on laboratory evidence.[15] Some selected occupational carcinogens for leukemia are benzene, ethylene oxide, and ionizing radiation; for malignant mesothelioma is asbestos; and for cancers of the trachea, lung, and bronchus are arsenic, asbestos, beryllium, cadmium, chromium, diesel exhaust, nickel, and silica.

5. **Specificity.** Specificity of association means an exposure is associated with only one disease, or that the disease is associated with only one exposure. Although this condition may support a causal hypothesis, failure to satisfy this criterion cannot rule out a causal hypothesis because many exposures are related to a given disease or many diseases are related to a given exposure. For example, increased risk of lung cancer is associated with cigarette smoking, diet, radon gas, and asbestos. On the other hand, cigarette smoking has been associated with several cancers, heart disease, and stroke. When diseases are grouped together or misclassified, specificity diminishes.

In 1965, Hill added two more important criteria that are often viewed as necessary today: biological plausibility and experimental evidence. Hill used these criteria to help him evaluate results of several studies he conducted with Doll concerning smoking and lung cancer.[9] Biologic plausibility is similar to biologic coherence, although it is broader in the sense that laboratory proof is not necessary; for instance, we might be able to say that it is biologically plausible that lung cancer is caused by smoking because cigarette smoke comes in direct contact with the surface of alveoli contained within the lungs. To obtain experimental evidence, an intervention study of some kind must be performed. Although a randomized, blinded controlled experimental study may be best for minimizing the effects of chance, bias, and confounding, ethical barriers limit the universality of this criterion.

In sum, these criteria provide evidence for causal relationships. It is important that the totality of the evidence be considered and the criteria weighed against each other to infer causal relationships.

Risk Factors

A term that is commonly used to describe a factor that is associated with disease is "risk factor." A **risk factor** is a variable that is associated with the increased probability of a human health problem. Risk factors are not necessarily causal because not everyone who has the risk factor will experience the health problem. The term "risk factor" was first introduced by researchers in 1961, where it was shown from data collected in the Framingham Study that high blood pressure, high cholesterol, and smoking increased the risk of heart disease.[16] Greater exposure to the factor is associated with increased probability of experiencing the outcome. For example, exposure to ionizing radiation is a risk factor for breast cancer. Risk factors are also referred to as at-risk behaviors. An at-risk behavior is an activity performed by persons who are healthy, but are at greater risk of developing a particular condition because of the behavior. For example, consumption of high levels of meat is a risk factor for colon cancer.

Selected factors have been proposed in order to better understand health problems: predisposing factors, enabling factors, precipitating factors, and reinforcing factors.[17,18]

1. **Predisposing factors.** These are the factors or conditions already present that produce a susceptibility or disposition in a host to a health problem without actually causing it. For example, there are several factors that increase susceptibility to ultraviolet radiation: skin with relatively little pigmentation, certain diseases (e.g., xeroderma pigmentosa, lupus erythematosus, pellagra, and porphyria), fungi growing on certain plants, fungi growing in celery (producing psoralen, a chemical that photosynthesizes the skin), and a number of medications and plant extracts.[19]

2. **Enabling factors.** These factors or conditions allow or assist the disease, condition, injury, disability, or death, letting the process begin and run its course. For example, lack of protection from sufficiently high levels of ultraviolet radiation can cause marked systemic effects (fever, nausea, and malaise), aging of the skin (from cumulative exposure), and premalignant and malignant tumors. People can protect themselves from ultraviolet radiation by using sunscreen, wearing dark glasses, and wearing protective clothing. Lack of education about the potentially harmful effects of high and extended exposure to ultraviolet radiation can also enable adverse health effects. Conversely, recommendations for the control of exposures from ultraviolet lamps used in tanning booths or from sun lamps can prevent, control, and facilitate recovery from skin damage. The obvious goal is to enable people to reduce the harmful effects from high and excessive exposure to ultraviolet radiation.

3. **Precipitating factors.** These are the factors essential to the development of health problems. For example, ultraviolet radiation can damage cell regulation resulting in uncontrolled growth of malformed cells. There are three types of genes that regulate and protect the cell, protooncogenes that regulate cell replication, tumor suppressor genes that lead to apoptosis (cell suicide), and DNA repair genes. The protooncogene may be thought of as the gas pedal on your car and the tumor suppressor gene as the brake. The DNA repair gene may be compared with the mechanic that can fix a gas pedal or brake if it is not working properly. If the gas pedal is stuck to the floor but the brake is able to stop the car, then you will be all right. If the gas pedal and brake are broken and you have the mechanic fix these before embarking on a drive in the French Alps, you will still be all right. However, if you discover on your drive that the gas pedal is stuck to the floor, the brake does not work, and there is no way to repair them, last rights might be in order. Similarly, mutated protooncogenes (called oncogenes), tumor suppressor genes, and DNA repair genes are precipitating factors in skin cancer.

4. **Reinforcing factors.** Like enabling factors, reinforcing factors have the ability to support the production of and transmission of health problems. For example, society may promote suntans as healthy and attractive, thereby supporting excessive sun exposure and tanning. Reinforcing factors can also support and improve a population's health status and help reduce health problems. For example, breaking down social forces that promote tanning can reduce skin damage. The factors that help aggravate and perpetuate diseases, conditions, disabilities, or deaths are negative reinforcing factors. Negative reinforcing factors are repetitive patterns of behavior that recur, perpetuate, and support a disease that is spreading and running its course in a population. Positive reinforcing factors are those that support, enhance, and improve the control and prevention of the causation of disease.

Four Types of Causal Factors

Types of causal factors include "sufficient" and/or "necessary." There are four combinations possible of these factors: necessary and sufficient, necessary but not sufficient, sufficient but not necessary, and neither sufficient nor necessary.

- Necessary and sufficient: The disease does not develop without the factor; for example, often necessary for the study of infectious diseases such as hepatitis B virus or human immunodeficiency virus (HIV).
- Necessary but not sufficient: The main factor is required, along with other factors; for example, HIV is necessary, along with one or several latent or newly acquired infectious cofactors (pneumocystis carinii, mycobacterium tuberculosis) to produce acquired immunodeficiency syndrome (AIDS).[20]
- Sufficient but not necessary: The factor has the potential of causing disease, but it is not necessary; for example, both asbestos and tobacco smoke are sufficient to cause lung cancer, but neither is necessary if the other is present.
- Neither sufficient nor necessary: Complex models of disease etiology; for example, high-fat diet and heart disease, hypertension, diabetes, breast cancer, etc.

Where a single exposure causes the disease, removal of the exposure should reduce or eliminate the disease risk, assuming irreversible damage has not occurred. Where multiple types of exposure contribute to a given disease, removal of one type of exposure may reduce disease risk, but it will not eliminate disease risk.

Web of Causation

Environmental epidemiology often aims to explain complex interactions of factors that explain injury or disease. Health-related states or events may involve a multifactorial etiology without continuous exposure to the contaminant. Further, causal associations between exposures and health outcomes are often influenced by specific economic, cultural, social, and political conditions. Identifying causal associations in the contexts of these other factors is not only useful for explaining causal associations but provides useful information for developing prevention and control programs. Because of the complexity of risk factors and variables contributing to environmental disease, a method of study is needed to effectively assess complex factors of causation. MacMahon and Pugh (1970) referred to the complex interaction of factors that explain disease as **webs of causation.**[10] Webs are graphic, pictorial, or paradigm representations of complex sets of events or conditions caused by an array of activities connected to a common core or common experience or event. In webs of causation the core or final outcome is the disease or injury. Webs have many arms, branches, sources, inputs, and causes that are somehow interconnected or interrelated to the core. Webs can also have a chain of events where some events must occur before others can take place.

Despite the complexity generally associated with webs of causation, two concepts universally apply. First, it is not necessary to have a complete understanding of the causal factors and mechanisms to develop effective prevention and control measures. Second, the production of a disease may be interrupted or stopped by cutting the chain of various factors and occurrences at strategic points. What often occurs in environmentally induced disease states is that individuals are subject to risk factors in small doses, sometimes in many doses and from many sources, all resulting in a chain of causation. The many risk factors and their various sources constitute a complex web of causation for a disease that may involve several sites in a single organ system and/or several organ systems. A single-line chain of events can be found within phases or parts of a web of causation. A single chain of events can be seen in some environmentally caused diseases or conditions. The complexity of environmentally caused diseases or conditions requires that all facets, risk factors, exposures, or contributing causes be understood and shown so that understanding is complete and the investigation is thorough.

Asthma Example

To illustrate a web of causation, consider the example of asthma (see Figure 6.1). Asthma is an environmentally induced disease that causes restricted breathing due to coughing, wheezing, and increased mucus production. In the United States, asthma affects approximately 29.8 million people, of which 9.1 million are children under the age of 18.[21] As identified by the Asthma and Allergy Foundation of America (AAFA) and the Centers for Disease Control and Prevention (CDC), the major triggers for asthma include exposure to allergens such as pet dandruffs, mold, dust mites, and pollen; air pollution, tobacco smoke, heredity, respiratory infections, and exercise.[22] Factors such as age, pregnancy, weather, and emotional states can also influence the occurrence of asthmatic attacks. However, asthma is not caused by any one source, but is rather the result of exposure to several risk factors. For example, many studies have shown that individuals with asthma often have family members who also suffer from asthma, indicating that asthma is hereditary. However, genetic disposition alone does not cause asthma. Instead, heredity increases an individual's risk for asthma, which is then triggered by allergens or other environmental irritants. Because asthma has a multifactorial etiology, it is important to consider all risk factors and exposures in asthma treatment.

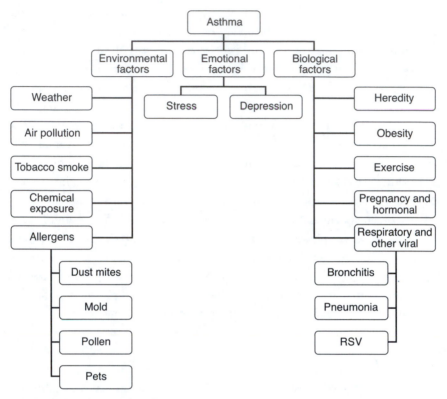

FIGURE 6.1   Example of a web of causation for asthma

Lead Poisoning Example

Another illustration of a web of causation involves the example of lead poisoning (see Figure 6.2). Lead poisoning is an environmentally induced disease caused by an elevated intake of lead by ingestion, inhalation, or absorption and results in damage to the body's vital organs and nervous system. However, as shown in Figure 6.1, there are several factors that influence or lead to the environment under which lead intake occurs. For example, individuals with low education levels and/or low income are often forced to live in older houses that may contain lead plumbing or lead-based paint. In turn, these poor housing conditions precipitate the ingestion of lead by individuals through drinking water or accidental eating of lead paint. Because lead poisoning is a preventable disease, the key to controlling lead poisoning is to understand its web of causation, especially underlying contributors.

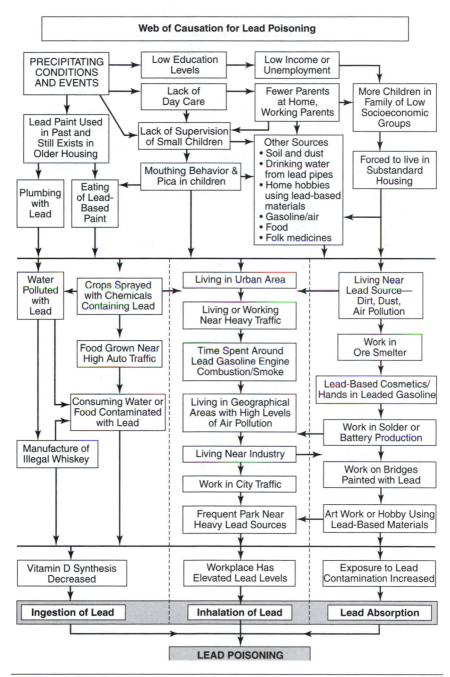

FIGURE 6.2   Example of a web of causation for lead poisoning

The End Goal

The primary purpose of an environmental epidemiologic investigation is to draw conclusions about the presence of a health problem and give reasons for its existence. In other words, with the use of study designs, statistical methods, and theory, causal inferences are made. Then, on the basis of causal inference, informed and effective individual and public health decisions can be made, with the intended results being to prevent and control the health problem.

Key Issues

1. The primary aim of environmental epidemiology is to identify environmentally caused public health problems and identify reasons for their existence. Identifying the existence of environmental health problems and their origins is at the heart of effective prevention and control efforts.
2. A causal inference is a conclusion about the presence of a disease and reasons for its existence.
3. A risk factor is a variable that is associated with the increased probability of a human health problem.
4. Causal criteria set forth in the 1964 Surgeon General's report are consistency, strength of association, temporality, biologic coherence, and specificity. Hill adds biologic plausibility and experimental evidence to these criteria.
5. A web of causation is useful in identifying the risk factors of the disease, and the chain of events and exposures necessary and/or sufficient to cause the disease.

Exercises

Key Terms

Define the following terms.

> Bias
> Biological coherence
> Causal criteria
> Causal inference
> Chance

Confounding

Consistency

Dose–response relationship

Enabling factors

Koch's postulates

Latency period

Precipitating factors

Predisposing factors

Reinforcing factors

Risk factor

Specificity

Statistical inference

Strength of association

Temporality

Webs of causation

Study Questions

1.1. What is causal inference?

1.2. Explain the weaknesses of Koch's postulates.

1.3. Describe five criteria for making causal inference.

1.4. Define "risk factor."

1.5. Discuss the four types of factors that have been proposed in order to better understand health problems. Give examples of each.

1.6. How are webs of causation used in environmental epidemiology?

1.7. Why is causal inference critical to preventing and controlling environmental health problems?

References

1. American Medical Association, Council on Scientific Affairs. *Stewardship of the Environment.* Chicago; 1989.

2. Weed DL. Causal and preventive inference (chapter 17). In: Greenwald P, Kramer BS, Weed DL, eds. *Cancer Prevention and Control.* New York: Marcel Dekker Inc; 1995.

3. Koch R. Über die Ätiologie der Tuberkulose. In: *Verhandlungen des Kongresses für Innere Medizin.* Erster Kongress, Wiesbaden; 1882.

4. Evans AS. Causation and disease: A chronological journey. *Am J Epidemiol.* 1978;108:249–258.
5. Lilienfeld AM. On the methodology of investigations of etiologic factors in chronic diseases—some comments. *J Chronic Dis.* 1959;10:41–46.
6. Sartwell PE. On the methodology of investigations of etiologic factors in chronic diseases—further comments. *J Chronic Dis.* 1960;11:61–63.
7. Surgeon General's Advisory Committee on Smoking and Health. Smoking and health: 1964. Rockville, MD: U.S. Public Health Service; 1964 (DHEW publication no. (PHS) 1103).
8. Susser M. *Causal Thinking in the Health Sciences.* New York, NY: Oxford University Press; 1973.
9. Hill AB. The environment and disease: association or causation? *Proc R Soc Med.* 1965;58:295–300.
10. MacMahon B, Pugh TF. *Epidemiology: Principles and Methods.* Boston, MA: Little, Brown and Company; 1970.
11. Choi BC, Noseworthy AL. Classification, direction, and prevention of bias in epidemiologic research. *J Occup Med.* 1992;34(3):265–271.
12. U.S. Department of Health and Human Services. A report of the surgeon general: the health benefits of smoking cessation. U.S. Department of Health and Human Services, Public Health Service, Centers for Disease Control, Center for Chronic Disease Prevention and Health Promotion, Office of Smoking and Health. DHHS Publ. No. (CDC) 90–8416; 1990.
13. Lee LAH, Merrill JM. Sunlight and the aetiology of malignant melanoma: a synthesis. *Med J Aust.* 1970;2:846–851.
14. Doll R. Mortality of lung cancer in asbestos workers. *Br J Ind Med.* 1955; 18:81–86.
15. International Agency for Research on Cancer. *IARC monographs programme on the evaluation of carcinogenic risks to humans.* Lyon, France: IARC; 2002.
16. Kannel WB, Dawber TR, Kagan A, Revotskie N, Stokes JI. Factors of risk in the development of coronary heart disease—six year follow-up experience; the Framingham Study. *Ann Intern Med.* 1961;55:33–50.
17. Evans AS. Causation and disease: The Henle-Koch postulates revisited. *Yale J Biol Med.* 1976;49:175–195.
18. Green L, Krueter M. *Health Promotion Planning.* 2nd ed. Mountain View, CA: Mayfield Publishing Company; 1991.
19. Moeller DW. *Environmental Health.* Cambridge, MA: Harvard University Press; 1992.
20. Haverkos HW. HIV necessary though not sufficient for AIDS. *J Biosci.* 2003; 28(4):365–366.
21. Asthma and Allergy Foundation of America. Available at: http://www.aafa.org/display.cfm?id=8&sub=17&cont=157. Accessed October 19, 2006.
22. Centers for Disease Control and Prevention. Available at: www.cdc.gov/asthma/faqs.htm. Accessed October 19, 2006.

Disease Clusters

LEARNING OBJECTIVES

After completing this chapter, you should be able to:

1. Define "cluster."
2. Define "cluster investigation" and discuss the process for investigating clusters.
3. Discuss the responsibility of public health officials in responding to a disease cluster.
4. Identify the primary challenges in detecting reported clusters.
5. Describe methods for assessing reported clusters.

Introduction

When environmental pollutants are geographically localized and there is a suspicion of higher than normal health problems, the tendency is to try to connect the pollutant with the problem. In the United States, every year there are over 1,000 calls placed to public health officials about suspected disease clusters.[1] The large number of reports from concerned citizens may be attributed, at least in part, to an increasingly high level of public awareness about environmental hazards. In a national survey, nearly 90% of Americans said they believed that health problems can be caused by environmental factors.[1]

In response to public concerns about disease clusters, **disease investigations** are performed to enable researchers to identify possible links between environmental exposures and injury or disease. These investigations may result in the discovery and cleanup of environmental hazards and help public health officials to more effectively utilize limited health resources for preventing and controlling health problems. However, cluster investigations often fail to find the putative disease cluster as real. Some states resolve as many as 99% of putative cluster reports during the initial phone conversation to the state health department.[1] In addition, suspected cluster investigations are often complicated by lack of access to high-quality health-tracking data, lack of exposure data, and lack of funding.

For some conditions, such as birth defects or cancer, monitoring and registry data are becoming more readily available for evaluating whether clusters exist. Currently, more than 70% of the 50 states, Puerto Rico, and the District of Columbia have some sort of birth defect monitoring or registry, which can provide case data and historical records for comparison.[2] To facilitate efforts of linking clusters of birth defects to environmental factors, approximately 33% of the 52 U.S. jurisdictions now have birth defect programs in collaboration with environmental exposure studies. Several notable studies exist of birth defect clusters that have been associated with environmental factors such as metam sodium, methyl bromide, and cyanazine.[3] Cancer data are routinely available among residents of 47 states (including 6 metropolitan areas) and the District of Columbia, with these areas reflecting about 96% of the U.S. population.[4] Hence, cancer clusters may be readily determined by a comparison of the rates with historical levels of the cancer. The study of several cancer clusters has identified carcinogenic agents such as polychlorinated biphenyls and pesticides.[5–8]

The purpose of this chapter is to define disease clusters, cluster investigations, and sentinel events; review the four-stage process for cluster investigation recommended by the Centers for Disease Control and Prevention (CDC); discuss the public health role of responding to cluster investigations; discuss statistical challenges associated with clusters in the search for a causal hypothesis; and present some alternative approaches for assessment when the cluster occurs before the causal hypothesis.

Disease Clusters, Cluster Investigations, and Sentinel Events

The term "epidemic" was defined in Chapter 1 as the increase of health-related states or events above what is normally expected in a specified population of interest. Epidemics are the result of change in the environment that results from exposure to a physical stress, contaminant, or social condition that is not typically encountered. A related term is **disease cluster**, which is defined by the CDC as "an unusual aggregation, real or perceived, of health events that are grouped together in time and space and that are reported to a health agency."[9] A disease cluster tends to occur when an agent is introduced into the human environment or when some event brings people into contact with an environmental contaminant or pathogen at levels not typically encountered. For example, the exposure of salmonella bacteria, characterized by symptoms of diarrhea, headaches, stomach cramps, nausea and vomiting, and fever, may affect a large number of people because of improperly prepared food. Natural disasters, occupational accidents, and social conflicts may also correspond with clusters of disease and injury.

A **cluster investigation** is "a review of an unusual number, real or perceived, of health events (for example, reports of cancer) grouped together in time and location."[10] Cluster investigations attempt to confirm reported disease cases; determine if there is a higher than expected level of the disease; and, if possible, identify causal relationships. Some well-known examples of disease cluster investigations are John Snow's study of the cholera outbreak in the Broad Street and Golden Square area of London in 1848,[11] the study of a pneumonia outbreak at the Bellevue-Stratford Hotel in Philadephia in 1976,[12] and the study of seven cases of *Pneumocystis carinii* pneumonia among young homosexual men in Los Angeles in 1981.[13] Many of the 50 cluster investigations of childhood leukemia and lymphoma in the United States during 1961 and 1977 implicated chemicals, but only eight showed evidence of an underlying infectious causal association.[14]

Investigations of noninfectious disease clusters have also been useful in identifying potential biological and environmental causes. For example, clusters of angiosarcoma have been found in vinyl chloride workers,[15] neurotoxicity and infertility have been found in kepone workers,[16] dermatitis and skin cancer have been found in individuals wearing contaminated gold rings,[17] and adenocarcinoma of the vagina has been found in women who consumed diethylstilbestrol during pregnancy.[18] These studies are characterized by clusters with definable health outcomes, either new or rare; a suspected environmental agent; a highly unusual situation confirmed by statistical testing; and a short-term public health impact that is immediate and self-evident.[9]

Selected organ or system events and their associated environmental risk factors are presented in Table 7.1. In the vast majority of cluster investigations, however, the putative cluster turns out to be not real, or if it is real, data limitations make it impossible to establish an association between the disease cluster and environmental contaminant.

It should be emphasized that disease clusters are different than sentinel events. A disease cluster involves the occurrences of seemingly unexpected events where no clearly recognized cause exists. On the other hand, **sentinel events** are occurrences of unexpected health-related states or events that occur from specific, recognized causes that are known to be associated with the health event.[20] For

TABLE 7.1   Selected Organ/System Events and Their Toxic Exposure Risks

Organ/system	Exposure risks
Respiratory	Asbestos, radon, cigarette smoke, glues
Dermatologic	Dioxin, nickel, arsenic, mercury, cement (chromium), polychlorinated biphenyls (PCBs), glues, rubber cement
Liver	Carbon tetrachloride, methylene chloride, vinyl chloride
Kidney	Cadmium, lead, mercury, chlorinated hydrocarbon solvents
Cardiovascular	Carbon monoxide, noise, tobacco smoke, physical stress, carbon disulfide, nitrates, methylene chloride
Reproductive	Methylmercury, carbon monoxide, lead, ethylene oxide
Hematologic	Arsenic, benzene, nitrates, radiation
Neuropsychologic	Tetrachloroethylene, mercury, arsenic, toluene, lead, methanol, noise, vinyl chloride

Source: From CDC, 2006.[19]

example, during March 5 through October 26, 1991, nine individuals were diagnosed with elevated blood lead levels at local hospitals in Alabama.[21] Although none of the patients had histories of occupational or other potential sources of lead exposure, an immediate investigation found that all had recently ingested illicit distilled alcohol (moonshine). The moonshine was made in two automobile radiators containing lead-soldered parts. Identification of the patients was made possible through review of notifiable disease surveillance data. These patients had blood lead levels much greater than the 15 ug/dL notifiable base level.

The framework for investigating sentinel events in occupational settings was established in the early 1980s by David Rutstein and colleagues at the National Institute for Occupational Safety and Health (NIOSH). The concept of a Sentinel Health Event (Occupational), SHE(O), was defined as "an unnecessary disease, disability, or untimely death that is occupationally related, with its occurrence yielding evidence of a failure in prevention."[22] For example, lead poisoning among persons working in occupations such as radiator repair, lead soldering, nonferrous smelting and casing, battery manufacturing, and so on, is a SHE(O) because it represents failure in prevention.

Case experiences can help us better understand failures and aid in the development of effective intervention strategies for preventing failures that may result elsewhere and in the future. An epidemiologist's role in the investigation of sentinel health events include assisting in recognition of the events; participating in their evaluation, often with the aid of an industrial hygienist; arranging for appropriate interventions; and summarizing and disseminating relevant information from the investigation to prevent similar cases elsewhere and in the future.[23] Sentinel health events are not restricted to occupational exposures but may apply in other settings where cases of known etiology are investigated.

Guidelines for Investigating Clusters

The CDC recommends a four-stage process to cluster investigation: (1) initial response, (2) assessment, (3) major feasibility study, and (4) etiologic investigation.[9] These stages are to be tailored according to the specific setting where the cluster is under investigation. The discretion and judgment of local health officials are critical in the investigation. Health agencies may also wish to select an advisory committee to provide consultation at critical decision points of the investigation.

Stage 1: Initial Contact and Response

The purpose of this stage is to collect information from those reporting the possible cluster. The recommended procedures follow:

1. Obtain identifying information on the caller.
2. Obtain initial data on the suspected cluster, including proposed health events, suspected exposure(s), number of cases, geographic area, and time period of concern.
3. Obtain identifying information on those affected.
4. Discuss initial impressions.
5. Obtain additional information on cases such as a follow-up time for contact, if necessary.
6. Ensure that a written response to their concern will be received.
7. Keep a log of initial and follow-up contacts.
8. Notify the public affairs office in the local health agency about the contact.

Some factors that may explain a reported disease cluster are presented in Table 7.2.

TABLE 7.2   Issues Frequently Associated with Reported Clusters

1. Assortment of unrelated diseases and disease processes means a common origin is unlikely.

2. If only women or only the elderly are affected, for example, this might indicate that an environmental pollutant is an unlikely cause.

3. For neoplasm, an implicated environmental carcinogen is only plausible if the affected residents have lived in the area for a sufficiently long period of time because of the long latency period that typically accompanies cancer.

4. Deceased cases may not provide useful information for linking exposure and disease because exposure may not be available and confounding factors may be present.

5. A rare disease cluster may be a result chance and not related to a given exposure.

6. New diagnostic procedures may explain a cluster.

7. Changes in reporting practices may explain a cluster.

8. Misdiagnoses by physicians may explain a suspected cluster.

9. Migration patterns (e.g., existence of a new military base, housing area, or retirement area) may explain a cluster.

10. Increased awareness in certain diseases may explain a cluster.

At the early stages of a cluster investigation, new environmental data may be required. However, existing data, if available, may also be useful in the investigation. Reasons for proceeding to Stage 2 include the presence of a single and rare disease, a plausible exposure, or a plausible clustering.

Stage 2: Assessment

There are three phases of the assessment stage: (1) preliminary evaluation to determine whether an excess of the health problem has occurred, (2) case evaluation to assure that a biological basis is present, and (3) a further evaluation of some or all of the suspected cases to describe the epidemiologic characteristics. These may be performed in order or concurrently.

Preliminary Evaluation

The purpose of a **preliminary evaluation** is to quickly estimate whether an excess of the health event has occurred and to provide a description of the characteristics of the cluster. The procedures involve (a) determining the geographic area and time period for study; (b) ascertaining those cases within the established time and space boundaries; (c) identifying an appropriate reference population; (d) determining if there is a sufficient number of cases for assessment and whether a denominator is available for calculating rates and other statistics; and (e) if small numbers prevent obtaining meaningful rates or if the denominator is not available, assess space, time, or space-time clustering. Computer software (e.g., SaTScan™) 2005) is now available for performing geographical surveillance of disease to detect spatial or space-time clustering, and to evaluate statistical significance.

Determining unusual aggregations of health events requires knowledge of what is usual based on the distribution of occurrences in the same location at an earlier time period or in other similar locations at the same time period.[24] What is considered usual may be determined from local health officials. These people often know if more disease is occurring than is expected based on ongoing disease surveillance data through local surveys or health data registries.

Although laboratory confirmations may not be initially available for some acute conditions, there may be sufficient evidence available to warrant an investigation. Examples of clusters can involve injury or death related to accidents (e.g., plane crashes, fires, worksite conditions); natural disasters (e.g., flooding, tropical cyclones, tornadoes, volcanic eruptions, earthquakes, drought); or political and social upheaval (e.g., unavailable health care, wars, racial discrimination); food poisoning due to improper food handling introducing bacterial contaminants; and birth defects or cancer associated with biological and chemical contaminants.

Cases that may not have been recognized or reported can sometimes be identified through physicians, clinics, health maintenance organizations, hospital emergency departments, public health clinics, migrant health clinics, and related facilities, which should be canvassed to ascertain if other people might have the disease or condition under investigation. Case identification should include specifications on the time period for incidence of cases or mortality, the geographic region, and the diagnostic group. A **case definition** involves a set of standard clinical criteria to establish if a person has a particular disease. Applying a standard case definition guarantees that every case is consistently diagnosed. In general, case definitions work best when information is available about a probable exposure (e.g., lead, radiation, cigarettes).

Following an acceptable case definition and confirmation of cases, the question is whether the putative cluster is actually unusual. This requires calculating rates. Rates are more meaningful than only counts because they take into account the population size and can be effectively compared with rates in other time periods or places. However, accurate population figures are required to avoid reporting misleading rates. **Person–time rates** are sometimes used because they allow each subject's contribution to the denominator of the rate calculation to be only as much time as observed in the at-risk population. However, cumulative incidence (also called the **incidence proportion** or the **attack rate**), where the denominator consists of only those people at the start of a given time interval, are more commonly used in cluster investigations.

When calculating rates, it is important to consider potential confounding effects. Adjusting the rates by potential confounders (e.g., age, sex, or race/ethnicity) allows for making more meaningful comparisons among groups. Stratifying the rates by age, sex, race/ethnicity, social class, and occupation, when the numbers are sufficiently large, will further allow us to identify high-risk groups. A potential problem arises when a disease cluster is confined to a small area with small numbers of people involved. In this situation disease rates tend to be unstable.

Statistical methods allow us to assess the probability that there is an excess of the health event being considered; this probability is the *P* value, as discussed in previous chapters. If the probability that the health event is due to chance is sufficiently low (generally less than 0.05), this causes us to doubt the null hypothesis of no association between the proposed cause and health outcome and we conclude otherwise. However, the interpretation of the conventional P value is dependent on whether the hypothesis is a priori or not. This will be discussed below in the section entitled "Statistical Challenges in Cluster Investigations." In addition, some standard statistical methods for assessment are presented. If an excess of the health problem is suggested from the preliminary evaluation, the next step is to do a case evaluation.

Case Evaluation

The purpose of a **case evaluation** is to verify the diagnosis because false positive results may cause considerable concern and present the impression that a suspected cluster is real. Because of the cost involved with verifying diagnoses, rates are typically calculated as a first step. Diagnosis verification then requires obtaining a referral to the responsible physician and permission to examine the patient's record, and access to pathology and medical examiner's reports, if possible; in addition, histological reevaluation may be warranted. However, obtaining confirmation and reevaluation may not be possible. Some conditions, injuries, or behaviorally caused occurrences have no laboratory tests that are applicable. Occupational or environmental disorders or conditions are often difficult to diagnose. If an excess of the health problem is supported by case confirmation, then proceed to the next step of occurrence evaluation. If some cases are not verified, the investigators may still proceed if biologic plausibility persists.

Occurrence Evaluation

In an **occurrence evaluation** the characteristics of the cluster are defined. This typically requires a field investigation. The procedures are to (a) identify the appropriate geographic and temporal boundaries, (b) ascertain all potential cases according to the specified time and space boundaries, (c) identify numerator and denominator data and their availability, (d) identify appropriate epidemiologic and statistical methods for describing and analyzing the data, (e) review the literature and consider biologic plausibility, (f) assess whether an exposure–event relationship can be established, (g) identify the public pulse (perceptions, reactions, needs), and (h) complete the descriptive investigation.

Particularly critical in this process is selecting appropriate geographic and temporal boundaries. The boundaries should correspond to the entire area that could have been exposed to the suspected environmental hazard. Improper selection of boundaries can greatly influence rate calculations used in the determination of whether a cluster exists.

To do this, epidemiologists should quickly become acquainted with the person-related issues and characteristics related to the health event under investigation. Line listings should include information that characterizes the population and that can be adjusted for in the analysis, including inherent characteristics of people (age, sex, race/ethnicity), acquired characteristics (immunity or marital status), activities (occupation, leisure, use of medications), and conditions (socioeconomic status, access to health care). The interactions of family, friends, fellow workers, and relatives also need to be considered. Certain person characteristics will have more relevance to some diseases or conditions than others. For example, if a cluster report involves brain cancer, the epidemiologist should include the characteristic occupation because occupational factors such as ionizing radiation, organic solvents, pesticides, and electromagnetic fields have been linked to brain cancer.[25–32]

Next, the epidemiologist should consider whether the disease cluster is associated with a common source or spread from person-to-person contact. A **common source outbreak** may be traced to an exposure at a point in time, an intermittent exposure, or a continuous exposure over days, weeks, or years. A **propagated outbreak** occurs as people transmit the disease from person to person. Classifying the disease cluster by type of outbreak can narrow the potential cause of disease. For example, diseases that are propagated from person to person are biologically based, while common source outbreaks that cannot be spread from person to person result from physical stressors or chemical contaminants.

The concentration of cases should be determined with regard to residence, birthplace, place of employment, school district, hospital unit, census tract, street address, map coordinates, and so on. This allows the epidemiologist to understand the geographic extent of disease and gain an understanding of where the environmental contaminant exists that causes a disease. A map is often an effective way to present these data pictorially. If possible, the epidemiologist might also plot on a map the locations of exposures, the locations of each case at the time of exposure, or when those exposed were identified as being a case.

Presenting each case by time of onset with an epidemic curve can provide important information about the disease outbreak. It is important to be familiar with the incubation or latency period and how time affects the disease. Chronologic events, step-by-step occurrences, chains of events tied to time, and time distribution of the onset of cases should be determined and plotted on charts and graphs. While doing this, epidemiologists should make sure to determine the nature of the course of the disease and ascertain if people were exposed and infected at about the same time or at different times, look for clustering of disease by both time and place, and use the information from incubation or latency periods to determine time factors in the course of the disease peaks and valleys in the epidemic curve.

If an excess of events is confirmed, along with compelling epidemiologic and biologic evidence, then investigators proceed to the next stage.

Stage 3: Major Feasibility Study

At this stage the potential for linking the putative exposure to the health event is assessed. The procedures follow:

1. Review the literature for putative exposures of the health event under consideration.
2. Select the appropriate study design and consider the attendant cost, sample size, use of previously identified cases, area and time dimensions, and selection of a control group.
3. Determine the required case and control data needed, which should include laboratory and physical measurements.
4. Consider the appropriate methods for assessment.
5. Outline the logistics for collecting and processing the data.
6. Determine the analysis plan (e.g., hypotheses to be tested, power to detect differences, etc.).
7. Consider the current social and political climate and the potential impact of decisions and outcomes.
8. Consider the resource requirements of the study.

After the number of observed cases is determined to be in excess of what is expected, a review of the literature is helpful to identify potential causes. Consideration is needed as to what environmental contaminants might have been present, the biological effects of these contaminants, and whether there are known or potential pathways by which the contaminants might affect the population at risk (e.g., air, water, soil, food). If the cluster is environmentally caused, the conditions of the environment in which the individuals spent time must be investigated (e.g., the air at a work site or skin exposure to chemicals). Once the exposure assessment is complete, the question is whether sufficient information is available to formulate a biologically plausible hypothesis. The research hypothesis is formulated by first identifying the most probable source for the cluster.

Accurate measurement of exposure, particularly at the appropriate time and place, is critical to evaluating dose–response relations within clusters. Quantified personal measurement of exposure on a continuous scale is best for assessing dose–response relationships, followed by data that reflect information obtained from quantifying concentration of toxic contaminants in a specific environment (air, water, soil, food), and then indirect proxy measures of exposure such as use of drinking water, distance from a site, duration of residence, and residence of employment (see Table 2.2). Confounding effects of age and other factors should also be considered when evaluating dose–response relationships. If exposure and disease data were available over a long period of time, stable estimates of association may be obtainable. Historical exposure is often difficult to measure or may not be available. Consequently, it may be impossible to define the exposed population, even ecologically, which is often true for populations located near potentially hazardous chemical sites.

Hypotheses should be developed for all aspects of the investigation. For example, in a foodborne outbreak, hypotheses should be developed for

- the source of infection;
- the vehicle of infection;
- the suspect foods;
- the mode of transmission;
- the type of pathogen (based on clinical symptoms, incubation periods);
- the time factors in the outbreak and course of the disease;
- the place factors in the outbreak;
- the person characteristics and factors in the outbreak;
- the outside sources of the infection;
- the transmission of the disease outside of the study population containing the exposed, unexposed, well, and ill cases/individuals; and
- whether the suspected sources are biologically plausible and should be considered when determining the time boundary of the investigation.

Although a foodborne outbreak constitutes a disease cluster, the focus of the investigation is on shared foods and personal contacts, not geography.

The study design, data, methods, logistics, and context are all factors that provide support in assessing the hypotheses. If resources are sufficient for investigation and an etiologic investigation is considered to be justified, proceed to Stage 4.

Stage 4: Etiologic Investigation

At this stage an etiologic investigation is performed for the hypothesized relationship between the exposure and the health event. This involves a standard epidemiologic study approach, with specific criteria for establishing a cause and effect relationship. A study of feasibility serves as a guide to developing a protocol and implementing the study. The results of the investigation should contribute to our knowledge of whether an association exists between the exposure and health event.

A report should follow the analysis, presenting a narrative of the investigation. Tables, graphs, charts, or any useful and helpful illustrations are presented as well as any pertinent epidemiologic data, tests, lab reports, information, and characteristics. A good epidemiologic report compares the hypotheses with the established facts.

Public Health Response

Public health officials have a responsibility to carefully consider the legitimacy of each reported disease cluster. Careful consideration of each of the stages of a cluster investigation is necessary to allay public concerns and to potentially link the putative exposure to the health event. The main purpose of etiologic investigations is to understand causes of health-related states or events so that public health prevention and control measures can be taken. Ideally, a cluster investigation not only identifies the source and mode of transmission, but it also identifies ways to remedy the health problem. Once the links to the continuance of the health problem are understood, then intervention can occur, the links can be broken, the course of the health problem can be stopped, and environmental cleanup can begin. Risk-factor prevention and health protection programs are the first line of defense in environmentally founded diseases. It is often where prevention and control measures have failed or were never adequately implemented that disease clusters arise.

When an event poses a risk or danger to the public, then those who are in a position to intervene and control the health problem should be informed. Communication with key individuals is critical to effective control efforts. Public health officials, related government agencies, physicians, hospitals, health maintenance organizations, medical clinics, schools, universities, and any group of people at risk should be informed. Unfortunately, many times public health officials know of a health concern but fail to inform those who need to know most. Public health officials have a responsibility to warn the public and the population at risk. Sometimes officials are fearful that such information will create a panic, but this is not a reason to withhold information from the public or at least from those who are at risk.

Covello and Allen proposed seven cardinal rules of risk communication, which are directly applicable in managing a cluster investigation: (1) accept and involve the public as a partner; (2) plan carefully and evaluate your findings; (3) listen to the public's specific concerns; (4) be honest, frank, and open; (5) work with other credible sources; (6) meet the needs of the media; and (7) speak clearly and with compassion.[33] In other words, the public should be informed of the potential health problem, possible risks, and progress made along the course of the investigation.[33] Actions taken by the investigative team should be tailored to the audiences and media involved. This requires knowing your public, including their concerns, attitudes, levels of interest, levels of involvement, levels of knowledge, opinions, reasons for interest, and types of involvement. Successful communication increases when you know those with whom you are communicating. Early in the investigation learn about the people involved, their concerns (health, safety, environment, fairness, process, legalities, etc.), their perceived risks (whether voluntary or imposed, under the individual's control or not, natural or humanmade, etc.), and whom they trust. Trust and credibility need to be established; once lost, it may be impossible to regain. Working with relevant groups and organizations and facilitating effective interaction among these bodies are critical. When interacting with the media, information should be communicated in a timely, accurate, simple, and understandable manner. Finally, in an effort to identify the scientific explanation for a cluster, maintain perspective of the human element of the public health problem.

Chess and colleagues point out the importance of involving the community, listening and responding to their needs, and learning from the information they can provide:[34]

1. To the extent possible, involve the community in the decision-making process.
   - Involve the community early in the investigation.
   - Clarify the community's role from the outset.
   - Acknowledge that there may be situations where the agency can only provide the community with limited decision-making power.
   - Identify the type of involvement the community prefers.

2. Identify and respond to the needs of different audiences.
   - Try to identify the various interests and key representatives.
   - Recognize the strengths and weaknesses of any citizen-represented groups.
   - Be fair and equitable.

3. When appropriate, develop alternatives to public hearings. In particular, hold smaller, more informal meetings.
   - If possible, break large groups into smaller ones.
   - Clarify the goals for the meeting.
   - In some situations, one-on-one communication may be more informative.

4. Recognize that people's values and feelings are a legitimate aspect of environmental health issues and that such concern may convey valuable information.
   - Provide a forum that allows people to express their feelings.
   - Listen.
   - Acknowledge people's concerns and feelings.
   - Respond with empathy and compassion, not necessarily with data and facts.
   - Show respect by responding to community questions and concerns promptly.
   - Recognize and be honest about values that may be incorporated into agency decisions.
   - Be sensitive to your own values and feelings and how they affect you.

Data Challenges in Cluster Investigations

Several types of data are useful in cluster investigations: accurate diagnostic information; case information according to person, place, and time; length of time cases lived in the area in question; potential changes in diagnostic or reporting procedures; migration patterns; and increased public awareness of the disease in question. In addition, a sufficient number of cases are needed in order to rule out chance as an explanation for the cluster finding. Not only are these data useful for ruling out a putative cluster as real (see Table 7.2), but they are also needed to support a disease cluster.

An example of an exposure history questionnaire developed in 1992 by the Agency for Toxic Substances and Disease Registry in cooperation with NIOSH is provided in Appendix IV. Such questionnaires often play a fundamental role in cluster investigation. However, the investigator should be sensitive to limitations of cross-sectional surveys (e.g., response bias and difficulty in establishing temporality of events).

Unavailable data limit all levels of a cluster investigation. Based on a review of several completed cluster investigations, a review of the literature, and interviews with state public health officials, Dutzik and Baumann concluded that lack of access to quality health-tracking data is a primary hindrance to cluster investigation and may (1) cause long delays in cluster investigations; (2) prevent public health officials from identifying disease trends; (3) inhibit the identification of true disease clusters; (4) reduce the number of cluster investigations carried out by states, meaning that some clusters go uninvestigated; and (5) deter communities from getting the information and help they need when a suspected cluster arises.[1]

Statistical Challenges in Cluster Investigations

Although cluster investigations appear straightforward, some basic epidemiologic and statistical challenges can further hinder cluster studies. The primary challenge to cluster investigation involves the fact that most cluster analyses involve post hoc (also called posteriori) rather than a priori hypotheses. **Post-hoc hypotheses** refer to formulation of the hypotheses after observation of an event such as an excess of cancer. Hypotheses of this type are problematic because the conventional P value is only interpretable with **a priori hypotheses**, that is, those hypotheses established without prior knowledge of the level of the health events in a specified population. Selectively choosing a suspected cluster for statistical testing is equivalent to multiple testing because the probability of finding a significant result increases as we become highly selective in testing only a given area out of many. For example, suppose there is a cluster reported in a region that has 20 subareas. We may conclude that the disease rate in the one area is statistically significant at the 5% level. However, because we selectively chose this area out of 20, we have in essence simultaneously conducted 20 tests. If the null hypothesis is true, we would expect 1 in 20 independent tests to be significant by chance alone at the 5% level of significance; in other words, the chance occurrence in the random variation of disease may be the sole explanation for the unusual events.

Another challenge with cluster investigations is that disease rates have the danger of being overestimated due to **boundary shrinkage** of the population where the cluster is assumed to exist. For example, a suspected cluster of childhood leukemia in the United Kingdom around a nuclear processing site at Windscale (later called Sellafield) was reported in 1983.[35] The report came from a journalist who suggested that the excess of leukemia could be associated with radiation discharged from the nuclear processing site. Initially, the journalist intended to make a documentary of health among employees at the plant. However, during his investigation he was informed by people in the area about a number of childhood leukemia cases in Seascale, a village close to the plant. Further study showed that the rate of childhood leukemia in the area containing the village was significantly higher than the national rate. Olsen and colleagues, however, interpreted the finding as statistically problematic because of multiple comparisons and boundary tightening.[36] These problems were related to post hoc testing of hypotheses. First, the journalist may have followed several leads before choosing to focus on the leukemia cases. In this situation multiple comparisons have been made (regardless of whether significance tests were made), thereby making the interpretation of the P value invalid. Second, boundary tightening is a potential problem because after the identification of a group of cases occurs, we subsequently define the underlying population corresponding to the suspected cluster. The narrower this underlying population is defined, the greater the estimated rate of the health event and the more pronounced the statistical significance. Rothman illustrates this situation by comparing it with the Texas sharpshooter who first fires his gun and then draws a target around the bullet hole.[37]

In those cases where a causal hypothesis is formulated prior to searching for a disease cluster, there is no longer the interpretive problem with the P value that exists with post hoc hypotheses. An example would be a study of coronary heart disease and acute myocardial infarction in relation to proximity to an organic pollution site, instigated because of previous epidemiologic research.[38] Another example would be that researchers hypothesize that increased elderly hospital admissions due to cardiovascular disease (cardiac disease, cardiac failure, ischemic heart disease, and myocardial infarction) are associated with comparatively high levels of carbon monoxide, based on previous such findings.[39]

Assessing Clusters

Although much of the material that follows is relevant to any possible disease outbreak, not simply clusters, the following approaches are presented here because of their useful application in cluster investigations.

Standardized Mortality (or Registration) Ratio

Observed and expected estimates of cases of mortality can be evaluated using the **standardized mortality ratio** (SMR). If incident events are being evaluated, the **standardized registration ratio** (SRR) should be used. The formula for calculating these statistics is the same—the only difference is whether mortality or incidence data are being considered:

$$\text{SMR, SRR} = \theta = \frac{\text{Observed}}{\text{Expected}}$$

To test whether the observed count is significantly different than the expected count for a selected area and time period, the z statistic is calculated based on the following formula:

$$z = 2(\sqrt{Observed} - \sqrt{Expected})$$

The observed number of cases is assumed to be Poisson distributed with mean (μ) $= \theta \times Expected$. The symbol θ (= SMR or SRR) represents the amount of excess risk (e.g., $\theta = 1$ means there is no excess risk). A one-sided P value for $\theta = 1$ is obtained from the probability of observing in a Poisson distribution, with $\mu = Expected$, at least the number of cases observed in the suspected cluster area. This is approximated by z, where z is the standard normal distribution.[40]

To obtain a 95% confidence interval of $\theta =$, calculate:

$$\left(\sqrt{Observed} \pm 1.96/2\right)^2 / Expected$$

For example, two pooled analyses of workers from 56 plants in North America and Europe provided cohort data for assessing the association between occupational exposure to vinyl chloride and selected cancers.[41] The results found that after excluding confirmed angiosarcomas, 60 deaths occurred from liver cancer compared with 44.35 expected. The SMR = 1.35 and, applying the above formula, a 95% confidence interval is obtained of 1.03–1.72. Hence, there appears to be an excess risk of liver cancer death associated with vinyl chloride. The SMRs for soft-tissue sarcoma, brain, lymphoid, and haematopoietic system cancers were also significantly different from unity. Note that the link between vinyl chloride and liver angiosarcoma was already well established.[42]

To illustrate how to calculate an SRR with an associated z score and 95% CI, consider the following hypothetical incidence data for disease X. Information is presented on age-specific rates for the putative cluster of disease. Reference rates are also available, representing what is typical or expected.

| | Disease Cluster | | | Regional Reference Rates | | |
Age	Counts	Population	Rate per 100,000	Counts	Population	Rate per 100,000
< 40	11	30,000	37	6,000	20,000,000	30
40–49	20	9,000	222	4,000	2,100,000	190
50–59	36	8,000	450	9,800	2,200,000	445
60–69	49	5,000	980	35,000	4,000,000	875
70–79	59	2,000	2,950	90,000	5,000,000	1,800
80+	53	1,000	5,300	150,000	6,000,000	2,500
Total	228	55,000	415	294,800	39,300,000	750

Expected age-specific counts in the suspected cluster area are obtained by taking the age-specific rates from the reference population and multiplying them by the age-specific population values in the cluster area.

Age	Population in Cluster Area	Expected Rate per 100,000	Expected Counts
< 40	30,000	30	9
40–49	9,000	190	17
50–59	8,000	445	36
60–69	5,000	875	44
70–79	2,000	1800	36
80+	1,000	2500	25
Total			167

The sum over the age groups of these expected counts represents the expected number of counts in the putative cluster area, assuming they had the same rate structure as found in the reference population. To calculate the SRR we divide the observed by the expected counts, as follows:

$$SRR = \frac{Observed}{Expected} = \frac{228}{167} = 1.40$$

This means the observed number of cases of disease X is 1.40 times (or 40%) higher than in the reference population. The elevated number of cases in the cluster area is statistically significant, based on the following:

$$z = 2(\sqrt{228} - \sqrt{167}) = 4.39$$

The P value corresponding to this z score is p < 0.0001, indicating that the observed number of cases is significantly higher than the expected, with almost zero probability that the result is due to chance. The 95% confidence interval for the SRR is

$$\left(\sqrt{Observed} \pm 1.96/2\right)^2 / Expected = \left(\sqrt{228} \pm 1.96/2\right)^2 / 167 = \left(1.2, 1.6\right)$$

Because this 95% confidence interval does not overlap 1, it also indicates a significantly greater number of cases than expected in the putative cluster area.

It is important to note that because the age distribution between the two populations is considerably different, it would have been inappropriate to base the analysis on the crude numbers. That is, suppose the age-specific information had been ignored and the overall rate in the reference population was multiplied by the overall population in the suspected cluster area. This would have yielded an estimate of 413 (= 0.00750 × 55,000) cases in the suspected cluster area. The SRR would then be 0.55 (or 45% lower) instead of 1.40 (or 40% higher) in the cluster area. This unusual result occurs because of differences in the age structure between the two groups.

When a Cluster Is in Search of a Cause

A way of dealing with cluster data, other than focusing on an isolated phenomenon, has been suggested by Olsen and colleagues.[36] They recommend testing for clustering as a feature of the disease pattern over an entire region. Consider the situation where data are categorized into subareas. The null hypothesis is that the disease or injury rate is the same in each of the subareas, the cases occur at random across the regions, the frequencies are proportional to the numbers at risk in each subarea, and variability is characterized by the Poisson distribution. In this context a summary measure for total variability of the rate can be derived across all subareas. The chi-square can be calculated for the i subareas as:

$$\chi^2 = \sum_{i=1}^{n} \frac{\left(O_i - E_i\right)^2}{O_i}$$

where O_i is the observed number of cases and E_i is the expected number of cases in each subarea. The chi-square value is related to how much the observed cases differ from the expected in the subareas. It is possible to assess the P value using this approach. A P value less than 5% indicates that variability in the disease rates across the subareas is higher than the Poisson model allows. In other words, there appears to be a clustering within one or more of the subareas. This test does not indicate, however, whether an underlying spatial distribution exists in the data, but only that the rates vary across subareas.

Although significant test results in a cluster investigation involving a post hoc hypothesis are not effective at proving that the cluster is real, statistical tests are useful for screening out potential clusters, which would not have been statistically significant even if the area had been selected a priori.[40]

Alternative Measures

With post hoc hypotheses where significance tests are inappropriate, alternative methods of assessment include:

1. Performing the study in a different location but with a similar exposure.
2. Excluding the cases in the original cluster and using new cases in the test of significance, assuming further case ascertainment occurred.
3. Looking for factors that distinguish the cases from others in the cluster, other than their residence.
4. Evaluating a dose–response relationship between the exposure and health event.[40]

In the final stage of a cluster investigation, the relation between the exposure and health event is assessed. This assumes that exposure information is measurable. Exploring whether there is a dose–response relationship with a putative cluster is independent of whether the study is based on a post hoc or a priori hypothesis. Common statistical techniques for assessing dose–response relationship were presented in Chapter 4. For example, using logistic regression, an Australian case-control study conducted in 2000–2001 identified a significant positive association between non-Hodgkin's lymphoma and the level of exposure to pesticides (OR =

3.09; 95% CI: 1.42, 6.70).[43] As discussed in Chapter 5, the stronger the statistical association between exposure and disease variables, the greater support there is for a causal association.

Key Issues

1. Disease cluster is an unusual aggregation, real or perceived, of health events that are grouped together in time and space and that are reported to a health agency.
2. Cluster investigations attempt to confirm reported disease cases, determine if there is a higher than expected level of the disease, and, if possible, identify causal relationships.
3. Sentinel events are occurrences of unexpected health-related states or events that occur from specific, recognized causes that are known to be associated with the health event.
4. CDC stages of cluster investigations are (1) initial contact and response, (2) assessment, (3) major feasibility study, and (4) etiologic investigation.
5. Unavailable data, poor quality data, and post hoc hypotheses (resulting in multiple comparisons and boundary shrinkage) limit cluster investigations.
6. For clusters reported prior to a causal hypothesis, the chi-square test considering the subareas of the region where the putative cluster exists may be used. Alternative approaches to studying clusters in search of a causal hypothesis include (1) performing the study in a different location but with a similar exposure; (2) excluding the cases in the original cluster and using new cases in the test of significance, assuming further case ascertainment occurred; (3) looking for factors that distinguish the cases from others in the cluster, other than their residence; and (4) evaluating a dose–response relationship between the exposure and health event.

Exercises

Key Terms

Define the following terms.

    A priori hypothesis
    Attack rate
    Boundary shrinkage

Case definition
Case evaluation
Cluster investigation
Common source outbreak
Disease Cluster
Disease investigation
Incidence proportion
Occurrence evaluation
Person–time rate
Post-hoc hypothesis
Preliminary evaluation
Propagated outbreak
Sentinel event
Standardized mortality ratio
Standardized registration ratio

Study Questions

7.1. Define each of the following as cluster, sentinel event, or neither.
  a. In Chicago during June, temperatures are higher than normal, and several dozen cases of heat stroke are reported.
  b. Following a severe tropical storm, there is a sharp rise in stomach cramps and dehydration.
  c. An industrial town with many factories experiences a rise in upper respiratory infection over a 10-year period.
  d. A researcher suspicious of a health risk caused by a chemical leak in the area searches out newly diagnosed pancreatic cancer cases and finds a fairly strong correlation with exposure to the leak.
  e. Flowers in bloom bring a rise in upper respiratory congestion during spring.
7.2. List and describe the four-stage process of cluster investigation as described by the CDC.
7.3. In which of the four-stage process are attack rates calculated?
7.4. What should a good epidemiologic report include?
7.5. What are two statistical challenges in cluster investigation?

Information is presented on age-specific rates for a putative cluster of leukemia. Reference rates are also available, representing what is typical or expected. Use the information to answer questions 7.6–7.10.

| Age | Leukemia Cluster 2004 | | | Leukemia Reference Rates 2003 | | |
	Counts	Population	Rate per 100,000	Counts	Population	Rate per 100,000
< 40	65	1,612,003		63	1,592,023	
40–49	26	299,056		11	296,284	
50–59	28	224,625		22	214,530	
60–69	56	135,299		44	129,739	
70–79	81	93,967		38	91,951	
80+	48	55,758		42	54,169	
Total	304	2,420,708		220	2,378,696	

Data source: Utah Cancer Registry. Hypothetical counts for 2004 are used to illustrate a possible cluster.

7.6. Calculate the age-specific rates.

7.7. Calculate the expected age-specific counts in the suspected cluster.

7.8. Calculate the SRR. Interpret.

7.9. Is the elevated number of leukemia cases statistically significant based on the z statistic?

7.10. Calculate the 95% confidence interval for the SRR and indicate whether the confidence interval shows statistical significance.

7.11. If a report were to come in to your office about a suspected disease cluster, what might be some good questions to ask before sending an epidemiologist out to investigate?

7.12. What are some approaches that may be taken for investigating post hoc hypotheses?

References

1. Dutzik T, Baumann J. *Health Tracking and Disease Clusters: The Lack of Data on Chronic Disease Incidence and Its Impact on Cluster Investigations.* Washington, DC: U.S. PIRG Education Fund; 2002.

2. Trust for America's Health. Available at: http://healthyamericans.org/state/birthdefects/. Accessed May 16, 2007.

3. Pew Environmental Health Commission, Healthy from the Start: Why America Needs a Better System to Track and Understand Birth Defects and the Environment, based on A. Aspelin, Pesticide Industry Sales and Usage, 1994 and 1995 Market Estimates, 1997.

4. U.S. Cancer Statistics Working Group. United States Cancer Statistics: 2003 Incidence and Mortality. Atlanta: U.S. Department of Health and Human

Services, Centers for Disease Control and Prevention and National Cancer Institute; 2006.

5. Unger M, Olsen J. Organochlorine compounds in the adipose tissue of deceased people with and without cancer. *Environment Res.* 1980;23:257–263.

6. Figa-Talamanca I, Mearelli I, Valente P, Bascherini S. Cancer mortality in a cohort of rural licensed pesticide users in the province of Rome. *Int J Epidemiol.* 1993;22(4):579–583.

7. Sinks T, Steele, G, Smith AB, Watkins K, Shults RA. Mortality among workers exposed to polychlorinated biphenyls. *Am J Epidemiol.* 1992;136:389–398.

8. Bertazzi PA, Riboldi L, Pesatori A, Radice L, Zocchetti C. Cancer mortality of capacitor manufacturing workers. *Am J Indust Med.* 1987;11:165–176.

9. Centers for Disease Control and Prevention. Guidelines for investigating clusters of health events. *MMWR.* 1990;39(RR-11):1–23.

10. Centers for Disease Control and Prevention. Glossary of Terms. Available at: http://www.atsdr.cdc.gov/glossary.html#G-A-. Accessed August 12, 2006.

11. Snow J. *On the Mode of Communication of Cholera.* New York, NY: Commonwealth Fund. (2nd edition, 1855); 1936.

12. Fraser DW, Tsai TR, Orenstein W, et al. Legionnaires' disease: description of an epidemic of pneumonia. *N Engl J Med.* 1977;297:1189–1197.

13. Centers for Disease Control. Pneumocystic pneumonia—Los Angeles. *MMWR.* 1981;30:250–252.

14. Heath CW Jr. Community clusters of childhood leukemia and lymphoma: evidence of infection? *Am J Epidemiol.* 2005;162(9):817–822.

15. Waxweiler RJ, Stringer W, Wagoner, JK, et al. Neoplastic risk among workers exposed to vinyl chloride. *Ann N Y Acad Sci.* 1976;271:40–48.

16. Cannon SB, Veazey JM Jr, Jackson RS, et al. Epidemic kepone poisoning in chemical workers. *Am J Epidemiol.* 1978;107:529–537.

17. Baptiste MS, Rothenberg R, Nasca PC, et al. Health effects associated with exposure to radioactively contaminated gold rings. *J Am Acad Dermatol.* 1984; 10:1019–1023.

18. Herbst AL, Ulfelder H, Poskanzer DC. Adenocarcinoma of the vagina: association of maternal stilbesterol therapy with tumor appearance in young females. *N Engl J Med.* 1971;284:878–881.

19. Centers for Disease Control and Prevention. Disease Clusters: An Overview Evaluating a Disease Cluster. Available at: http://www.atsdr.cdc.gov/HEC/ CSEM/cluster/evaluating.html. Accessed August 18, 2006.

20. Joint Commission on Accreditation of Healthcare Organizations. Setting the standards for quality in health care. *Sentinel event.* Available at: http://www. jointcommission.org/SentinelEvents/. Accessed November 22, 2006.

21. Centers for Disease Control and Prevention. Elevated blood lead levels associated with illicitly distilled alcohol—Alabama, 1990–1991. *MMWR.* 1992; 41(17):294–295.

22. Rutstein D, Mullan R, Frazier T, et al. The sentinel health event (occupational): a framework for occupational health surveillance and education. *J Am Public Health Assoc.* 1983;73:1054–1062.

23. Halperin WE. Field investigations of occupational disease and injury. In: Gregg MB, ed. *Field Epidemiology.* 2nd ed. New York, NY: Oxford University Press; 2002.

24. Hertz-Picciotto I. Environmental epidemiology. In: Rothman KJ, Greenland S, eds. *Modern Epidemiology.* Philadelphia, PA: Lippincott-Raven Publishers; 1998.

25. Blair A, Grauman DJ, Lubin JH, Fraumeni JF Jr. Lung cancer and other causes of death among licensed pesticide applicators. *J Natl Cancer Inst.* 1983; 71:31–37.

26. Lin RS, Dischinger PC, Conde J, Farrel KP. Occupational exposure to electromagnetic fields and the occurrence of brain tumors. *J Occup Med.* 1985; 27:413–419.

27. Thomas TL, Waxweiler RJ. Brain tumors and occupational risk factors: a review. *Scand J Work Environ Health.* 1986;12:1–15.

28. Cordier S, Poisson M, Gerin M, Varin J, Conso F, Hemon D. Gliomas and exposure to wood preservatives. *Br J Ind Med.* 1988;45:705–709.

29. Musicco M, Sant M, Molinari S, Fillippini G, Gatta G, Berrino F. A case-control study of brain gliomas and occupational exposure to chemical carcinogens: the risk to farmers. *Am J Epidemiol.* 1988;128:778–785.

30. Schlehofer B, Kunze S, Sachsenheimer W, Blettner M, Niehoff D, Wahrendorf J. Occupational risk factors for brain tumors: results from a population-based case-control study in Germany. *Cancer Causes Control.* 1990;1(3): 209–215.

31. Mack W, Preston-Martin S, Peters JM. Astrocytoma risk related to job exposure to electric and magnetic fields. *Bioelectromagnetics.* 1991;12:57–66.

32. National Radiologic Protection Board. *Electromagnetic Fields and the Risk of Cancer.* Chilton: Her Majesty's Stationery Office; 1992.

33. Covello V, Allen F. *Seven Cardinal Rules of Risk Communication.* Washington, DC: Environmental Protection Agency, Office of Policy Analysis; 1988.

34. Chess C, Hance BJ, Sandman PM. *Improving Dialogue with Communities: A Short Guide to Government Risk Communication.* New Jersey Department of Environmental Protection; 1988.

35. Gardner JM. Review of reported increases of childhood cancer rates in the vicinity of nuclear installations in the UK. *J Royal Stat Soc, Ser A.* 1989;152: 307–325.

36. Olsen SF, Martuzzi M, Elliott P. Cluster analysis and disease mapping—why, when, and how? a step by step guide. *Br Med J.* 1996;313:863–866.

37. Rothman KJ. A sobering start for the cluster busters' conference. *Am J Epidemiol.* 1990;132(suppl):S6–S13.

38. Sergeev AV, Carpenter DO. Hospitalization rates for coronary heart disease in relation to residence near areas contaminated with persistent organic pollutants and other pollutants. *Environ Health Perspect.* 2005;113:6.

39. Barnett AG, Williams GM, Schwartz J, Best TL, Neller AH, Petroeschevsky AL, et al. The effects of air pollution on hospitalizations for cardiovascular disease in elderly people in Australian and New Zealand cities. *Environ Health*

Perspect. 2006;144:1018–1023. Available at: http://www.ehponline.org/docs/2006/8674/abstract.html. Accessed September 18, 2006.

40. Wilkinson, P, ed. *Environmental Epidemiology.* New York, NY: Open University Press; 2006.
41. Bosetti C, La Vecchia C, Lipworth L, McLaughlin JK. Occupational exposure to vinyl chloride and cancer risk: a review of the epidemiologic literature. *Eur J Cancer Prev.* 2003;12(5):427–430.
42. Creech JL, Johnson MN. Angiosarcoma of liver in the manufacture of polyvinyl chloride. *J Occup Med.* 1974;16(3):150–151.
43. Fritschi L, Benke G, Hughes AM, et al. Occupational exposure to pesticides and risk of non-Hodgkin's lymphoma. *Am J Epidemiol.* 2005;162(9):849–857.

Mapping and Geographic Information Systems

LEARNING OBJECTIVES

After completing this chapter, you should be able to:

1. Describe disease mapping.
2. Describe the components of geographic information systems (GIS).
3. Describe implicit and explicit geographic reference.
4. Describe and distinguish between vector and raster format data in GIS.
5. Discuss why rates may be preferred to counts in mapping and GIS.
6. Describe the use of global positioning system (GPS) in environmental epidemiology.

Introduction

In order to identify and depict relevant patterns of health-related states or events in the population, counts or rates of the health event should be organized according to person, place, and time. Mapping and geographic information systems (GIS) are descriptive methods that are useful for describing disease patterns by person and place. Specifically, GIS is a technique that combines spatial information with layers of attribute information. **Attributes** may refer to demographic characteristics of those affected, socioeconomic status, education, and other personal variables, or features of a suspected source of disease (e.g., types and amounts of chemicals produced by a plant). Mapping and GIS methods can assist us in identifying and verifying disease clusters, and in identifying potential causes of disease clusters and modes of transmission. This chapter will present mapping and GIS for assessing the relationship between disease clusters and environmental contaminants. In the next chapter we will discuss time–trend analysis.

Disease Mapping

Mapping of disease counts or rates is a useful approach for identifying patterns of disease according to geographic location. Disease patterns can also be shown in relation to the potential source of the disease. An example of this is the investigation conducted by John Snow of the 1848 cholera epidemic in London.[1] Snow investigated the epidemic by determining where persons with cholera lived and worked. This information was used to create a spot map (also called a dot map) of the distribution of cases (see Figure 8.1). Snow believed that contaminated water was the source of cholera, so he marked the location of water pumps on his spot map. He was then able to assess the relationship between the distribution of cholera cases and the location of the water pumps. A clustering of cases was observed around the Broad Street pump, thus implicating it as the primary source of the cholera epidemic.

Maps may involve discrete or continuous data. Snow applied discrete events to a geographical map of the Golden Square area of London. Continuous data may involve disease rates, life expectancy, temperature, and so on. When disease rates or arithmetic means are mapped, geographic areas are first selected (e.g., census tracks, zip code areas, states). Rates or means are grouped into typically 5 to 10 categories that reflect the range of data, with colors or shading schemes increasing or decreasing in intensity (brightness or color) to represent the ordered categories. Maps can

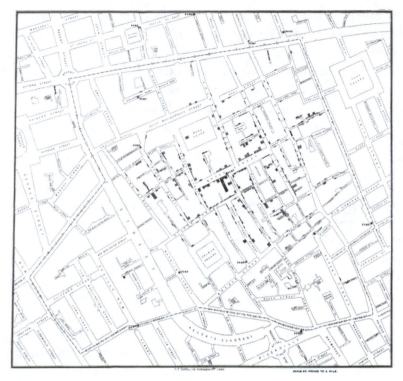

FIGURE 8.1 Distribution of cholera cases in the Golden Square area of London. (*Source:* Courtesy of Frerichs, R. R. John Snow website: http://www.ph.ucla.edu/episnow.html, 2006.)

produce misleading information if the size of the underlying population within selected geographic areas is small such that the rates are unstable or even zero. Some methods for addressing small and unequal population densities across geographic areas are presented elsewhere.[2–5] For a presentation of the historical evolution of disease mapping techniques applied to geographical and demographic base maps, the reader can refer to Howe.[6]

Spatial comparisons using maps typically require information on events as well as data on the underlying population (e.g., age, sex, race/ethnicity, and size distributions). Maps can be influenced by confounding factors that cluster spatially; that is, a correlation of disease rates between adjacent areas may be the result of factors other than those we are interested in studying. For example, the age distribution, smoking patterns, diagnostic coding, and reporting practices may all be related to location, as well as to customs and socioeconomic status, which can influence seeking medical care. Stratification of analyses by potential confounders or multiple regression techniques for spatial data may be effective approaches for spatially controlling for confounders.

Maps of disease counts or rates can then be used to construct ecologic epidemiologic studies where maps of disease patterns are linked with spatial information on geographic and demographic type maps. GIS are commonly used to assess disease data in relation to environmental contaminants. This is a rapidly growing technology.

Geographic Information System

A **geographic information system (GIS)** is a computer system used to store, view, edit, and analyze geographical information. Its intent is to assess real-world problems by incorporating graphical features with tabular data. GIS is a useful screening tool for evaluating whether cluster alarms warrant further investigation or appear to be chance occurrences.[7] When a cluster investigation is warranted, GIS allows health researchers to explore the complex interplay between human health data and potential environmental contaminants. Hidden patterns and relationships are often more apparent using spatial analysis than with other methods.

Geographic information systems originated around 1960, when maps began to be programmed and stored in computers, creating the potential to more easily make modifications. This was an important and welcomed advancement over the era when maps were created by hand. Initially, GIS was called **computer cartography**, with simple lines used to represent geographic features; it was thought of as a high-tech equivalent of a map. As it evolved, map features were overlaid on top of each other to identify patterns and potential causes of special phenomenon. GIS can also calculate distances, define adjacency of features, and carry out complex analyses. Easily accessible, digitally formatted maps now enable complex analysis and modeling not possible in the past.[8]

The components of GIS include hardware, software, and data. The hardware refers to the equipment that supports the activities of GIS, from data collection to analysis. The computer workstation is the central piece of equipment that runs the GIS software. A digitizer may be required for conversion of hard-copy data to digital data. Handheld field technology can also be useful for data collection in GIS. In addition, Web-enabled GIS require the use of Web servers. GIS software makes it possible to create, edit, and analyze spatial and attribute data. Different software packages contain a large range of GIS functions. Geographic information software capabilities can also be extended using extensions or add-ons (e.g., an extension that adds more editing capabilities). At the core of any GIS are data. The two primary types of data used in GIS are geologic data that reference location using some coordinate system and attribute data that refer to additional information that can then be connected with the spatial data.[8]

In GIS, geographical space is called land. Spatial data are often combined with data referred to as attribute data. **Spatial data** pertain to the space occupied by objects. **Attribute data** are generally defined as additional information on the characteristics of the object under investigation. This additional information can be combined with spatial data. An example of this would be a chemical plant. The spacial data show the actual location of the plant. Additional data such as the plant name, types of chemicals produced, and the amount of chemicals produced make up the attribute data. Partnership of these two data types enables GIS to be an effective problem-solving tool.

Geographic reference may be explicit or implicit. Explicit refers to geographic information absolutely tied to the earth; it is described in terms of geographic coordinates (latitude and longitude or some national grid coordinates). On the other hand, implicit geographic reference refers to geographic information being described as a street address, census track, postal code, or forest-stand identifier. GIS is effective at translating implicit geographic data into explicit map location. A GIS process for converting implicit information (e.g., street addresses) into explicit map images (i.e., displayed features on a map) is called **geocoding**.

GIS store data as vectors or in raster format. A **vector** is a quantity having both direction and magnitude that determines the position of one point in space relative to another. Two-dimensional data are stored according to x and y coordinates. Political boundaries, census boundaries, zip code boundaries, streets, and rivers are examples of what can be described by a series of x and y coordinates. Some possible vector layers may include points, lines, and polygons. For example, polygons representing the cumulative number of West Nile virus cases in 2006 are shown according to county in Figure 8.2. Darker shaded counties represent at least one confirmed case. There are 3,498 cases represented on the map.

Raster data are an abstraction of the real world, where the raster is a form of spatial data stored as a matrix of cells or pixels. Raster data are represented by a grid of rectangular cells covering a given area. For example, a scanned image or photograph constitutes raster data. Each pixel reflects the smallest unit of information

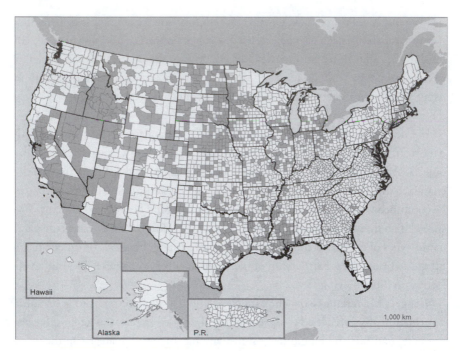

FIGURE 8.2   West Nile virus in year end of 2006, United States, according to county. Areas of darker gray indicate countries with positive test results for West Nile virus, while lighter areas indicate countries that either did not perform surveillance or did not report any positive results from their surveillance. (*Source:* Courtesy of USGS Disease Maps Website.)

(e.g., color) in the raster map. A raster data model reflects characteristics as a matrix of cells in continuous space. Each layer represents a unique phenomenon or attribute. Raster layers allow topography to be spatially associated with health data. For example, the global sea-surface temperature in May 2001, shown in Figure 8.3, is based on raster data. Most GIS make use of data in both vector and raster format.

Combining Cases with Population Data

John Snow's spot map showed the Broad Street and Golden Square area of London, location of the water pumps, cases of cholera (dots) in the area, and a clustering of cases around a specific pump. Unfortunately, some characteristics of the population at risk were not considered. For example, the population density would certainly

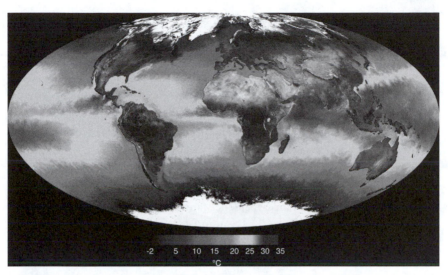

FIGURE 8.3   Global sea-surface temperature, May 2001. (*Source:* Courtesy of NASA Goddard Space Flight Center (NASA-GSFC).)

influence the distribution of cases. Perhaps a cluster around the pump was because that area was more densely populated than around other pumps. Snow could have linked these cases to population data to obtain disease rates. These rates could then be compared among the affected areas or with neighboring areas. However, population data were likely not available at the time, especially since a large portion of the population fled the area when the cholera outbreak began.

An alternative would have been for Snow to obtain data on a control group that would reflect the population distribution. These data would have the advantage of providing a comparison with the location of cases and selected characteristics that may not be available otherwise and yield more flexible options in the analysis. Although direct measure of water use from the various pumps in the Broad Street and Golden Square area would have been ideal, Snow did not have this information. He needed to rely on proximity to the water pumps as a measure of exposure. Had Snow elected to do a case–control study, he would have selected a control group that did not have cholera. Because the location was used to categorize exposure (water from pump A), it would have been inappropriate for him to select controls from the nondisease group around pump A because it is the difference in location that reflects exposure. However, it would have been reasonable for Snow to match on potential confounders like age, sex, and socioeconomic status—not just on location.

Survey data could have been used to collect information on these and other potential confounders, which, in turn, could be used for matching or for adjustment at the analysis level of the study. Census track or zip code may also provide information that could be included in GIS as a proxy for socioeconomic status.

Since the late 1990s, the U.S. National Cancer Institute has used GIS techniques to examine the geographic distribution of cancer incidence across the country and compare the magnitude of differences among states. Age-adjusted incidence rates are used to account for variability in population sizes and differences in the age-distribution across areas. Smoothed maps of county-level incidence make it possible to see differences among geographic subareas other than by states. For example, a clustering of female lung cancer incidence rates is evident along the northern Pacific coast (see Figure 8.4). Smoothed county-level maps may allow for correlation with environmental data to help provide causal associations.

Global Positioning System

The **global positioning system (GPS)** is a global navigation system of at least 24 satellites that orbit the earth twice a day at approximately 12,000 miles above the earth's surface.[12] These satellites broadcast high-frequency radio signals that contain satellite position and precise time data. Handheld GPS receivers process signals from at least four satellites to accurately determine latitude, longitude, altitude, velocity, and time. GPS is an effective method for locating features too numerous or dynamic to be mapped by traditional approaches. For example, GPS mapping can locate pests, insects, soil types, power lines, rivers, and hazardous-waste sites. It can be used to measure the number of insects in a field, measure the area of a soil type, or create a map of sampled locations. In some studies, GPS is being used to measure the arctic ice sheets, volcanic activity, and the earth's tectonic plates.

Scientists are increasingly using GPS in environmental research. For example, small receivers can be attached to people to relate their location with environmental factors such as particulate matter or carbon monoxide. Evolution of personalized exposure assessment has involved miniaturization of sensors and widespread availability of GPS receivers, which allow for an accurate record of individual time-location and linear velocity. One group of researchers used GPS to measure dynamic air-pollution exposure patterns of children living in urban areas. The GPS

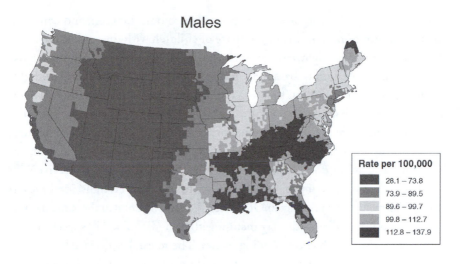

Males

Rate per 100,000

28.1 – 73.8
73.9 – 89.5
89.6 – 99.7
99.8 – 112.7
112.8 – 137.9

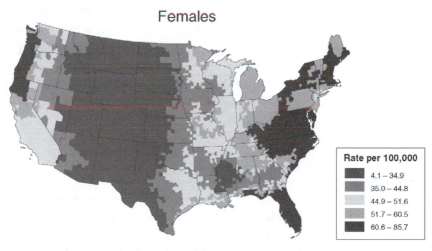

Females

Rate per 100,000

4.1 – 34.9
35.0 – 44.8
44.9 – 51.6
51.7 – 60.5
60.6 – 85.7

FIGURE 8.4   Smoothed predicted lung cancer incidence rates by county, males and females, 1999. (*Source:* Courtesy of Pickle LW, Feuer EJ, Edwards BK. US Predicted Cancer Incidence, 1999: Complete Maps by County and State From Spatial Projection Models. NCI Cancer Surveillance Monograph Series, Number 5. Bethesda, MD: National Cancer Institute, 2003. NIH Publication No. 03-5435.)

Personal Exposure Tracker can simultaneously record time, location, and contaminant concentration in the breathing space of children with the sensor mounted to the lapel of a lightweight vest.[13] Other uses of GPS include tracking study participants in a community-based environmental exposure assessment study;[14] mapping urban air pollution by using mobile carbon monoxide sensors, where GPS receivers were used to track the sensors and explore carbon monoxide variations at a fine geographic scale;[15] and examining exposure to particulate matter, volatile organic compounds, and other air pollutants inside patrol cars, where location and activity information of the cars were identified using GPS receivers.[16]

Data collected by a simple, handheld GPS receiver can be transferred into a suitable format for data display in GIS. The GPS data must be in the same datum and projection in order to display them together in GIS. The GPS receiver can record vector data with corresponding names. The researcher decides how he or she wants to collect the data (i.e., as a point, line, or polygon). If a researcher is studying hazardous-waste runoff, it would be useful to collect the data as a polygon. If one wants to show the location of selected waste sites, points would suffice. Attribute information (e.g., characteristics or properties associated with a waste facility) must be manually recorded. In order to take GPS data and display it using GIS, you will need a personal computer, a GPS receiver with a personal computer (PC) interface cable, a GIS data viewer, and PC interface software. Online tutorials for this process are available (e.g., at http://cse.pdx.edu/forest/conduct_gps_gis_walk_through.pdf).

Conclusion

GIS provides an effective way to identify a spatial trend or aggregation of high rates of disease or injury in one area compared with another, and to combine such information with the location and attributes of a suspected cause. GIS-generated data can then be formally assessed using statistical methods (see Chapters 5 and 6). GIS can be useful for generating data that can be downloaded and assessed statistically. However, a cluster investigation, whether involving GIS data or not, requires consideration of whether a suspected cluster is in search of a cause or a causal association is in search of a disease cluster. GPS has been used to improve exposure assessment and for locating features too numerous or dynamic to be mapped by traditional approaches.

Key Issues

1. The spot map employed by Snow was an effective descriptive approach for describing the cluster of disease cases and their association with selected water pumps.
2. Maps are useful for stimulating etiologic research.
3. Mapping is a useful approach in environmental epidemiology that often relies on ecologic data. This descriptive approach can provide exposure and disease information for analytic study designs where models are used to relate regional attributes with disease outcomes.
4. GIS make it possible to effectively map health events and corresponding population information, as well as proximity to the suspected source.
5. To identify whether a cluster exists, we begin by determining the relevant geographic area and time period for study. The boundaries should correspond to the entire area that could have been exposed to the suspected environmental hazard.
6. Expected numbers of events used for comparison with the observed counts require known population figures.
7. Data generated using GIS methods for conducting cluster investigation are formally investigated using statistical methods (see Chapter 4).
8. Scientists are increasingly using GPS in environmental research to improve exposure assessment and locate features too numerous or dynamic to be mapped by traditional approaches.

Exercises

Key Terms

Define the following terms.

Attributes
Attribute data
Computer cartography
Geocoding
Geographic reference
Geographic information system (GIS)
Global positioning system (GPS)

Mapping
Raster data
Spatial data
Vector

Study Questions

8.1. Why is GIS a useful tool in exploring the relationship between adverse health problems and environmental contaminants?

8.2. List and describe the three components of GIS.

8.3. What are the two types of data used in GIS?

8.4. List two ways that potential confounders may be controlled for in a spatial analysis.

8.5. Why is it important to combine case and population data?

8.6. Suppose you are interested in evaluating selected environmental influence on rheumatoid arthritis. You are not looking to solve the problem but simply to identify variables associated with the disease. How might GIS be useful?

8.7. Discuss the differences between vector and raster data. Which type of data would likely take up the most space as a computer file? Are there any advantages that raster data have over vector data?

8.8. Provide an example for each of the following: (a) spatial data; (b) attribute data; (c) explicit reference; and (d) implicit reference.

8.9. List some ways that mapping can be a useful tool in an environmental epidemiologic investigation.

8.10. How can GPS be useful in evaluating exposure?

References

1. Frost WH. *Snow on Cholera: being a reprint of two papers by John Snow, M.D. together with a biographical memoir by BW Richardson and an introduction by Wade Hampton Frost, M.D.* The Commonwealth Fund, New York; 1936.

2. Hertz-Picciotto I. Environmental epidemiology. In: Rothman KJ, Greenland S, eds. *Modern Epidemiology.* Philadelphia, PA: Lippincott-Raven Publishers; 1998.

3. Diehr P, Cain K, Connell F, Volinn E. What is too much variation? the null hypothesis in small-area analysis. *Health Serv Res.* 1990;24:741–771.

4. Elliott P, Kleinschmidt I, Westlake AJ. Use of routine data in studies of point sources of environmental pollution. In: Elliott P, Cuzick UJ, English D, Stern R, eds. *Geographical and Environmental Epidemiology: Methods for Small Studies.* New York, NY: Oxford University Press; 1992.

5. McMahon LF, Wolfe RA, Griffith JR, Cutherbertson D. Socioeconomic influence on small area hospital utilization. *Med Care.* 1993;31(5):YS29–YS36.

6. Howe GR. Historical evolution of disease mapping in general and specifically of cancer mapping. *Recent Results Cancer Res.* 1989;1141:21.

7. Kulldorff M, Athas WF, Feuer EJ, Miller BA, Key CR. Evaluating cluster alarms: A space-time scan statistic and brain cancer in Los Alamos, New Mexico. *Am J Public Health.* 1998;88:1377–1380.

8. Geographic Information Systems Lounge. What Is GIS? Available at: http://gislounge.com/library/introgis.shtml. Accessed October 2, 2006.

9. U.S. Department of Interior. US Geological Survey. Available at: http://diseasemaps.usgs.gov/wnv_us_human.html. Accessed December 8, 2006.

10. Descloitres J. MODIS Land Rapid Response Team. NASA/GSFC. Global sea surface temperature. Available at: http://visibleearth.nasa.gov/view_rec.php?id =2366. Accessed November 24, 2006.

11. Pickle LW, Feuer EJ, Edwards BK. *US predicted cancer incidence, 1999: complete maps by county and state from spatial projections models. NCI Cancer Surveillance Monograph Series, Number 5.* Bethesda, MD: National Cancer Institute; 2003.

12. Kennedy M. *The Global Positioning System of GIS: An Introduction.* Chelsea, MI: Ann Arbor Press Inc; 1996.

13. Elgethun K, Yost M. Integrated GPS/pollution-sensor datalogger for personal exposure measurements of children. *Epidemiology.* 2006;17(6):S37–S38.

14. Phillips ML, Hall TA, Esmen NA, Lynch R, Johnson DL. Use of global positioning system technology to track subject's location during environmental exposure sampling. *J Exp Anal Environ Epidemiol.* 2001;11(3):207–215.

15. Milton R, Steed A. Mapping carbon monoxide using GPS tracked sensors. *Environ Monit Assess.* 2007;124(1–3):1–19.

16. Riediker M, Williams R, Devlin R, Griggs T, Bromberg P. Exposure to particulate matter, volatile organic compounds, and other air pollutants inside patrol cars. *Environ Sci Technol.* 2003;37(10):2084–2093.

Time Series

LEARNING OBJECTIVES

After completing this chapter, you should be able to:

1. Identify time–series designs.
2. Identify main concepts in time series.
3. Describe the function of age-period-cohort analyses.
4. Define "epidemic curve."
5. Distinguish between secular and seasonal trend data.
6. Be familiar with selected statistical methods for assessing time–series data.

Introduction

In the preceding chapter, the geographic information system was presented as a means of evaluating counts and rates of health-related states or events by person and place. The focus of this chapter is on organizing counts or rates of health-related states or events by time to identify the nature of the phenomenon represented by the sequence of observations. Once a time–series pattern is established, it can be combined with other data (e.g., exposure) as a useful means for identifying incubation or latency periods and for better understanding possible causal relationships.

Time–Series Designs

Time–series designs involve a sequence of measurements of some numerical quantity made at or during two or more successive periods of time. The simple time–series design involves the collection of quantitative observations made at regular intervals through repeated observations, such as air temperature measured at noon every day, number of hospital admissions per day, number of deaths per day, or air pollution levels per day. Analysis of time–series data requires statistical consideration of autocorrelation.

Time–series analysis may involve the assessment of a group of people who have experienced an event at roughly the same time, such that these individuals may be thought of as a cohort. Time–trend analysis of cohort data allows researchers to study the pattern of illness or injury for a group of people who experienced an exposure at roughly the same time. A histogram can be used to depict this, with the horizontal axis representing time and the vertical axis representing frequency. The time begins at the point of exposure and extends over the course of the outbreak. If the duration time of the epidemic is reflected, the histogram is called an **epidemic curve**. Time intervals may reflect hours, days, weeks, or longer. A sufficient lead period should be reflected on the graph between the suspected exposure and clinical manifestations of the disease to demonstrate the incubation period. **Incubation period** and **latency period** both refer to the time from exposure until clinical manifestations of the health event occur. The term "incubation period" is used with acute conditions and "latency period" is used with chronic conditions. For example, the maximum incubation period for severe acute respiratory syndrome is ten days.[1] On the other hand, the latency period for lung cancer or malignant mesothelioma associated with asbestos dust is generally 20 to 40 years.[2]

The shape of the epidemic curve is influenced by whether the source of exposure is at a point in time or continuous over time. In a **point source** epidemic, persons are exposed to the same exposure over a limited time period. Because incubation or latency period influences the rate of increase and decrease in the epidemic curve, a point source epidemic tends to show a clustering of cases in time, with a sharp increase and a trailing decline. In a **continuous source** epidemic where exposure is continuous over time but at relatively low levels, the epidemic curve tends to increase more gradually than it does for a point source exposure, then it plateaus, and finally it decreases. The rate of decrease depends on the latency period and whether the exposure is removed gradually or suddenly.

If a health event is identified and the source is unknown, the time from a presumed exposure until the manifestation of symptoms of disease can help focus the causal hypothesis. If a causal agent is suspected, then estimating the incubation or latency period can support or dispel a suspicion. For example, if several people attending a picnic become ill, the incubation period can help identify the specific cause of disease. Salmonella has an incubation period from 6 to 72 hours, botulism has an incubation period of 12 to 36 hours, and *E. coli enteritis* has an incubation period of 24 to 72 hours. If several cases occur within 12 hours of eating, then salmonella food poisoning is the likely cause of illness. Another example is lung cancer, where asbestos exposure from a local plant is only a possible cause if cases have been employed for a sufficiently long period of time because of the long latency period that typically accompanies asbestos and lung cancer.

In an outbreak of infectious diarrhea among U.K. tourists staying in a Greek hotel between May 22 and June 9, 1997, epidemic curves for both diarrhea and vomiting indicated a point-source outbreak (see Figure 9.1). The peak of illness occurred during June 5–7. The investigators did not know the date of exposure, so they could not calculate the exact incubation period. However, they were able to estimate the upper limit of the incubation time by calculating the interval between checking into the hotel and the onset of disease (see Figure 9.2). Most people became ill within three days of arriving. The high proportion of people reporting vomiting indicated that some illness was caused by a viral gastroenteropathic pathogen. Laboratory testing of definite cases found the primary pathogen involved was *Giardia lamblia* (86% of cases), followed by *Cryptosporidium parvum* (16% of cases).

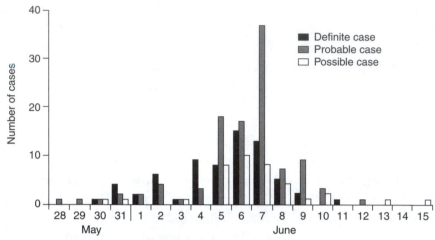

FIGURE 9.1 Epidemic curve showing diarrhea according to category of case. (*Source:* Hardie et al., 1999.)[3]

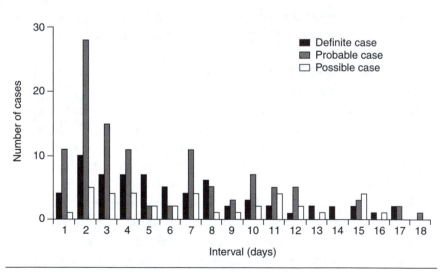

FIGURE 9.2 Interval between arrival at the hotel and symptoms of vomiting or diarrhea according to category of case. (*Source:* Hardie et al., 1999.)[3]

Not only are ecologic (group level) data used in time–series analyses, but longitudinal (individual level) data are used. Specifically, **longitudinal data** refer to the same sample of respondents being observed in each period. Longitudinal data avoid some of the concern regarding confounding in ecologic studies. Factors that change little over time do not confound time–series studies, but confounding could occur from time varying environmental factors (e.g., secular trend; carryover effect/residual influence of the intervention on the outcome).[4]

Time–Series Concepts

In studies investigating patterns in time–series data, three potential effects are generally considered: age, period, and cohort. The **age effect** is the change in rate of a condition according to age. This effect is irrespective of birth cohort or calendar time. A **cohort effect** is the change in the rate of a condition according to birth year. This effect is irrespective of age and calendar time. A **period effect** is a change in the rate of a condition affecting an entire population at a given point in time. This effect is irrespective of age and birth cohort. Environmental factors contribute to both cohort and period effects. When investigators observe cohort and/or period effects, this can help in the investigation of the causes of health-related states or events.

The birth cohort effect results from health-influencing lifetime experiences of individuals born at a given time. Numerous studies have demonstrated disease rates to be correlated with the period of birth. For example, the incidence of testicular cancer increased 51% (3.6 to 5.4 per 100,000) between 1973 and 1995 in the United States. Poisson regression models showed a strong birth cohort effect on the risk of testicular cancer ($p < 0.001$), with peak age at diagnoses decreasing with each successive birth cohort.[5] In Canada researchers observed a 50% increase (2.8 in 1969–1971 to 4.2 in 1991–1993 per 100,000) in testicular cancer. This study also found a strong birth cohort effect, with a steady increase in risk among men born since 1945.[6] The epidemiological patterns observed in these studies implicate higher exposure to environmental factors in more recent birth cohorts.

A period effect involves a shift or change in the trends in rates that affect all birth cohorts and age groups. Period effects are responses to phenomenon that occur at a period of time across the entire population. A period effect may result from the introduction of a new antibiotic, vaccine, or disease-prevention program that affects various age groups and birth cohorts in a similar manner. A period effect may also result from adverse physical stresses or social conditions (e.g., earthquake, flood, terrorism, war, and economic collapse) that affect the whole population irrespective of age group or birth cohort. For example, the Great Depression started a world-wide economic downturn in 1929. In Australia, for instance, approximately 29% of the work force was unemployed in 1932, and suicide rates among males rose to unprecedented levels across all age groups.[7]

In addition to these three time–series effects, important concepts used in time series are dependence, stationarity, differencing, and specification. **Dependence** in a time series refers to the correlation of observations of a variable at one point in time with observations of the same variable at prior points in time. **Stationarity** in a time series results when the mean value of the series remains constant over time (i.e., there is no trend). **Differencing** is a step taken to detrend data in order to control autocorrelation and achieve stationarity. If the trend of a series is a straight line, the first differences of the series will have no trend; if the trend is quadratic, taking the second difference will have no trend; and so on. Finally, **specification** refers to testing for linear versus nonlinear dependence, followed by selection of the model (e.g., autoregressive moving average, threshold autoregressive, exponential autoregressive, etc.).

General Aspects of Time–Series Patterns

Analysis of time series involves searching for patterns of disease over time and attempting to explain their underlying causes. A simple yet powerful method of identifying whether the data consist of a systematic pattern is to create a visual display of a series. Time–series patterns can be described according to secular trend and seasonality. The secular trend is the general systematic linear or nonlinear component that changes over time. Seasonality is the component that repeats itself in a systematic manner over time. Temporal comparisons may appropriately involve just event data if there is no temporal change in baseline risk factors or in the size of the population of interest. The time scale used will depend on the exposure and the disease, varying from hours to days to weeks to years. The population size, the disease rate, and the time scale will all influence the stability of measures of association between exposure and disease. Shorter time scales require larger population sizes to obtain stable rates.

A **secular trend** is a long-term trend typically lasting more than one year. Changes in disease trends seen over extended periods of time, even several decades in certain diseases, are a concern in epidemiology. Long-term secular trends can also be informative about causal factors. For example, trends in lung cancer and heart disease, compared with trends in cigarette smoking in the United States, implicated a causal association between smoking and these health outcomes (see Figures 9.3 and 9.4). The trends show about a 20- to 25-year latency period for lung cancer compared with a very short latency period for diseases of the heart.

Several diseases are characterized by seasonal patterns. A **seasonal trend** represents periodic increases and decreases in the occurrence, interval, or frequency of disease. These patterns tend to be predictable. A number of explanations have been given for the occurrence of seasonal patterns. Some disease cycles are seasonal, while other disease cycles may be influenced by cyclic factors such as the school calendar, immigration patterns, migration patterns, duration and course of diseases, placement of military troops, wars, famine, and popular tastes in food. Some

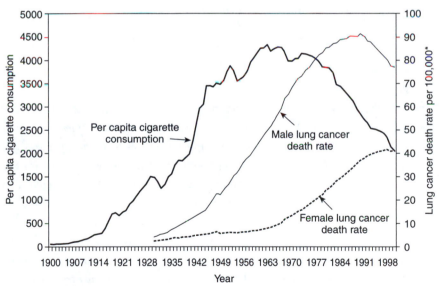

FIGURE 9.3   Lung cancer death rates and per capita cigarette consumption for males and females in the United States 1900–2000. (*Source:* U.S. Mortality Public Use Data, 2002.)[8]

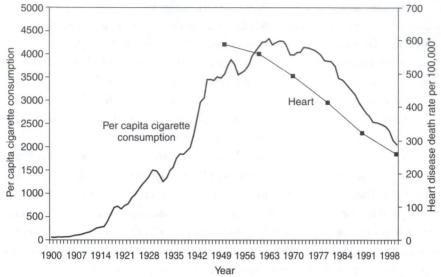

Per capita cigarette consumption

Heart

Per capita cigarette consumption

Heart disease death rate per 100,000*

1900 1907 1914 1921 1928 1935 1942 1949 1956 1963 1970 1977 1984 1991 1998

Year

*Age-adjusted to 2000 U.S. standard population.

FIGURE 9.4   Death rates for all causes and diseases of the heart and per capita cigarette consumption for males and females in the United States 1900–2000. (*Source:* NCHS, 2004.)[9]

disease outbreaks occur only at certain times, but in predictable time frames or intervals over long terms. Hence, epidemiologists track cyclic changes over time. Cyclic patterns in disease incidence may implicate an infectious agent. However, temperature, sunlight, behaviors, and environmental factors associated with the season, such as pesticide use for agricultural purposes, may also be considered. The study approach is straightforward; cases of the disease are followed and tabulated by time of onset according to a diagnosis or proof of occurrence.

Certain pathogen-borne diseases have a seasonal pattern that corresponds with changes in the vector populations, which, in turn, are influenced by environments where the vectors live and multiply. In 2005, for example, nationally reported West Nile virus began late in May, peaked in the third week of August, and then lasted through November (see Figure 9.5). This cyclic pattern that corresponds with season is consistent with infected mosquitoes being the primary source of spreading the virus to humans.

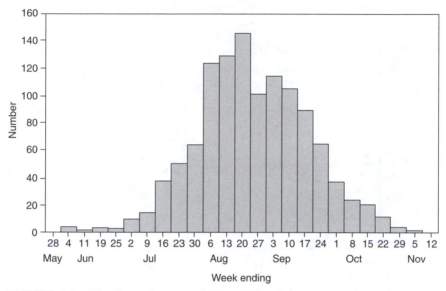

FIGURE 9.5   Number of reported West Nile virus neuroinvasive disease cases in humans, by week of illness onset—United States, 2005 (1,165 cases). (*Source:* CDC, 2005.)[11]

Cyclical disease patterns have also been associated with extreme temperatures, seasonal patterns in diet, physical activity, and environmental factors (e.g., agricultural pesticides). For example, evaluation of daily deaths in England and Wales and in New York has found a relationship between temperature and deaths from myocardial infarction, stroke, and pneumonia. Death rates rise with extreme cold and hot temperatures. The influence of temperature on deaths is much stronger in the elderly.[10]

Consider further the annual cycles of respiratory complaints (e.g., bronchiolitis, chest congestion, chest pain, cold, cough, croup, flu, headache, laryngitis, pneumonia, respiratory, sinus, stuffy nose, sore throat) for people reporting to emergency departments. Figure 9.6 demonstrates these cycles for data from the Emergency Center of the University Hospital, Albuquerque, New Mexico, with peaks occurring in weeks in January and February of the years 2000, 2001, and 2002.[12]

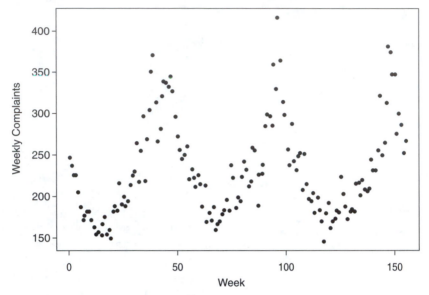

FIGURE 9.6   Annual cycle of respiratory complaints, New Mexico (United States). (*Source:* From Brillman et al., 2005.)[12]

Time–Series Graphs

To illustrate some of the types of time–series graphs, we will use malignant melanoma skin cancer incidence data for males and females from the U.S. National Cancer Institute. The series consists of annual rates for the nine surveillance, epidemiology, and end results (SEER) areas (San Francisco–Oakland, Connecticut, Metropolitan Detroit, Hawaii, Iowa, New Mexico, Seattle–Puget Sound, Utah, and Metropolitan Atlanta) from 1975 through 2003.[13] A plot of the rates by calendar time t is shown in Figure 9.7. This simple plot provides a history of the data, undistorted by data transformations, and is useful for searching for trends and patterns. Because the vertical axis is scaled in the same units of measurements as the rates, change in rates reflects the actual change in the series that corresponds to a unit change in time. The plot is on an arithmetic scale.

The plot of the log rate of time t of malignant melanoma of the skin among whites by time t is shown in Figure 9.8. In this plot, the vertical scale no longer reflects the same units as the original series, but a log scale is used. The difference in heights at two points is proportional to the corresponding percent change in the original series. A fairly stable percentage growth in the series is shown from year to

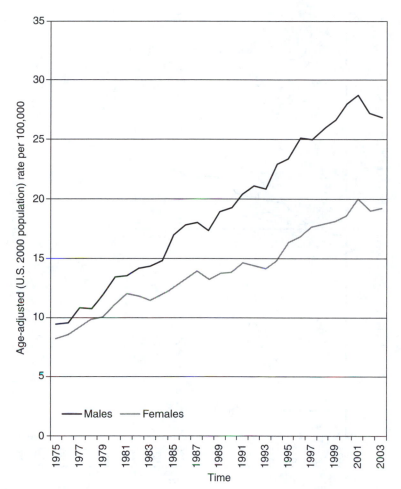

FIGURE 9.7   Plot of rates of malignant melanoma of skin among whites by calendar time. (*Source:* Data from SEER, 2006.)[13]

year for both males and females. The log scale can be used to compare two time series. The series is changing at a slightly higher percentage each period for males than females. Note that the arithmetic scale was less similar between males and females.

The plot of the rate of time t divided by the rate of time $t − 1$ versus t is shown in Figure 9.9. A point on this graph shows how much the current value of the series has changed relative to the previous value. The ratios are typically multiplied by 100 when constructing the vertical scale for this graph. This allows the scale to be interpreted as period-to-period percent changes. For example, the rates increase

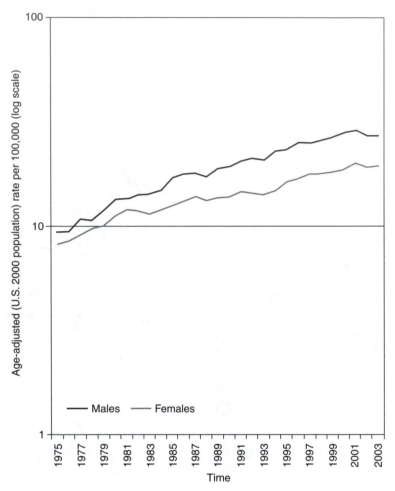

FIGURE 9.8 Plot of the log rates of malignant melanoma of the skin among whites by calendar time. (*Source:* Data from SEER, 2006.)[13]

by 15% in males and 5% in females from 1984 to 1985. Overall, because the ratios are generally greater than 100% but trending downward slightly over time, the rates are constantly increasing, but at a decreasing rate. The actual magnitude of annual growth averaged across calendar years is 4% for males and 3% for females (see Table 9.1). The information presented in the table would be harder to obtain from the log plot displayed in the previous figure.

A plot of the rate of time t minus the rate of time $t-1$ versus t is shown in Figure 9.10. The plot of the series of first differences versus t shows the actual changes

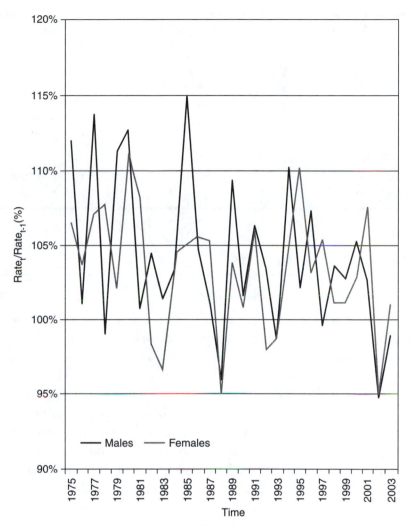

FIGURE 9.9 Plot of $Rate_t/Rate_{t-1}$ of malignant melanoma of the skin among whites by calendar time. (*Source:* Data from SEER, 2006.)[13]

in magnitude of the rates between successive time periods. For example, from 1984–1985 the rate per 100,000 increased 2.2 for males and 0.6 for females. Overall, the actual changes in rates per 100,000 people between successive time periods, averaged across selected time periods, were 0.64 for males and 0.40 for females (see Table 9.2). The differencing process may be extended beyond first differences to second, third, or higher differences.

TABLE 9.1 Percent Change in Annual Growth Averaged Across Calendar Years

Years	Males	Females
1975–1979	7%	5%
1980–1984	5%	4%
1985–1989	5%	3%
1990–1994	4%	2%
1995–1999	3%	4%
2000–2003	0%	2%
1975–2003	4%	3%

Statistical Analysis

Presenting Rate Data over Time

Age-adjusted rates are a weighted average of the age-specific rates, where the weights are the proportions of persons in the corresponding age groups of a standard population. These rates are often preferred over crude rates because they can be compared between groups or over time without the differences influenced by the confounding effect of differences or changes in the age distribution. The standard error of the age-adjusted rate can be approximated using the standard error of a crude rate SE(Rate) = Rate/[Number of cases]$^{1/2}$.[14] **Percent change** in rates over the entire time period covered by a study is obtained by subtracting the ending rate by the beginning rate and then dividing the difference by the beginning rate and finally multiplying by 100. Sometimes, for greater stability, the last two rates are averaged and subtracted by the average of the first two rates. The difference is then divided by the average of the first two rates and multiplied by 100.

The **estimated annual percent change** (EAPC) is another measure commonly used to describe change in trend data. It is calculated by fitting a regression line to the natural logarithm of the rates (r) using calendar year as a regressor variable.

$y = mx + b$ where $y = \ln(r)$ and x = calendar year.
EAPC = $100 \times (e^m - 1)$

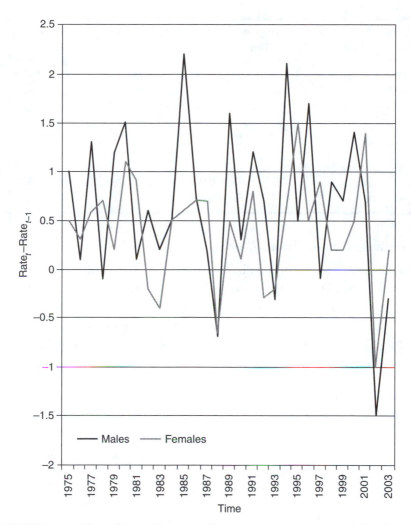

FIGURE 9.10   Plot of $Rate_t/Rate_{t-1}$ of malignant melanoma of the skin among whites by calendar time. (*Source:* Data from SEER, 2006.)[13]

To test whether the annual percent change is equal to zero, we test the hypothesis that the slope of the line (m) equals zero. This hypothesis is evaluated using the t distribution of m/SE_m and the degrees of freedom the number of calendar years minus 2, where SE_m is obtained by the fit of the regression line.[15]

TABLE 9.2 Annual Change in Rates (per 100,000) between Successive Time Averaged across Selected Time Periods

Years	Males	Females
1975–1979	0.70	0.46
1980–1984	0.58	0.38
1985–1989	0.82	0.36
1990–1994	0.80	0.22
1995–1999	0.74	0.66
2000–2003	0.07	0.27
1975–2003	0.64	0.40

Piecewise Linear Trend Models

In some cases trends in rates may be best represented by piecewise linear lines fit to the data, such as the trend for prostate cancer incidence in the United States (see Figure 9.11). Statistical software is available for analyzing such trends using join-point models where two or more different lines are connected together. Cancer trends reported by National Cancer Institute publications use this Joinpoint Re-

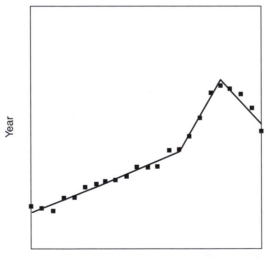

Prostate Cancer Incidence per 100,000

FIGURE 9.11 Piecewise linear models fit to the prostate cancer incidence trend for men in the United Staes. (*Source:* From NCI, 2005.)[17]

gression Program to analyze rates.[16] The methods and software for performing joinpoint regression are available at http://srab.cancer.gov/software/.

Application of Regression Methods to Time Series

Regression plays an important role in time–series analysis. In order to test hypotheses about the regression parameters, probabilistic assumptions are required. These assumptions are as follows:

1. Zero mean: For any fixed combination of levels of the independent variables, the expected value of the error term is zero.
2. Normality: For any combination of levels of the independent variables, the distribution of the dependent variable is normally distributed.
3. Homoskedasticity: The standard deviations of the outcomes of the dependent variable do not change across the values of the independent variable.
4. Independence: The outcomes of the dependent variable are independent.

In time–series analysis, these latter two assumptions are likely to be violated. If assumption 3 is violated, hypothesis tests and prediction intervals based on a regression analysis would be invalid and potentially misleading. A remedy would be to transform the data to obtain constant variance and then proceed with estimating the regression model. If assumption 4 is violated such that positive correlation exists, for example, hypothesis tests fitting a regression model would result in inflated significance levels and prediction intervals that are too narrow.

For time–series data, regression needs to be adapted. If the response variable is a time series, the independent variable used in the model can be the time variable t. Modeling y_t as a function of t is useful for identifying the nature of a trend in a series. Some commonly used models involving time t as an independent variable include:

$$y_t = \beta_0 + \varepsilon_t \qquad\qquad \text{No trend model}$$

$$y_t = \beta_0 + \beta_1 t + \varepsilon_t \qquad\qquad \text{Linear trend}$$

$$y_t = \beta_0 + \beta_1 t + \beta_2 t^2 + \varepsilon_t \qquad \text{Quadratic trend}$$

$$y_t = \beta_0 \times \beta_1^t + \varepsilon_t \qquad\qquad \text{Exponential trend}$$

Autoregressive models are typically used to assess time–series data. Such models have the form

$$y_t = \beta_0 + \beta_1 y_{t-1} + \beta_2 y_{t-2} + \ldots + \beta_p y_{t-p} + \varepsilon_t$$

The subscript p, the number of lagged terms, is the *order* of the model. The autoregressive model is appropriate when the current level of the series is likely dependent on the recent history of the series. For example, measuring surface ozone concentrations often uses the autoregressive process because the ozone level one day often affects the ozone level in the next day.

Three problems arise with autoregressive models: (1) if y_t has a trend, so will $y_{t-1}, y_{t-2}, \ldots$; (2) assumption 4 above is violated because the independent variables are previous values of the dependent variable; and (3) the order of the model p has to be selected.[18]

If the first problem occurs, then the regression on $y_{t-1}, y_{t-2}, \ldots, y_{t-p}$ can result in misleading results. It is important that y_t is stationary before using an autoregressive model. If not, differencing or another detrending method should be used; then the stationary series fit using an autoregressive model. In addition, violation of assumption 4 can result in estimated regression coefficients that are biased downward (underestimated). However, a large number of data points make this problem negligible. Finally, the appropriate number of lags to use (order p of the model) can be determined by assessment of the partial autocorrelation coefficients of the series. This process is described in detail by Farnum and Stanton.[18]

Other modeling techniques, such as autoregressive integrated moving average models and the four phases of Box-Jenkins modeling can be used to effectively handle seasonal time series. Development of these models is beyond the scope of this book. Interested readers are encouraged to refer elsewhere for this information, such as in Farnum and Stanton.[18]

Key Issues

1. Time–series designs involve a sequence of measurements of some numerical quantity made at or during two or more successive periods of time.
2. The shape of the epidemic curve is influenced by whether the source of exposure is at a point in time or continuous over time.
3. The epidemic curve can be instructive about the incubation period.

4. Age-period-cohort analyses can provide clues as to the cause of the health-related state or event.

5. Cyclical or secular trends can provide clues as to the cause of the health-related state or event.

6. Commonly used functions in time–series graphs are the original series, logarithms of the original series, the "link relative" series, and the series of "first differences."

7. Time series can provide exposure and disease information for analytic study designs where models are used to relate time–period attributes with disease outcomes. Selected methods for assessing time–series data are presented.

Exercises

Key Terms

Define the following terms.

Age-adjusted rate
Age effect
Cohort effect
Continuous source
Dependence
Differencing
Epidemic curve
Estimated annual percent change
Incubation period
Latency period
Longitudinal data
Percent change
Period effect
Point source
Regression
Seasonal trend
Secular trend
Specification
Stationarity
Time–series designs

Study Questions

9.1. Describe the difference between a graph that has *y*-axis values given as the natural log of the reported data observation, and those that graph only the real data on the *y*-axis. What is the relationship between an incremental change in *y* and a change in *x* (dependent vs. independent) in each of these cases?

9.2. Why is the following statement true? "Shorter time scales require larger population sizes to obtain stable rates." Is there an advantage to having a greater time span with only a fixed number of observations available? Why or why not?

9.3. You are an epidemiologist who has just been made aware of some interesting surveillance data collected by a local county health department. It was noticed that during the months of June through August the rate of respiratory-related illnesses is higher than at other times of the year.

　　a. In order to perform a time–series analysis, how would you set up your model? What must you control for?

　　b. Is there a possibility of dependence in this data? How might differencing help correct this problem?

　　c. Based on what you know from the passage about the increasing annual rate, would the effect likely be an age effect, period effect, or cohort effect? Why?

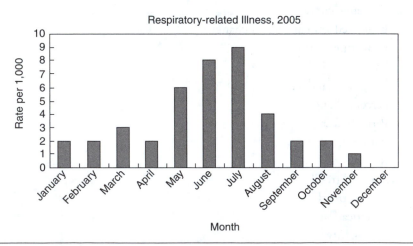

FIGURE 9.12   Respiratory related illness, 2005.

9.4. In the following hypothetical scenarios, state whether each would be best evaluated as an age effect, a cohort effect, or a period effect.

    a. A magazine article reports on a 10-year cohort study that particulate matter respiratory problems and eye irritation are three times more prevalent for people over 60 than for those under 60.

    b. Another report on the same issue as that in "a" suggests that, in light of new data, 20 years ago those over 40 were three times more likely to have respiratory and eye irritation problems than those under 40.

    c. All those living in Las Vegas, Nevada, in 1995 onward have showed a higher incidence of colon cancer than those living there up to 1995 but not afterward.

    d. A strange occurrence of brain cancer among adults in their late 40s, higher than in the past, has been coined "Boomer Tumors" by the media.

    e. A recent academic publication finds a statistically significant positive correlation between male baldness and mean age among various communities in the southeast United States.

9.5. Discuss how confounding may be a problem in longitudinal data.

References

1. U.S. Department of Agriculture, 1900–2000 (cigarette consumption). WHO. Update 49 - SARS case fatality ratio, incubation period. 2003. Available at: http://www.who.int/csr/sarsarchive/2003_05_07a/en/. Accessed August 4, 2006.

2. Selikoff IJ, Hammond EC, Seidman H. Latency of asbestos disease among insulation workers in the United States and Canada. *Cancer.* 1980;46(12): 2736–2740.

3. Hardie RM, Wall PG, Gott P, Barhan M, Bartlett CLR. Infectious diarrhea in tourists staying in a resort hotel. *Emerg Infect Dis.* 1999;5(1). Available at: http://www.cdc.gov/ncidod/eid/vol5no1/hardie.htm#figs. Accessed October 22, 2006.

4. McKiernan JM, Goluboff ET, Liberson GL, Golden R, Fisch H. Rising risk of testicular cancer by birth cohort in the United States from 1973 to 1995. *J Urol.* 1999;162(2):361–363.

5. Brown BW Jr. Statistical controversies in the design of clinical trials—some personal views. *Control Clin Trials.* 1980;1:13–28.

6. Liu S, Wen SW, Mao Y, Mery L, Rouleau J. Birth cohort effects underlying the increasing testicular cancer incidence in Canada. *Can J Pub Health.* 1999; 90(3):176–180.

7. Snowdon J, Hunt GE. Age, period and cohort effects on suicide rates in Australia, 1919–1999. *Acta Psychiatr Scand.* 2002;105(4):265. Available at: http://www.blackwell-synergy.com/links/doi/10.1034/j.1600–0447.2002.1193.x/full/. Accessed October 20, 2006.

8. U.S. Mortality Public Use Data Tables 1960–2001, U.S. Mortality Volumes 1930–1959, National Center for Health Statistics, Centers for Disease Control and Prevention, 2002 (death rates).

9. National Center for Health Statistics. *Health, United States, 2004 with Chartbook on Trends in the Health of Americans.* Table 36. U.S. Department of Agriculture, 1900–2000 (cigarette consumption). Hyattsville, MD: NCHS; 2004.

10. Bull GM, Morton J. Environment, temperature and death rates. *Age and Aging.* 1978;7(4):210–224.

11. Centers for Disease Control and Prevention. West Nile virus activity—United States. *MMWR.* 2005;54(49):1253–1256. Available at: http://www.cdc.gov/mmwr/preview/mmwrhtml/mm5449a1.htm. Accessed September 18, 2006.

12. Brillman JD, Burr T, Forslund D, Joyce E, Picard R, Umland E. Modeling emergency department visit patterns for infectious disease complaints: results and application to disease surveillance. *BMC Med Inform Decis Mak.* 2005. Available at: http://www.biomedcentral.com/1472–6947/5/4. Accessed August 23, 2006.

13. Surveillance, Epidemiology, and End Results (SEER) Program (www.seer.cancer.gov) SEER*Stat Database: Incidence - SEER 9 Regs Public-Use, Nov 2005 Sub (1973–2003) - Linked To County Attributes - Total U.S., 1969–2003 Counties, National Cancer Institute, DCCPS, Surveillance Research Program, Cancer Statistics Branch, released April 2006, based on the November 2005 submission.

14. Kayfitz N. Sampling variance of standardized mortality rates. *Human Biology.* 1966;38:309–317.

15. Kleinbaum DG, Kupper LL, Muller KE. *Applied Regression Analysis and Other Multivariable Methods.* North Scituate, MA: Duxbury Press; 1988.

16. Ries LAG, Harkins D, Krapcho M, et al. (eds). *SEER Cancer Statistics Review, 1975–2003, National Cancer Institute.* 2006. Available at: http://seer.cancer.gov/csr/1975_2003/, based on November 2005 SEER data submission, posted to the SEER Web site, 2006. Bethesda, MD. Accessed June 12, 2007.

17. National Cancer Institute. U.S. National Institutes of Health. Statistical research applications. Available at: http://srab.cancer.gov/joinpoint. Accessed November 24, 2006.

18. Farnum NR, Stanton LW. *Quantitative Forecasting Methods.* Boston, MA: PWS-Kent Publishing Company; 1989.

Indoor and Ambient Air Quality and Health

LEARNING OBJECTIVES

After completing this chapter, you should be able to:

1. Define "air pollution" and discuss six common air pollutants.
2. Identify how time–series studies can be used to monitor ambient air.
3. Identify how geographical studies can be used to monitor ambient air.
4. Identify common sources of indoor air pollution.
5. Discuss standards and methods used to reduce indoor air pollution.

Introduction

Epidemiologic evidence, primarily from time–series studies, has associated air pollution with a lower quality of life, shorter life expectancy, and less productivity and time at work.[1–4] Air pollution increases the risk of stroke,[5] cardiovascular diseases,[6–8] asthma,[9,10] chronic respiratory diseases,[11,12] and possibly lung cancer.[13,14] In addition, ambient air pollution can adversely affect agricultural products, buildings, and monuments.[15–18]

On the basis of epidemiologic findings, most countries now have legislation in place to monitor and control air pollution. For example, the U.S. **Clean Air Act** **(CAA)** is a comprehensive federal law that regulates all sources of air pollutant emissions. In 1970, the CAA authorized the U.S. Environmental Protection Agency (EPA) to establish national ambient air quality standards (NAAQS) to protect the environment and the public's health. In 1977, the CAA was amended to set new goals and dates for achieving NAAQS. Regulations were also established to prevent any deterioration in air quality above an established baseline level. In 1990, the CAA was further amended to meet problems such as acid rain, ground-level ozone, stratospheric ozone depletion, and air toxics. Six common ambient air pollutants regulated by the EPA are ozone, particulate matter, carbon monoxide, nitrogen dioxide, sulfur dioxide, and lead.[19] Protecting the public's health, especially asthmatics, children, and the elderly, requires low levels of these air pollutants in the environment.

Each state's Division of Air Quality is responsible for monitoring concentrations of air pollutants in the state and providing results of its assessment to the EPA. When monitored concentrations exceed the EPA standards a given number of times over a 3-year period, the area is designated by the EPA as a **nonattainment area**. Regulatory consequences occur for nonattainment areas.

If an industry that produces air emissions wants to locate in a nonattainment area, it faces a new source review, which may require the industry to install the strictest pollution controls available. It must also purchase pollution offset credits from other industries in the area. Because of these strict requirements, industries are often discouraged from locating or expanding into a nonattainment area.

In addition, all nonattainment areas are required to prove that their long-range transportation plan will not increase pollution levels. Proving this is called **transportation conformity**. Modeling conducted by the Metropolitan Planning Organization is used to show this result. If transportation conformity cannot be shown, then the area is no longer eligible for new federal highway funds. Finally, in nonattainment areas, the state Division of Air Quality is required to submit a State Implementation Plan to the EPA. This plan details how the state intends to reduce air pollution to comply with the EPA standard.

The purpose of this chapter is to present common forms of air pollution, discuss standards and methods for monitoring ambient air pollution, present common forms of indoor air pollution, and discuss standards and methods for monitoring indoor air pollution.

Air Pollution

Air pollution is a broad term applied to "chemical, physical (e.g., particulate matter), or biological agents that modify the natural characteristics of the atmosphere."[20] Air pollution is an undesirable state of the natural environment where the air is contaminated with substances harmful to human health. Industrial air pollution results from an industrial plant discharging contaminants into the atmosphere. **Acid precipitation (rain)** occurs when acids are formed in the atmosphere when industrial gas emissions (primarily sulfur dioxide and nitrogen oxides) combine with water. **Small-particle pollution** is caused by fine particles of soot produced by power plants or diesel engines. Finally, **smog** is air pollution that is a mixture of smoke and fog.

Scientists have established six common air pollutants dangerous to human health and environmental conditions: carbon monoxide (CO), lead, nitrogen dioxide, ozone, particulate matter (PM), and sulfur dioxide. These are referred to as **criteria pollutants**. They are monitored and highly regulated. Burning of fossil fuels (coal, oil, natural gas) or wood causes four of the six pollutants. Major sources of the criteria pollutants, along with volatile organic compounds (VOCs), and their estimated time in the atmosphere, is presented in Table 10.1.

Carbon Monoxide

Carbon monoxide is a colorless, odorless gas that forms when carbon in fuel is not completely burned. Sources of such carbon include on-road motor vehicles (56%), nonroad engines and vehicles (22%), industrial process (4%), fuel combustion (6%), and miscellaneous (12%). In cities, CO emissions from motor vehicle exhaust may be as high as 85% to 95%. The highest levels of CO tend to be during the winter months when inversions trap CO near the earth's surface. CO is

TABLE 10.1   Sources of Selected Pollutants and Estimated Time in the Atmosphere

Pollutant	Nature	Major sources Human-made	Estimated time in atmosphere	May damage or contribute to the following
Carbon monoxide	Forest fires, photochemical reactions	Transportation, kerosene and gas space heaters, leaking chimneys and furnaces, gas stoves, gas water heaters, wood stoves, and fireplaces	1–3 months	Headaches, nausea, fatigue, brain damage, heart damage, death
Methane gas	Wetlands, termites, oceans, and hydrates	Rice cultivation, biomass burning, and cattle and sheep ranching, fossil fuel production; decaying material in landfills, coal mining, oil drilling, and other power-producing processes	12 years	Fatigue, dizziness, headaches, premature mortality
Lead	Wind-blown soil	Transportation, fuel combustion, lead smelting and refining, storage-battery manufacturing	Minutes to a few days	Heart, blood, organs, osteoporosis, brain and nerves, seizures, mental retardation, behavioral disorders, memory problems, mood changes
Nitrogen oxides	Lightning, biogenic processes in soil	Combustion	2–5 days	Respiratory infection, asthma, chronic lung disease

TABLE 10.1   Sources of Selected Pollutants and Estimated Time in the Atmosphere (continued)

Pollutant	Nature	Major sources Human-made	Estimated time in atmosphere	May damage or contribute to the following
Ozone (ground-level)	Chemical reaction between oxides of nitrogen (NO_x) and volatile organic compounds (VOCs) in sunlight and hot weather	60% of ozone's ingredients come from vehicle emissions; 40% come from industry and consumer products	Peak concentrations may last up to 2–3 hours	Aggravated asthma, reduced lung capacity, pneumonia and bronchitis, permanent lung damage
Particulate matter	Volcanoes, wind, erosion, pollens, forest fires	Industrial processes, combustion, transportation; diesel-powered vehicles and engines contribute over half the mobile source of particulate emissions	Minutes to a few days	Lungs, heart, premature death
Sulfur dioxide	Volcanoes, reactions of biogenic sulfur emissions	Fossil fuel combustion, processing of some minerals	1–4 days	Respiratory illness, aggregation of existing heart and lung diseases
Volatile organic compounds	Biogenic processes in soil and vegetation	Combustion, transportation	Hours to a few days	Eye, nose, and throat irritation; headaches; loss of coordination, nausea; damage to liver, kidney, and central nervous system; cancer

Source: Columns 1-4 reprinted by permission of the publisher from *Environmental Health* by Dade W. Mueller, pp. 18–19, Cambridge, Mass.: Harvard University Press, Copyright 1992 by the President and Fellows of Harvard College.[21] Column 5 obtained from EPA, 2006;[22-28] Dockery, 2001;[29] Pope et al., 2002;[30] West et al., 2006.[31]

poisonous, can adversely affect people with heart disease, and can affect the central nervous system.[22]

Lead

Lead is a metal found in manufactured products and in the environment. With leaded gasoline being phased out, the major sources of lead emissions are metal processing (52%), nonroad engines and vehicles (13%), fuel combustion (13%), waste disposal (16%), and other (6%). People are generally exposed to lead by breathing and ingesting it in food, water, soil, or dust. Lead can accumulate in various parts of the body (i.e., in the blood, bones, muscles, and fat). Infants and children are most sensitive to lead—even low levels. Lead exposure may damage organs including kidneys, liver, brain and nerves; lead to osteoporosis; affect the brain and nerves causing seizures, mental retardation, behavioral disorders, memory problems, and mood changes; affect the heart and blood causing high blood pressure and increased heart disease or anemia; affect animals and plants with same effects as in humans; and affect reproductive and neurological function in fish.[24]

Nitrogen Oxides

Nitrogen oxides (NO_x) are gases that contain nitrogen and oxygen in varying amounts. They may be colorless and odorless. However, nitrogen dioxide (NO_2) is a common pollutant that combines with particles in the air to produce a reddish-brown appearance. A layer of NO_2 can be seen in many urban settings. NO_x forms from fuel burned at high temperatures. Although NO_x can form naturally, the primary sources are from motor vehicles; electric utilities; and industrial, commercial, and residential sources. NO_x is also a primary ingredient in ground-level ozone and contributes to the formation of acid rain, nutrient overload that deteriorates water quality, atmospheric particles, global warming, and toxic chemicals formed through reactions. Indoor sources of nitrogen oxides include gas stoves and gas or wood heaters. Elevated levels of exposure to NO_2 can increase one's susceptibility to and the severity of respiratory infections and asthma. Chronic lung disease may result from long-term exposure to high levels of NO_2.[25]

Ozone

Ground-level ozone and ozone located miles above the earth's surface have the same chemical structure. Ozone that forms naturally in the stratosphere, 10 to 30 miles above the surface of the earth, is considered good because it acts as a protective layer against harmful rays from the sun. However, ground-level ozone is considered dangerous, leading to a variety of health problems, including aggravated asthma, reduced lung capacity, increased risk of pneumonia and bronchitis, and permanent lung damage after long-term exposure. Ozone also interferes with photosynthesis in plants. **Ground-level ozone** is created by a chemical reaction between oxides of nitrogen (NO_x) and VOCs in sunlight and hot weather.

$$VOC + NO_x + Sunlight = Ozone$$

Sources of VOCs and NO_x include motor vehicle exhaust, industrial emissions, gasoline vapors, and chemical solvents. Because sunlight and hot weather help catalyze the formation of ozone and industrialized processes are sources of VOCs and NO_x, ozone is known as a summertime air pollutant and high levels tend to form in urban areas. Ozone, VOCs, and NO_x can be carried considerable distances by wind, affecting downwind rural areas as well.[23]

In Chapter 14, Climate Change and Health, ozone is discussed further.

Particulate Matter

Particulate matter consists of a complex mixture of extremely small particles and liquid droplets suspended in air. It is made up of acids (e.g., nitrates and sulfates), organic chemicals, metals, soil and dust particles, and allergens (e.g., fragments of pollen or mold spores). PM smaller than 10 micrometers represents airborne particles, which pose the greatest health problems. $PM_{2.5}$ is a commonly used term referring to particulate matter that is 2.5 micrometers or smaller in size, or approximately 1/30 the size of human hair. These particles can penetrate into the deepest parts of the lungs and even into the bloodstream. Smaller particles also can stay in the air longer and travel farther. Larger particles are of less concern, although they can adversely affect the eyes, nose, and throat. PM_{10} particles can stay in the air for minutes or hours whereas $PM_{2.5}$ particles, such as found in smoke and haze, can stay in the air for days or weeks. PM_{10} particles can travel up to 30 miles and $PM_{2.5}$ particles may travel up to hundreds of miles. PM can affect both the lungs and heart, leading to irritation of respiratory airways, coughing, wheezing, or difficulty breathing; decreased lung function; aggravated asthma; chronic bronchitis; irregular heartbeat; nonfatal heart attacks; and premature death in people with heart or lung disease. People most affected by PM are those with heart or lung diseases, children (whose immune and respiratory systems are still developing), and the elderly (whose immune system is weaker because of their age).[26]

Sulfur Dioxide

Sulfur dioxide (SO_2) forms when fuel containing sulfur, such as coal and oil, is burned. Extraction of gasoline from oil or metals in ore also produces SO_2. In turn, acid can form when SO_2 dissolves in water vapor, leading to acid rain, which has the potential to damage trees and crops and to make soils, lakes, and streams acidic. Sulfates and other products harmful to people and their environment are also formed as SO_2 interacts with gases and particles in the air. Sources of SO_2 are fuel combustion for electrical utilities (67%), fuel combustion for industrial and other purposes (18%), metal processing (3%), nonroad engines and vehicles (5%), and all other (7%). SO_2 released in the air by electrical utilities alone represents over 13 million tons per year. SO_2 contributes to respiratory illness, the aggregation of existing heart and lung diseases, and the formation of acid rain and atmospheric particles. People with asthma, children, and the elderly are particularly susceptible to respiratory illness.[27]

Volatile Organic Compounds

VOCs are gases emitted from certain solids or liquids. These gases can persist in the air for long periods. Organic chemicals are widely used ingredients in household products and fuels. Literally thousands of products emit VOCs, including paints, varnishes, wax, cleaning supplies, degreasing products, disinfecting cosmetics, pesticides, building materials, copiers and printers, permanent markers, photographic solutions, and glues and adhesives. Concentrations of VOCs are generally higher indoors than outdoors. The EPA's Total Exposure Assessment Methodology studies have identified numerous common organic pollutants to be two to five times higher inside homes than outside, notwithstanding whether the homes were in rural or industrial locations. Adverse health effects associated with VOCs are influenced by the level of exposure and the time exposed and include irritation to the eyes, nose, and throat; headaches; allergic skin reactions; dyspnea; declines in serum cholinesterase levels; nausea; emesis; epistaxis; fatigue; loss of coordination; damage to liver, kidney, and central nervous system; and cancer.[28]

Monitoring Ambient Air Pollution

Ambient (outdoor) air pollution has been shown in many epidemiologic studies to adversely affect health (see Table 10.1). Infants, children, the elderly, and those with cardiopulmonary disease are most susceptible to criteria air pollutants.[32–36] In 1970, as a response to the growing concern of air pollution in this country, the CAA became law. The EPA's responsibilities under the CAA, as amended in 1990, include:

1. Setting NAAQS for those pollutants shown to be harmful to the public health
2. Ensuring that the air quality standards are met
3. Ensuring control of sources of toxic air pollutants
4. Evaluating the effectiveness of the Ambient Air Monitoring Program[37]

The EPA's Ambient Air Monitoring Program is conducted by state and local agencies. There are three categories of monitoring stations: State and Local Air Monitoring Stations (SLAMS), National Air Monitoring Stations (NAMS), and Special Purpose Monitoring Stations (SPMS). Each monitoring station measures the criteria pollutants. Additionally, the Photochemical Assessment Monitoring Stations (PAMS) measure ozone precursors, which include approximately 60 volatile hydrocarbons and carbonyl.[37] The U.S. locations of approximately 4,000 SLAMS, 1,080 NAMS, and 90 PAMS are shown in Figures 10.1, 10.2, and 10.3, respectively. The SPMS are not permanently established, but are used to supplement the fixed monitoring networks as needed.

When monitoring and assessment of air quality standards reveal violations, identifying the source of the problem, choosing control options with evaluation of the choice considered, and implementing the controls follow.

Monitoring air pollution involves studies of air pollution trends over time and patterns of those diseases causally associated with air pollution. Air pollution studies are made possible because of extensive data collection on those pollutants for which monitoring data are routinely collected. Specifically, data are frequently collected on the six main criteria air pollutants to ensure that emissions in all areas of the United States are within EPA regulations. Table 10.2 shows EPA acceptable limits, or primary standards, for the six main criteria pollutants.

On the basis of monitoring these standards, the EPA produces county-level area maps showing nonattainment and attainment areas. For example, nonattainment

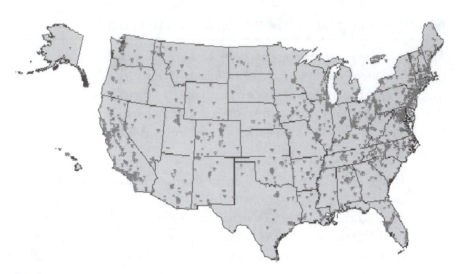

FIGURE 10.1   State and local air monitoring (SLAMS) network. (*Source:* From EPA, 2006.)[37]

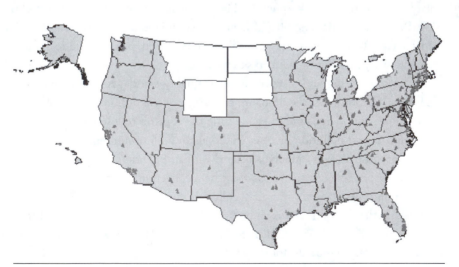

FIGURE 10.2   National air monitoring (NAMS) network. (*Source:* From EPA, 2006.)[37]

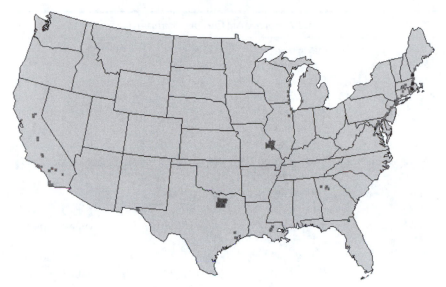

FIGURE 10.3   Photochemical assessment monitoring (PAMS) network. (*Source:* From EPA, 2006.)[37]

and attainment areas for 8-hour ozone in the United States are shown according to county in Figure 10.4. Another example, counties designated as nonattainment for particulate matter ($PM_{2.5}$), are shown in Figure 10.5. For these two criteria pollutants, nonattainment areas are primarily in Southern California and the Eastern part of the United States.

Because of the standards established by the EPA, the monitoring of air pollution by state agencies, and the penalties imposed for nonattainment areas, air quality in the United States has dramatically improved in recent years. Significant reductions in emissions of leading air pollutants in the United States between 1970 and 2005 are shown in Figure 10.6. National air pollution from major pollutants combined decreased by 53% (ranging from a 29% decrease for nitrogen oxides to a 99% decrease for lead). Not only are current emissions of air pollutants in the United States below previously predicted values, but continued EPA state-monitoring efforts have also resulted in substantial improvements to estimates of future air pollution (see Table 10.3).

TABLE 10.2   National Ambient Air Quality Standards

Pollutant	Primary standards	Averaging times	Secondary standards
Carbon monoxide	9 ppm (10 mg/m^3)	8-hour[a]	None
	35 ppm (40 mg/m^3)	1-hour[a]	None
Lead	1.5 mcg/m^3	Quarterly average	Same as primary
Nitrogen dioxide	0.053 ppm (100 mcg/m^3)	Annual (arith. mean)	Same as primary
Particulate matter (PM$_{10}$)	Revoked[b] 150 mcg/m^3	Annual[b] (arith. mean) 24-hour[c]	
Particulate matter (PM$_{2.5}$)	15.0 mcg/m^3 35 mcg/m^3	Annual[d] (arith. mean) 24-hour[e]	Same as primary
Ozone	0.08 ppm	8-hour[f]	Same as primary
	0.12 ppm	1-hour[g] (applies only in limited areas)	Same as primary
Sulfur oxides	0.03 ppm	Annual (arith. mean)	—–––
	0.14 ppm	24-hour[a]	—–––
	—–––	3-hour[a] (1300 mcg/m^3)	0.5 ppm

[a]Not to be exceeded more than once per year.

[b]Due to a lack of evidence linking health problems to long-term exposure to coarse particle pollution, the agency revoked the annual PM$_{10}$ standard in 2006 (effective December 17, 2006).

[c]Not to be exceeded more than once per year on average over 3 years.

[d]To attain this standard, the 3-year average of the weighted annual mean PM$_{2.5}$ concentrations from single or multiple community-oriented monitors must not exceed 15.0 mcg/m^3.

[e]To attain this standard, the 3-year average of the 98th percentile of 24-hour concentrations at each population-oriented monitor within an area must not exceed 35 mcg/m^3 (effective December 17, 2006).

[f]To attain this standard, the 3-year average of the fourth-highest daily maximum 8-hour average ozone concentrations measured at each monitor within an area over each year must not exceed 0.08 ppm.

[g](a) The standard is attained when the expected number of days per calendar year with maximum hourly average concentrations above 0.12 ppm is < 1.

(b) As of June 15, 2005, EPA revoked the 1-hour ozone standard in all areas except the fourteen 8-hour ozone nonattainment areas.

(*Source:* From EPA, 2006.)[38]

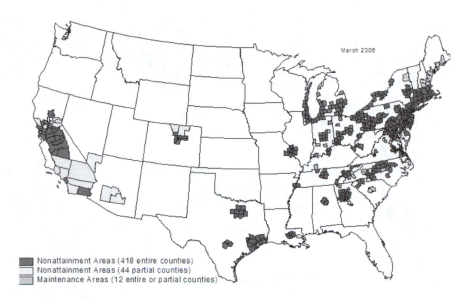

FIGURE 10.4 Nonattainment and attainment areas in the United States, 8-hour ozone standard. (*Source:* From EPA, 2006.)[39]

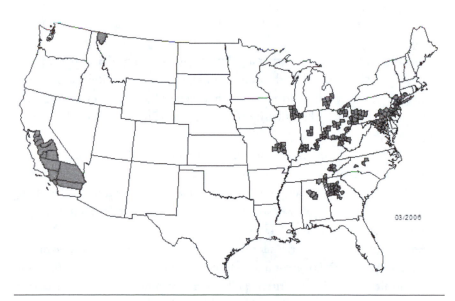

FIGURE 10.5 Nonattainment counties for $PM_{2.5}$. (*Source:* From EPA, 2006.)[40]

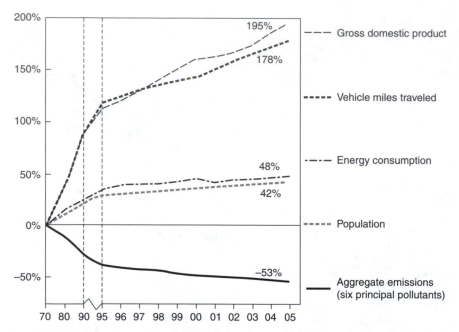

FIGURE 10.6　Comparison of growth areas and emissions. (*Source:* From EPA, 2006.)[41]

In addition to the tons of criteria pollutants released into the ambient air, air pollution may be reflected by the number of reports of noncompliance for emissions releases, vehicle miles driven per capita, average fuel efficiency among registered motor vehicles, and the density of the population in areas exposed to criteria air pollutants.

The EPA's Air Quality Index is a tool for monitoring daily air quality. It is used to issue public reports on actual levels of particles, ground-level ozone, and other air pollutants. The Air Quality Index's color-coded scale is useful for identifying unhealthy levels of air quality in your area. The Air Quality Index for particle pollution is presented in Table 10.4.

An example of a time–series plot shows $PM_{2.5}$ and troposphere ozone for Los Angeles, California, 2006, according to health classification (see Figure 10.7). The EPA classifies air quality for criteria pollutants according to health. This classification for assessing air quality is made available by the EPA for selected cities in the United States (http://www.epa.gov/airexplorer/).[42]

TABLE 10.3   National Air Pollutant Emissions Estimates (Fires and Dust Excluded) for Major Pollutants

Millions of tons per year

Carbon monoxide (CO)	1970	1975	1980	1985[a]	1990	1995	2000[a]	2005[b]
Nitrogen oxides (NO_x)[c]	197.3	184.0	177.8	169.6	143.6	120.0	102.4	89
Particulate matter (PM)[d]								
PM_{10}	12.2[1]	7.0	6.2	3.6	3.2	3.1	2.3	2
$PM_{2.5}$[e]	NA	NA	NA	NA	2.3	2.2	1.8	2
Sulfur dioxide (SO_2)	31.2	28.0	25.9	23.3	23.1	18.6	16.3	15
Volatile organic compounds (VOCs)	33.7	30.2	30.1	26.9	23.1	21.6	16.9	16
Lead[f]	0.221	0.16	0.074	0.022	0.005	0.004	0.003	0.003
Totals[g]	301.5	275.8	267.2	249.2	218.2	188.0	160.2	141

[a]In 1985 and 1996 EPA refined its methods for estimating emissions. Between 1970 and 1975, EPA revised its methods for estimating particulate matter emissions.

[b]The estimates for 2005 are preliminary.

[c]NO_x estimates prior to 1990 include emissions from fires. Fires would represent a small percentage of the NO_x emissions.

[d]PM estimates do not include condensable PM, or the majority of the $PM_{2.5}$ that is formed in the atmosphere from "precursor" gases such as SO_2 and NO_x.

[e]EPA has not estimated $PM_{2.5}$ emissions prior to 1990.

[f]The 1999 estimate for lead is used to represent 2000 and 2005 because lead estimates do not exist for these years.

[g]$PM_{2.5}$ emissions are not added when calculating the total because they are included in the PM_{10} estimate.

Source: From EPA, 2006.[41]

TABLE 10.4 Air Quality Index for Particle Pollution

Air Quality Index	Air Quality	Health Advisory
0–50	Good	None.
51–100	Moderate	Unusually sensitive people should consider reducing prolonged or heavy exertion.
101–150	Unhealthy for Sensitive Groups	People with heart or lung disease, older adults, and children should reduce prolonged or heavy exertion.
151–200	Unhealthy	People with heart or lung disease, older adults, and children should avoid prolonged or heavy exertion. Everyone else should reduce prolonged or heavy exertion.
201–300	Very Unhealthy	People with heart or lung disease, older adults, and children should avoid all physical activity outdoors. Everyone else should avoid prolonged or heavy exertion.

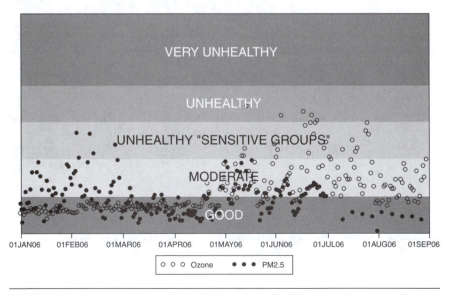

FIGURE 10.7 Daily ozone and $PM_{2.5}$ values for Los Angeles–Long Beach, California, 2006. (*Source:* From EPA, 2006.)[43]

Time Series and Geographical Studies for Monitoring Ambient Air Standards

Two epidemiologic methods for studying air pollution are time series and geographical studies. In this section both of these methods are presented. **Time–series studies** are designed to compare the same population over short periods of time. Their findings relate to short-term (e.g., day-to-day) changes in a contaminant, such as air pollution, on health events (morbidity or mortality counts). **Geographic studies** involving air pollution compare the health events of populations that have had various long-term exposure levels to ambient air pollution. It is also possible to compare the health effects of air pollution in the same population, only at different time periods over an extended length of time.

Time Series

Time–series studies examine how short-term changes in exposures influence health events, such as how daily particulate matter pollution levels are related to daily hospitalization or mortality. For example, time–series studies have found that air pollutants are positively associated with hospitalization for respiratory disease in the neonatal period,[44] hospital admissions,[45] respiratory disease and asthma medication,[46] and premature mortality.[47] Because the unit of analysis is on the group level, usually a city or region, time–series studies are ecologic. However, there is less a concern with confounding than in most ecologic studies because of the temporal nature of time–series studies. Potential confounders operating at short time scales, such as temperature, humidity, influenza, and day of the week, can be controlled by including them as covariates in the regression analysis.[48] Further, because the focus in time–series studies is generally on acute effects resulting in a few days or weeks for the same population, the effect of long-term changes (trends in mortality or climate) have little effect on the results. For example, many risk factors, such as smoking habits, use of gas for cooking, and social class, are unlikely to change over short durations of time because these types of risk factors do not depend on variables such as air pollution levels. However, births, migration, and deaths will change slowly over time and are therefore not considered in the denominators of time–series studies. Hence, daily counts of the health outcome are typically used rather than rates.

Time–series data are commonly used in regression analysis to describe the short-term health effects of air pollution, with possible adjustment for covariates and previous values in the series.[49] The Poisson multiple regression model is commonly used to evaluate time–series data (see Chapter 4). Statistical modeling of time–series data requires special consideration of temporal autocorrelation, over-dispersion, the shape of the exposure–response function, and lags. Temporal autocorrelation occurs when outcome data are correlated from day-to-day; over-dispersion occurs when that outcome data have more variation than predicted by the model; a linear exposure–response function is usually assumed when studying air pollution, but other exposure–response functions may be considered; and lags refer to the time for a pollutant to affect health. Studies investigating the association between PM air pollution and mortality tend to assume a linear dose–response relationship. On the other hand, temperature–mortality relationships are often found to deviate substantially from nonlinearity and lag times up to as much as 2 weeks may be appropriate.[50] In a recent study assessing urban air pollution and respiratory emergency visits at pediatric units in Reggio Emilia, Italy, the strongest associations were observed at lag 3 for 10-mcg/m^3 increase of total suspended particulates and PM_{10}, and at lag 4 for a 10-mcg/m^3 increase of NO_2.[51]

In a study assessing the association between school absenteeism and PM_{10} for six school years, 1985 through 1990, an increase in 28-day moving average PM_{10} equal to 100 mcg/m^3 was associated with an increase in overall absences of approximately 40%.[52] A relationship was observed for all grades, albeit generally greater for grades 1–3 compared with grades 4–6. Associations between absenteeism and PM_{10} pollution occurred with levels below 150 mcg/m^3. In a related study assessing the association between daily changes in respiratory health and PM_{10}, fifth- and sixth grade children who were symptomatic and asymptomatic for respiratory problems were observed.[53] A negative association was observed between peak expiratory flow and PM_{10} for both symptomatic and asymptomatic children, although the association was greater for symptomatic children. Increased PM_{10} concentrations were positively associated with respiratory symptoms, especially coughing. Both immediate and delayed PM_{10} effects were observed on peak expiratory flow and occurred with PM_{10} concentrations below 150 mcg/m^3.

Some challenges to time–series studies include measurement error that results from assuming that every person in a group has the same exposure level and uncontrolled confounding factors, which may bias the results. Bias may also result if people are asked to recall their exposure. The risk of recall bias or differential misclassification is especially present if a group knows it is in a high exposure category. In addition, lack of standardization of equipment for monitoring air pollutants may result in biased results.

Although acute health effects of air pollution can be effectively examined using time–series analysis it is not effective at identifying chronic health effects of air pollution. A difficulty of identifying the overall health effect of air pollution from time–series studies may result from a harvesting effect (mortality displacement), which is when very ill people die only a few days earlier because of the environmental pollution. Over the long term, time–series analysis cannot tell us whether more deaths occur because of the pollution.

The case–crossover design, as presented in Chapter 4, is becoming an increasingly used approach, where the analytic unit of time is the time just preceding the acute event compared with some other time. These time events are referred to as the "case" time and the "control" time, respectively. The design is a good alternative to the conventional time–series design when the exposure is intermittent, the effect on the risk is immediate and transient, and occurrence of the outcome is abrupt.[54,55] To estimate relative risk, exposure frequency during a specified time just before the outcome event occurred is compared with exposure frequency during an earlier time. Here exposure frequencies involve control times instead of control persons. Each person experiencing an event provides one or more control times. A good review of case–crossover studies is provided by Maclure and Mittleman.[54]

In a study assessing the influence of ambient coarse particulate matter on asthma hospitalization in children ages 6 to 12 years old living in Toronto between 1981 and 1993, both case–crossover and time–series analyses were performed. In this study, both analyses revealed that coarse particulate matter averaged over five to six days was significantly associated with asthma hospitalization.[56] Relative risk estimates using case–crossover analysis tended to be more pronounced compared with time–series analysis.

Geographical Studies

Chronic health effects from ambient air pollution cannot be determined from time–series studies because they do not capture long-term trends of disease. Designs appropriate for assessing the long-term health effects of air pollution are cross-sectional and cohort studies where ecologic assignment of exposure is used, based on fixed-site ambient monitors. However, care must be given to their greater susceptibility for confounding. For example, a cross-sectional study involving a random sample of adults ages 18 to 60 years in eight study sites in Switzerland in the 1990s gathered information on respiratory symptoms, and annual mean concentrations of air pollutants were assessed.[57] The study adjusted for the potential confounding effects of age, body mass index, gender, parental asthma, parental atopy, low education, and foreign citizenship. A positive association was found between annual mean concentrations of NO_2, total suspended particulates, and particulates less than 10 micrometers in aerodynamic diameter and reported prevalence of chronic phlegm production, chronic cough or phlegm production, breathlessness at rest during the day, breathlessness during the day or at night, and dyspnea on exertion. Dockery and colleagues examined the relation between particulate air pollution and daily mortality, adjusting for individual risk factors (e.g., smoking).[58] The exposure was classified for each city using air pollution monitoring stations. The study found that fine-particulate air pollution, or a more complex pollution mixture involving fine particulates, contributed to excess mortality in selected U.S. cities. In an extension of this study involving 8 more years of follow-up, cardiovascular, lung cancer, and total mortality were each found to be positively associated with ambient $PM_{2.5}$ concentrations.[59] Pope and colleagues also found a positive association between ambient air pollution and mortality, based on data from 151 metropolitan areas in the United States.[60] In a study conducted by Katsouyanni and colleagues, daily measurements of particulate matter less than 10 micrometers in aerodynamic diameter (PM_{10}) and/or black smoke from 29 European cities were associated with mortality.[61] Ambient particles were shown to increase the risk of mortality.

In their review of epidemiologic studies on the long-term effects of ambient air pollution, Kunzli and Tager found that cohort study designs are most frequently used to measure the relationship between community-based ambient air pollution concentrations and health outcomes such as disease incidence and prevalence and mortality.[62] In general, several people are enrolled in the study from selected communities. Long-term exposure to ambient air pollution is determined using fixed-site monitors. Average levels of community-level pollution are associated with health effects, adjusted for risk factors for individuals measured on the individual level. Studies combining ecologic and individual level data have been termed **semi-ecologic cohort** designs. These studies more readily provide valid inferences to individuals and should not be labeled as ecologic studies.

The "six cities" study referred to above is an example of a semi-ecologic cohort design because air pollution monitoring stations in each city classified the level of air pollution exposure for individuals in the same city. This information was associated with mortality on the individual level. Cox proportional hazards regression modeling was used to compare the mortality experience among the cities while adjusting for potential confounding factors. The results of that study found that the adjusted mortality risk was 26% higher for those in the most polluted city compared with the least polluted city.[58]

Indoor Air Pollution

Over half of the world's population is exposed to indoor air pollution.[63] This is mainly due to burning solid fuels for cooking and heating, such as firewood, charcoal, and cow dung. The most serious indoor air pollutants are particulates, carbon monoxide, polycyclic organic matter, and formaldehyde. Approximately 36% of lower respiratory infections and 22% of chronic obstructive pulmonary disease is attributed to indoor air pollution.

Indoor air pollution is on the rise in many urban areas. Indoor air pollution may originate from within a building or be brought in from outside. The main household sources of VOCs are hair sprays, furniture polish, glues, air fresheners, moth repellents, wood preservatives, and many others. Health effects of household air pollutants include irritation of the eyes, nose, and throat. Headaches, nausea, and loss of coordination occur in more severe cases. Liver damage and harm to other body organs may also occur. In addition, construction of more tightly sealed buildings, reduced ventilation, use of chemical products, pesticides, household-care products, and synthetic materials for building and furnishing can add to or cause "sick building syndrome." Common symptoms of sick building syndrome include headaches, fatigue, inability to concentrate, and mild inflammation of the eyes and pharynx.

Tobacco is one of the largest contributors to indoor air pollution. Tobacco smoke contains more than 60 carcinogens. Many health effects of tobacco smoke occur in the nonsmoking population. This is due to **environmental tobacco smoke (ETS)**, which is that portion of tobacco smoke to which individuals, excluding the smoker, are exposed. ETS has been found to increase cancer rates among nonsmokers.[64] In addition to cancer, ETS can cause burning eyes, nose, and throat; bronchitis; severe asthma; and a decrease in lung function. ETS in homes with children has been shown to be particularly dangerous. ETS increases the prevalence of asthma, wheezing, and chronic bronchitis in children two months to five years of age.[65] The exposure to ETS in children 4 to 12 years of age increased wheezing, the number of children who missed six or more days of school in a year's time, and two lung function measurements (forced expiratory volume and maximal mid-expiratory flow).[66]

Indoor biological pollutants can also cause asthma, hay fever, and other allergic diseases. Biological pollutants include pollen, bacteria, viruses, spores, mold, and parasites. Formaldehyde, a gas that comes mostly from carpets, particle boards, and insulation foam, may also cause irritation to the eyes and nose and allergies. In addition, asbestos, used in building materials, is a risk factor for lung cancer. Finally, radon, a colorless and odorless gas emitted naturally by the soil and found in many homes, is also a risk factor for lung cancer.[67] Selected indoor air pollutants, with their major sources and health effects, are presented in Table 10.5.

TABLE 10.5   Selected Indoor Air Pollutants, Sources, and Health Effects

Indoor air pollutant	Major sources	Health effects
Nitric oxide, nitrogen dioxide	Fuel burning	Lung cancer
Carbon monoxide	Fuel burning	Lung cancer
Carbon dioxide	Metabolic activity, combustion	Asphyxiation in high concentrations, nausea, respiratory problems[a,b]
Pollens/allergens	Trees, grass, weeds, plants, house dust, animal dander, insect parts	Rhinitis,[c] conjunctivitis[c,d]
Particles	Resuspension condensation of vapors, combustion products	Respiratory tract irritation
Water vapor	Biological activity, combustion evaporation	N/A
Organic substances	Combustion, paint, metabolic action, pesticides, adhesives, solvents, cooking, cosmetics	Birth defects,[e] cancer[e,f]
Spores	Fungi, molds	Conjunctivitis, rhinitis[c]
Radon	Underlying soil, water supply, building construction materials (concrete, stone)	Lung cancer[g]
Asbestos, mineral, and synthetic fibers	Fire-retardant materials, insulation	Airway obstruction[h]

TABLE 10.5 Selected Indoor Air Pollutants, Sources, and Health Effects (continued)

Formaldehyde	Particle board, insulation, furnishings, tobacco smoke	Respiratory tract irritation[i]
Ammonia	Metabolic activity, cleaning products, cement	Respiratory tract irritation, pulmonary edema, chemical pneumonitis, eye irritation[a,b]
Polycyclic hydrocarbons, arsenic, nicotine, acrolein, etc.	Tobacco smoke, water	Increased risk of skin, internal organ, and lung cancers; cardiovascular disease; neuropathy; fetal loss, premature delivery, and decreased birth weights; decrease in verbal IQ and long-term memory and suppression of hormone regulation and hormone-mediated gene transcription[j]
Lead	Automobiles, paint	Impaired neurobehavioral development, lower intelligence, reduced birth weight, decreased nerve conduction velocity, anemia[k]
Mercury	Fungicides, paints, spills in dental-care facilities or labs, thermometer breakage	Neurological, nephrological, immunological, cardiac, motor, reproductive, and genetic dysfunction[l]
Aerosols	Consumer products	Respiratory tract irritation, eye irritation, central nervous system damage[m,n]
Infectious agents/ pathogens (viruses, bacteria, parasites)	People, animals, plants	Health effects vary depending on pathogen

[a]MSDS safety data for ammonia, 2006; [b]MSDS ammonia, 2006; [c]Cakmak et al., 2002; [d]Bacsi et al., 2005; [e]Richter & Chlamtac, 2002; [f]Garcia, 2003; [g]Taylor & Taylor, 1997; [h]Delpierre et al., 2002; [i]Arts et al., 2006; [j]Kapaj et al., 2006; [k]Kwong et al., 2004; [l]Zahir et al., 2005; [m]Lectra Clean II Aerosol MSDS, 2006; [n]MSDS aerosol, 2006.[68-81]

In terms of indoor air, the EPA has conducted studies in Baltimore, Maryland, and other cities and observed that the measured indoor air concentration of gasoline constituents (e.g., benzene, toluene, xylene) and other agents were higher in indoor air than in that measured in ambient air immediately outside of the home.[82] In a study involving 112 homes in 56 high-rise apartment buildings with 10 or more stories, both the outdoor and the indoor air concentrations of three VOCs (methyl-tertiary butyl ether [MTBE], benzene, and toluene) were significantly higher for the low-floor apartments than for the high-floor apartments.[83] Further, the indoor concentrations of the target VOCs were higher than the outdoor air concentrations, regardless of the floor level. Specifically, for the low-floor apartments, median outdoor concentrations were 5.4 mcg/m^3 for MTBE, 6.8 mcg/m^3 for benzene, and 29.1 mcg/m^3 for toluene, whereas median indoor concentrations for these VOCs were 6.3, 9.4, and 44.8 mcg/m ^{3}. For the high-floor apartments, median outdoor concentrations were 4.4, 4.3, and 21.9 mcg/m^3, compared with 5.1, 7.6, and 38.8 mcg/m^3 for inside the apartments. As for fine particles, a study comparing median indoor, outdoor, and personal PM$_{2.5}$ mass concentrations for Houston, Texas; Los Angeles, California; and Elizabeth, New Jersey, found slightly lower levels indoors than outdoors or personal (14.4, 15.5, 31.4 mcg/m^3, respectively).[84]

Standards

One of the reasons so many individuals suffer exposure to indoor air pollution is the lack of standards to control indoor pollutants. Because most exposures occur in the home, it is hard to establish clear regulations. Therefore, the EPA has instead suggested several guidelines for controlling indoor air pollution. Because indoor air pollutants pose substantial health risks, these EPA guidelines or standards are aimed at minimizing air pollutants. EPA initiatives include eliminating the use of lead paint, reducing the production and use of carpets containing formaldehyde, banning several asbestos-containing products, encouraging smoke-free homes, and promoting individuals to seek professional help monitoring carbon monoxide, mold, and other air pollutants. Methods to monitor indoor air pollutants will be discussed in the next section.[85–91]

In addition to EPA initiatives, there are a few standards that do exist. These standards include regulations on building specifications and smoking in indoor public places. Because poor ventilation is one of the major causes of indoor air pollution, federal regulations have been established to ensure that adequate ventilation is installed in new buildings. In addition, several states and cities have enacted or are now enacting laws to ban smoking in all indoor public places, including bars, restaurants, and, in some cases, workplaces. Such restrictions are intended to protect all individuals from the ills of secondhand smoke.

Monitoring Indoor Air Pollution

Like standards for indoor air pollution, monitoring indoor air pollution is largely an individual responsibility. However, there are several fairly easy ways to monitor air pollutants indoors. A commonly used way to measure carbon monoxide levels indoors is to install carbon monoxide monitors. Carbon monoxide monitors range from expensive infrared radiation and electrochemical instruments to affordable real-time monitors. Because carbon monoxide is colorless and odorless, these monitors are not only effective in measuring carbon monoxide levels, but warning individuals when levels pose a hazard. The Consumer Product Safety Commission recommends that every home have a carbon monoxide alarm.[88]

Small instruments to measure the level of humidity in indoor spaces are also available to consumers for around $10 to $50. Because high humidity is often the cause of pollutants such as mold and dust mites, monitoring moisture levels in indoor places is an effective way to control air pollutants. The EPA recommends that relative indoor humidity be kept between 30% and 60%. Because mold is also commonly caused by leaky pipes, the EPA recommends that homeowners frequently check around pipes for mold growth. If mold is growing, individuals can isolate the leak and then remove the mold by scrubbing with bleach and water. However, if there is substantial mold or individuals wish to test for mold, professionals should be hired to isolate the mold and analyze it using methods established by the American Industrial Hygiene Association and the American Conference of Governmental Industrial Hygienists.[85,87]

Professionals should be hired when individuals wish to test for asbestos, and possibly radon. However, there are now available to consumers many kinds of low-cost, do-it-yourself radon test kits. Each state has a radon contact that can help arrange radon testing. Often when a home is sold, professionals are hired to check mold, asbestos, and radon levels.[92–93] The EPA has also launched a computer software program to analyze air pollution in large indoor places such as office buildings. The Indoor Air Quality Building Education and Assessment Model, or I-BEAM I, is used by building professionals to assess air pollutants and subsequent health conditions in commercial buildings and then explore ways to mitigate indoor air pollution.[93]

Key Issues

1. The Clean Air Act is a comprehensive federal law that regulates all sources of air pollutant emissions.
2. When monitored concentrations exceed the EPA standards a given number of times over a 3-year period, the area is designated by the EPA as a nonattainment area.
3. Six common air pollutants dangerous to human health and environmental conditions (carbon monoxide, lead, nitrogen dioxide, ozone, particulate matter, and sulfur dioxide) are referred to as criteria pollutants. They are highly regulated and monitored.
4. Time–series studies are designed to compare the same population over short periods of time. Their findings relate to short-term (e.g., day-to-day) changes in a contaminant such as air pollution on health events (morbidity or mortality counts).
5. Geographical studies involving air pollution compare the health events of populations that have had various long-term exposure levels to ambient air pollution.
6. Over half of the world's population is exposed to indoor air pollution. Primary causes are burning solid fuels for cooking and heating, such as firewood, charcoal, and cow dung. The most serious indoor air pollutants are particulates, carbon monoxide, polycyclic organic matter, and formaldehyde.

Exercises

Key Terms

Define the following terms.

> Acid precipitation (rain)
> Air pollution

Carbon monoxide
Clean Air Act
Criteria pollutants
Environmental tobacco smoke
Geographical studies
Ground-level ozone
Lead
Nitrogen oxides
Nonattainment areas
Particulate matter
Semi-ecologic cohort
Small-particle pollution
Smog
Sulfur dioxide
Time–series studies
Transportation conformity

Study Questions

10.1. What is air pollution and what are the six common ambient air pollutants?

10.2. What is the Clean Air Act and how has it evolved in recent years?

10.3. How is ground-level ozone formed? Include the chemical reaction for ground-level ozone and sources of NO_x and VOCs in your discussion.

10.4. Match the following air pollutants with the appropriate description.

Air Pollutants	Description
Ozone _____	a. A colorless, odorless gas that forms when carbon in fuel is not completely burned.
Particulate matter _____	b. A metal found in manufactured products and in the environment.
Carbon monoxide _____	c. A gas that contains nitrogen and oxygen in varying amounts, which often combines with particles in the air to produce a reddish-brown appearance.

    Nitrogen dioxide ____   d. A gas that forms naturally in the stratosphere, but forms from nitrous oxides and volatile organic compounds on the ground.

    Sulfur dioxide ____   e. A complex mixture of extremely small particles and liquid droplets including acids (e.g., nitrates and sulfates), organic chemicals, metals, and soil and dust particles.

    Lead ____   f. A gas that forms when fuel containing sulfur, such as coal and oil, is burned.

10.5. Compare and contrast the two epidemiologic methods for studying air pollution.

10.6. List some common indoor air pollutants and then describe the sources and health outcomes associated with them.

10.7. How can individuals monitor carbon dioxide, mold, and radon levels in their home?

References

1. Blanc PD, Eisner MD, Katz PP, et al. Impact of the home indoor environment on adult asthma and rhinitis. *J Occup Environ Med.* 2006;47(4):362–372.
2. Forsberg B, Hansson HC, Johansson C, Areskoug H, Persson K, Jarvholm B. Comparative health impact assessment of local and regional particulate air pollutants in Scandinavia. *Ambio.* 2005;34(1):11–19.
3. Mendell MJ, Fisk WJ, Kreiss K, et al. Improving the health of workers in indoor environments: priority research needs for a national occupational research agenda. *Am J Public Health.* 2002;92(9):1430–1440.
4. Yu-Peng C, Lin CG, Jong TC. Emissions of particulate and gaseous pollutants within the Keelung Harbor region of Taiwan. *Environ Monit Assess.* 2005; 109(1–3):37–56.
5. Maheswaran R, Haining RP, Pearson T, Law J, Brindley P, Best NG. Outdoor NO_x and stroke mortality: adjusting for small area level smoking prevalence using a Bayesian approach. *Stat Methods Med Res.* 2006;15(5):499–516.
6. Gehring U, Heinrich J, Kramer U, et al. Long-term exposure to ambient air pollution and cardiopulmonary mortality in women. *Epidemiology.* 2006; 17(5):545–551.

7. Inoue K, Takano H, Sakurai M, et al. Pulmonary exposure to diesel exhaust particles enhances coagulatory disturbance with endothelial damage and systemic inflammation related to lung inflammation. *Exp Biol Med (Maywood)*. 2006;231(10):1626–1632.

8. Martins LC, Pereira LA, Lin CA, et al. The effects of air pollution on cardiovascular diseases: lag structures. *Revista de Saude Publica*. 2006;40(4): 677–683.

9. Pattenden S, Hoek G, Braun-Fahrlander C, et al. NO_2 and children's respiratory symptoms in the PATY study. *Occup Environ Med*. 2006;63(12):828–835.

10. Watts J. Doctors blame air pollution for China's asthma increases. *Lancet*. 2006;368(9537):719–720.

11. LeVan TD, Koh WP, Lee HP, Koh D, Yu MC, London SJ. Vapor, dust, and smoke exposure in relation to adult-onset asthma and chronic respiratory symptoms: the Singapore Chinese health study. *Am J Epidemiol*. 2006;163(12): 1118–1128.

12. Viegi G, Maio S, Pistelli F, Baldacci S, Carrozzi L. Epidemiology of chronic obstructive pulmonary disease: health effects of air pollution. *Respirology*. 2006;11(5):523–532.

13. Chiu HF, Cheng MH, Tsai SS, Wu TN, Kuo HW, Yang CY. Outdoor air pollution and female lung cancer in Taiwan. *Inhal Toxicol*. 2006;18(13): 1025–1031.

14. Edwards R, Pless-Mulloli T, Howel D, et al. Does living near heavy industry cause lung cancer in women? a case control study using life grid interviews. *Thorax*. 2006;61(12):1076–1082.

15. Ghedini N, Sabbioni C, Bonazza A, Gobbi G. Chemical-thermal quantitative methodology for carbon speciation in damage layers on building surfaces. *Environ Sci Technol*. 2006;40(3):939–944.

16. Giles J. Hikes in surface ozone could suffocate crops. *Nature*. 2005;435 (7038):7.

17. Lorusso S, Marabelli M, Troili M. Air pollution and the deterioration of historic monuments. *J Environ Pathol Toxicol Oncol*. 1997;16(2–3):171–173.

18. Poma A, Arrizza L, Picozzi P, Spano L. Monitoring urban air particulate matter (fractions PM 2.5 and PM 10) genotoxicity by plant systems and human cells in vitro: a comparative analysis. *Teratog Carcinog Mutagen*. 2002;22(4): 271–284.

19. U.S. Department of the Interior. Environmental compliance: Clean Air Act. Available at: http://www.mms.gov/eppd/compliance/caa/index.htm. Accessed November 28, 2006.

20. Wikipedia: The free encyclopedia. Air pollution. Available at: http://en .wikipedia.org/wiki/Air_pollution. Accessed November 28, 2006.

21. Mueller DW. *Environmental Health*. Cambridge, MA: Harvard University Press; 1992.

22. Environmental Protection Agency. Six common air pollutants: CO: how carbon monoxide affects the way we live and breathe. Available at: http://www .epa.gov/air/urbanair/co/index.html. Accessed July 10, 2006.

23. Environmental Protection Agency. Six common air pollutants: ground-level ozone. Available at: http://www.epa.gov/air/ozonepollution/index.html. Accessed July 10, 2006.

24. Environmental Protection Agency. Six common air pollutants: lead: how lead affects the way we live and breathe. Available at: http://www.epa.gov/air/urbanair/lead/index.html. Accessed July 10, 2006.

25. Environmental Protection Agency. Six common air pollutants: NO_x: how nitrogen oxides affect the way we live and breathe. Available at: http://www.epa.gov/air/urbanair/nox/index.html. Accessed July 10, 2006.

26. Environmental Protection Agency. Six common air pollutants: particulate matter. Available at: http://www.epa.gov/air/particlepollution/index.html. Accessed July 10, 2006.

27. Environmental Protection Agency. Six common air pollutants: SO_2: how sulfur dioxide affects the way we live and breathe. Available at: http://www.epa.gov/air/urbanair/so2/index.html. Accessed July 10, 2006.

28. Environmental Protection Agency. An introduction to indoor air quality: organic gases (volatile organic compounds—VOCs). Available at: http://www.epa.gov/iaq/voc.html#Health%20Effects. Accessed May 30, 2007.

29. Dockery DW. Epidemiologic evidence of cardiovascular effects of particulate air pollution. *Environ Health Perspect.* 2001;109(suppl 4):483–486.

30. Pope CA 3rd, Burnett RT, Thun MJ, et al. Lung cancer, cardiopulmonary mortality, and long-term exposure to fine particulate air pollution. *JAMA.* 2002;287(9):1132–1141.

31. West JJ, Fiore AM, Horowitz LW, Mauzerall DL. Global health benefits of mitigating ozone pollution with methane emission controls. *Proceedings of the National Academy of Sciences U.S.A.* 2006;103(11):3988–3993.

32. American Thoracic Society, Committee of the Environmental and Occupational Health Assembly. Health effects of outdoor air pollution. Part 1. *Am J Respir Crit Care Med.* 1996a;153:3–50.

33. American Thoracic Society. Committee of the Environmental and Occupational Health Assembly. Health effects of outdoor air pollution. Part 2. *Am J Respir Crit Care Med.* 1996b;153:477–498.

34. Bates DV. The effects of air pollution on children. *Environ Health Perspect.* 1995;103(suppl 6):49–53.

35. Environmental Protection Agency. Air quality criteria for ozone and related photochemical oxidants, Vol. III. Publication No. EPA/600/P-93/004a-cF. Research Triangle Park, NC: Environmental Protection Agency; 1996.

36. Environmental Protection Agency. Air quality criteria for particulate matter, Vol. II. Publication No. EPA/600/P-99/002bB. Research Triangle Park, NC: Environmental Protection Agency; 2001.

37. Environmental Protection Agency. The ambient air monitoring program. Available at: http://www.epa.gov/air/oaqps/qa/monprog.html. Accessed June 4, 2007.

38. Environmental Protection Agency. Air and radiation: national ambient air quality standards (40 CFR part 50). Available at: http://www.epa.gov/air/criteria.html. Accessed November 29, 2006.

39. Environmental Protection Agency. Green book: map 8. Available at: http://www.epa.gov/air/oaqps/greenbk/map8hrnm.html. Accessed November 29, 2006.

40. Environmental Protection Agency. Green book: map 25. Available at: http://www.epa.gov/air/oaqps/greenbk/mappm25.html. Accessed November 29, 2006.

41. Environmental Protection Agency. Air trends: air emissions trends: continued progress through 2005. Available at: http://www.epa.gov/airtrends/econ-emissions.html. Accessed November 29, 2006.

42. Environmental Protection Agency. Air quality guide for particle pollution. Available at: http://airnow.gov/index.cfm?action=static.aqguidepart. Accessed June 11, 2007.

43. Environmental Protection Agency. Air explorer. Available at: http://www.epa.gov/airexplorer/. Accessed November 29, 2006.

44. Dales RE, Cakmak S, Doiron MS. Gaseous air pollutants and hospitalization for respiratory disease in the neonatal period. *Environmental Health Perspectives*. 2006;114(11):1751–1754.

45. Gouveia N, Freitas CU, Martins LC, Marcilio IO. Respiratory and cardiovascular hospitalizations associated with air pollution in the city of Sao Paulo, Brazil. *Cadernos de Saude Publica*. 2006;22(12):2669–2677.

46. Pope CA, Dockery DW, Spengler JD, Raizenne ME. Respiratory health and PM10 pollution. a daily time series analysis. *Am Rev Respir Dis*. 1991;144(3 Pt 1):668–674.

47. Bell ML, Peng RD, Dominici F. The exposure-response curve for ozone and risk of mortality and the adequacy of current ozone regulations. *Environ Health Perspect*. 2006;114(4):532–536.

48. Wilkinson P, ed. *Environmental Epidemiology*. New York: Open University Press; 2006.

49. Zeger SL, Irizarry R, Peng RD. On time series analysis of public health and biomedical data. *Annu Rev Public Health*. 2006;27:57–79.

50. Armstrong B. Models for the relationship between ambient temperature and daily mortality. *Epidemiology*. 2006;17(6):624–631.

51. Bedeschi E, Campari C, Candela S, et al. Urban air pollution and respiratory emergency visits at pediatric unit, Reggio Emilia, Italy. *J Toxicol Environ Health A*. 2007;70(3–4):261–265.

52. Ransom MR, Pope CA 3rd. Elementary school absences and PM10 pollution in Utah Valley. *Environ Res*. 1992;58(2):204–219.

53. Pope CA 3rd, Dockery DW. Acute health effect of PM10 pollution on symptomatic and asymptomatic children. *Am Rev Respir Dis*. 1992;145(5):1123–1128.

54. Maclure M, Mittleman MA. Should we use a case-crossover design? *Annu Rev Public Health*. 2000;21:193–221.

55. Jaakkola JJK. Case-crossover design in air pollution epidemiology. *Eur Respir J*. 2003;21:81S–85S.

56. Lin M, Chen Y, Burnett RT, Villeneuve PJ, Krewski D. The influence of ambient coarse particulate matter on asthma hospitalization in children:

case–crossover and time-series analyses. *Environ Helath Perspect.* 2002;110(6): 575–581.

57. Zemp E, Elsasser S, Scindler C, et al. Long-term ambient air pollution and respiratory symptoms in adults (SAPALDIA study). The SAPALDIA team. *Am J Respir Crit Care Med.* 1999;159(4 Pt 1):1257–1266.

58. Dockery DW, Pope CA 3rd, Xu X, et al. An association between air pollution and mortality in six U.S. cities. *N Engl J Med.* 1993;329(24):1753–1759.

59. Laden F, Schwartz J, Speizer FE, Dockery DW. Reduction in fine particulate air pollution and mortality: extended follow-up of the Harvard six cities study. *Am J Respir Crit Care Med.* 2006;173(6):667–672.

60. Pope CA 3rd, Thun MJ, Namboodiri MM, et al. Particulate air pollution as a predictor of mortality in a prospective study of U.S. adults. *Am J Respir Crit Care Med.* 1995;151(3 Pt 1):669–674.

61. Katsouyanni K, Touloumi G, Samoli E, et al. Confounding and effect modification in the short-term effects of ambient particles on total mortality: results from 29 European cities within the APHEA2 project. *Epidemiology.* 2001;12(5):521–531.

62. Kunzli N, Tager IB. The semi-individual study in air pollution epidemiology: A valid design as compared to ecologic studies. *Environ Health Perspect.* 1997;105(10):1078–1083.

63. World Health Organization. *World Health Report 2002: Reducing Risks, Promoting Healthy Life.* Geneva; 2002.

64. Hecht S. Tobacco carcinogens, their biomarkers and tobacco-induced cancer. *Cancer.* 2003;3:733–745.

65. Gergen PJ, Fowler JA, Maurer KR, Davis WW, Overpeck MD. The burden of environmental tobacco smoke exposure on the respiratory health of children 2 months through 5 years of age in the United States: Third National Health and Nutrition Examination Survey, 1988 to 1994. *Pediatrics.* 1998; 101(2):8–14.

66. Mannino D, Moorman J, Kingsley B, Rose D, Repace J. Health effects related to environmental tobacco smoke exposure in children in the United States. *Arch Pediatr Adolesc Med.* 2001;155(1):36–41.

67. Indoor Air Pollution. Available at: http://edugreen.teri.res.in/explore/air/indoor.htm. Accessed November 29, 2006.

68. MSDS 841—aerosol. Available at: http://www.lessemf.com/285.html. Accessed December 1, 2006.

69. MSDS for ammonia. Available at: http://www.vngas.com/. Accessed December 1, 2006.

70. Cakmak S, Dales RE, Burnett RT, Jadek S, Coates F, Brook JR. Effect of airborne allergens on emergency visits by children for conjunctivitis and rhinitis. *Lancet.* 2002;359(9310):947–948.

71. Bacsi A, Dharajiya N, Choudhury BK, Sur S, Boldogh I. Effect of pollen-mediated oxidative stress on immediate hypersensitivity reactions and late-phase inflammation in allergic conjunctivitis. *J Allergy Clin Immunol.* 2005; 116(4):836–843.

72. Richter E, Chlamtac N. Ames, pesticides, and cancer revisited. *International Journal of Occupational and Environmental Health.* 2002;8(1):63–72.

73. Garcia A. Pesticide exposure and women's health. *Am J Indust Med.* 2003; 44:584–594.

74. Taylor D, Taylor S. Environmental uranium and human health. *Rev Environ Health.* 1997;12:147–157.

75. Delpierre S, Delvolgo-Gori M, Faucher M, Jammes Y. High prevalence of reversible airway obstruction in asbestos-exposed workers. *Arch Environ Health.* 2002;57(5):441–447.

76. Arts J, Rennen M, De Heer C. Inhaled formaldehyde: evaluation of sensory irritation in relation to carcinogenicity. *Regul Toxicol Pharmacol.* 2006;44(2): 144–160.

77. Kapaj S, Peterson H, Liber K, Bhattacharya P. Human health effects from chronic arsenic poisoning—a review. *Journal of Environmental Science and Health Part A—Toxic/Hazardous Substances and Environmental Engineering.* 2006;41(10):2399–2428.

78. Kwong WT, Friello P, Semba RD. Interactions between iron deficiency and lead poisoning; epidemiology and pathogenesis. *Sci Total Environ.* 2004;330 (1–3):21–37.

79. Zahir F, Rizwi SJ, Haq SK, Khan RH. Low dose mercury toxicity and human health. *Environ Toxicol Pharmcol.* 2005;20(2):351–360.

80. Lectra Clean II Aerosol MSDS. Available at: http://msds.ehs.cornell.edu/msds/msdsdod/a177/m88247.htm#Section3. Accessed December 1, 2006.

81. MSDS—Safety data for ammonia (anhydrous). Available at: http://physchem.ox.ac.uk/MSDS/. Accessed December 1, 2006.

82. Payne-Sturges DC, Burke TA, Breysse P, Diener-West M, Buckley TJ. Personal exposure meets risk assessment: a comparison of measured and modeled exposure and risks in an urban community. *Environ Health Perspect.* 2004; 112(5):589–598.

83. Jo WK, Kim KY, Park KH, Kim YK, Lee HW, Park JK. Comparison of outdoor and indoor mobile source-related volatile organic compounds between low- and high-floor apartments. *Environ Res.* 2003;92(2):166–171.

84. Meng QY, Turpin BJ, Korn L, et al. Influence of ambient (outdoor) sources on residential indoor and personal PM2 concentrations: analyses of RIOPA data. *J Expo Anal Environ Epidemiol.* 2005;15(1):17–28.

85. Environmental Protection Agency. A brief guide to mold, moisture, and your home. Available at: http://www.epa.gov/mold/preventionandcontrol.html#Testing%20or%20Sampling%20for%20Mold. Accessed November 30, 2006.

86. Environmental Protection Agency. An introduction to indoor air quality: asbestos. Available at: http://www.epa.gov/iaq/asbestos.html. Accessed November 30, 2006.

87. Environmental Protection Agency. An introduction to indoor air quality: biological pollutants. Available at: http://www.epa.gov/iaq/biologic.html. Accessed November 30, 2006.

88. Environmental Protection Agency. An introduction to indoor air quality: carbon monoxide. Available at: http://www.epa.gov/iaq/co.html#Steps%20to%20Reduce%20Exposure%20to%20Carbon%20Monoxide. Accessed November 30, 2006.

89. Environmental Protection Agency. An introduction to indoor air quality: formaldehyde. Available at: http://www.epa.gov/iaq/formalde.html. Accessed November 30, 2006.

90. Environmental Protection Agency. An introduction to indoor air quality: lead. Available at: http://www.epa.gov/iaq/lead.html#Steps%20to%20Reduce%20Exposure%20to%20Lead. Accessed November 30, 2006.

91. Environmental Protection Agency. An introduction to indoor air quality: nitrogen dioxide. Available at: http://www.epa.gov/iaq/no2.html#Standards%20or%20Guidelines. Accessed November 30, 2006.

92. Environmental Protection Agency. Who can test or fix your home for radon? Available at: http://www.epa.gov/radon/radontest.html. Accessed November 30, 2006.

93. Environmental Protection Agency. Overview of I-BEAM text modules and visual reference modules. Available at: http://www.epa.gov/iaq/largebldgs/i-beam_html/ibeam.htm. Accessed November 30, 2006.

Soil and Food Contaminants and Health

LEARNING OBJECTIVES

After completing this chapter, you should be able to:

1. Identify soil-contaminating chemicals.
2. Identify soil-contaminating biologic agents.
3. Identify the effects of acid rain on soil, the environment, and human health.
4. Identify some monitoring efforts to avoid soil contamination.

Introduction

Identifying the influence of contaminated soil on human health is often difficult given that direct ingestion of soil is typically rare. However, certain occupations may result in direct exposure to contaminated soil, such as contaminated dust in the air being inhaled. Contaminated soil may further serve as a vehicle to contaminate plants and animals that, in turn, are ingested by people. For example, lead is a pollutant that enters the environment through automobile and industrial emissions, lead-based paint, solder, and old lead pipes.[1,2] Once in the atmosphere, lead eventually deposits in water and on soil. Lead deposited on soils can bind to other dusts, clays, hydrous oxides, and humic and fulvic acids. Lead-polluted soil has the potential to be absorbed and recycled into plants (home gardening, general agriculture), then animals (grazing animals), and eventually humans.[3] For example, lead may be present in topsoil, hay, silage, and the blood of cows from farms located near a former lead mine or a smelting plant operating without filters.[4,5] Children are most susceptible to direct lead exposure through contact with contaminated soil while playing, or from exposure to lead dust from lead-based paint.[6] Even low levels of lead exposure over a long period of time can be dangerous to children.

Food contaminants harmful to human health involve two broad groups of chemicals and biologic agents. Chemicals such as lead, cadmium, mercury, sodium, phosphates, nitrites, nitrates, and organic compounds and biologic agents such as bacteria, viruses, parasites, mold, and toxins may contaminate food at various stages: growing, processing, preparation, and storage. Chemicals, including toxins, may occur naturally or be introduced by human activities of food production and processing. Bacterial and viral infections and fungi may directly contaminate food or produce toxins harmful to human health. During 1998–2002, 6,647 outbreaks of foodborne diseases were reported in the United States to the Centers for Disease Control and Prevention (CDC).[7] These outbreaks corresponded to 128,370 people becoming ill. The etiology of disease was identified in 33% of the reported outbreaks. Bacterial pathogens were associated with 55% of the outbreaks, viral pathogens (mainly norovirus) were associated with 33% of the outbreaks, chemical agents caused 10% of the outbreaks, and parasitic pathogens were associated with 1% of the outbreaks.

Contaminants to soil can be physically or chemically attached to soil particles or be trapped between soil particles. Soil contamination can result from a hazardous substance that is spilled or buried in the soil or migrates to the soil from elsewhere. In addition, a factory may release hazardous substances into the air that are subsequently deposited on surrounding soil. Sewage is another example of a hazardous substance that can contaminate soil. Once soil is contaminated, plants may take up the hazardous contaminants through their roots, which, in turn, can adversely affect the health of animals and humans as previously described. The purpose of this chapter is to identify hazardous substances that may contaminate soil and affect the health of animals and humans.

Chemical Contaminants

Chemical contaminants may be defined as chemicals that pose an unacceptable threat to human health and/or the environment. Epidemiologic research has identified certain chemicals as sources of foodborne illness, including metals, fertilizers, pesticides, intentional food additives, and other chemical residues. Although some chemicals are beneficial to food production, abnormally high levels of beneficial chemicals can contaminate food and be harmful to humans. Chemical foodborne illness is called **chemical poisoning**.

Metals

Metals often identified as potential causes of chemical poisoning include arsenic, antimony, cadmium, lead, and mercury. Source of metal poisoning has been traced primarily to food-handling equipment and utensils, although hazardous metals can be absorbed directly into plants and animals. Most of these metal poisonings manifest themselves with digestive disorders such as nausea and abdominal pain. Lead and mercury poisoning cause neurological symptoms rather than digestive disorders. Common **heavy metals** that can adversely affect human health because of their toxicity at certain concentrations are discussed here.

Arsenic is a semimetal element that is odorless and tasteless and is widely distributed throughout the earth's crust. Arsenic tends to bind strongly to soil and can remain near the surface for hundreds of years. High levels of arsenic may be found in soil where crops were treated with arsenic pesticides, as well as some waste sites. Most exposure to arsenic occurs by swallowing arsenic in water, soil, dust, or food. Children are sometimes exposed to arsenic by eating dirt, or putting arsenic-contaminated pacifiers, toys, hands, and other items in their mouths. Arsenic-contaminated soil and dust may also be ingested through activities like gardening, mowing, construction work, and dusting. In addition, arsenic can be ingested by eating vegetables with soil on them that contains arsenic. Currently, arsenic is the top-ranked hazardous substance on the Agency for Toxic Substances and Disease Registry/Environmental Protection Agency [EPA] priority list.[8,9]

Several epidemiologic studies have reported health effects associated with arsenic. For example, subchronic arsenic exposure in young children, primarily from drinking water in developing countries, generally results in gastrointestinal, neurological, and skin effects. Some cases also experience facial edema and cardiac arrhythmia. Dermatoses (cutaneous abnormality) are consistently reported in adults and children with subchronic exposure. The severity of the disease typically increases with length of exposure and arsenic dose.[10] Arsenic has also been linked to cancer of the bladder, lung, skin, kidneys, nasal passages, liver, and prostate.[11,12]

Reliable data on arsenic exposure are rarely available, but many locations have concentrations of arsenic in their drinking water greater than the EPA maximum arsenic contaminant level in drinking water of 0.01 mg/L, including Argentina, Australia, Bangladesh, Chile, China, Hungary, India, Mexico, Peru, Thailand, and the United States. For example, 7 of 16 districts of West Bengal, India, have been reported to have groundwater arsenic concentrations exceeding 0.05 mg/L. The population using arsenic-rich water is greater than 1 million for 0.05 mg/L and 1.3 million for levels above 0.01 mg/L.[13,14] A 1998 British geological survey of shallow tube-wells in 61 of 64 districts in Bangladesh shows that 46% were above 0.1 mg/L and 27% were above 0.5 mg/L. An estimated 46 to 57 million people were exposed to arsenic concentrations above 0.01 mg/L, and 28 to 35 million people were exposed to concentrations above 0.05 mg/L in 1999.[15] In the United States, an estimated 13 million people, primarily in the western states, are exposed to arsenic at 0.01 mg/L. The EPA has required that water systems must comply with the 0.01 mg/L standard by January 23, 2006.[16] A more complete discussion of arsenic in drinking water is provided by the World Health Organization.[17]

Antimony is a metallic element used in alloys that often enters soil or sediment, where it attaches strongly with particles such as iron, manganese, or aluminum. However, some antimony is weakly attached to particles and can therefore be taken up by plants and animals. Exposure to antimony can be through eating foods, drinking water, breathing air contaminated by it, or being exposed by skin contact with contaminated soil, water, or other substances. The fate of antimony once released to soil is unclear (i.e., whether it is highly mobile in soils or strongly absorbs to soil). Antimony poisoning is similar to arsenic poisoning. It is toxic and irritating to skin and mucous membranes, and in the short term may cause headaches, dizziness, depression, nausea, vomiting, and diarrhea. The primary effects from chronic exposure to antimony are respiratory (i.e., inflammation of the lungs, chronic bronchitis, and chronic emphysema). Studies are inconclusive regarding its relation to cancer, and the EPA has not classified antimony for carcinogenicity.[18,19]

Everyone is exposed to antimony at low levels throughout the environment. Exposure levels are highest near factories where antimony ores are converted into metal. In the United States in 2006, antimony uses were estimated to be 40% flame retardants; 22% transportation, including batteries; 14% chemicals; 11% ceramics and glass; and 13% other. There was no domestic mine production of antimony in 2006. In 2006, recycling of lead-acid batteries was the only antimony production from domestic source materials in this country. In 2004, antimony smelters in New Jersey and Texas were closed and now only one domestic smelter, in Montana, makes antimony products. In the United States, resources of antimony are primarily located in Alaska, Idaho, Montana, and Nevada, and in some antimony resources in Mississippi Valley–type lead deposits in the eastern part of the country. Worldwide, principal resources of antimony are in Bolivia, China, Mexico, Russia, and South Africa.[20]

Low concentrations of antimony are generally found in soil (i.e., less than 1 part per million), although higher concentrations have been identified at hazardous-waste sites and antimony-processing sites. Personal exposure to antimony can be measured in the urine, feces, and blood.[21]

Cadmium is a metallic element that is primarily the result of burning fossil fuels. It can also be emitted into the air from zinc, lead, or copper smelters. Cadmium can bind with soil and be taken up in plants that are later ingested by people.[22,23] Smoking also increases exposure to cadmium. Among nonsmokers, food is a primary source of cadmium, with increased levels in foods grown with phosphate fertilizers or sewage sludge applied to farm fields. In addition to these potential exposure sources, discarded batteries may be a point of exposure.[21] Acute inhalation exposure at high levels can affect the lungs, potentially resulting in long-lasting impairment.[21,24,25] Chronic exposure to cadmium can result in kidney disease, respiratory disease, reduction of sperm count, and decreased birth weights in children of exposed women.[21] Cadmium also increases the risk of kidney cancer and is a possible prostate carcinogen.[26–29]

In a U.S. study of cadmium based on data from the Third National Health and Nutrition Examination Survey (NHANES III 1988–1994), urine cadmium increased with age and with smoking. Approximately 2.3% of the U.S. population has urine cadmium concentrations greater than 2 mcg/g creatinine, and 0.2% has concentrations greater than 5 mcg/g creatinine, which are the World Health Organization health-based exposure limits.[30]

Lead is another natural element harmful to humans if inhaled or ingested, as discussed previously. Exposure may result from lead-contaminated water, soil, paint chips, or dust; ingestion of food that contains lead from soil or water; or inhalation of lead-containing particles of soil or dust in air. Drinking water may be contaminated by lead pipes, metal vessels, pottery glazes, fungicides, lead-based paint, and leaded gasoline. Lead may also be deposited in water and on soil where it can be absorbed and recycled into plants (home gardening, general agriculture), then animals (grazing animals), and eventually humans. Lead poisoning has been associated with many health problems. Early symptoms may include persistent fatigue, irritability, loss of appetite, stomach discomfort and/or constipation, and reduced attention span. Long-term damage in adults can include poor muscle coordination, nerve damage, high blood pressure, hearing and vision impairment, reproductive problems, kidney cancer, and retarded fetal development, even at low exposure levels. In children, brain damage and/or mental retardation, behavioral problems, anemia, liver and kidney damage, hearing loss, hyperactivity, developmental delays, and death may occur.[11,12,31]

Eliminating blood lead levels greater than or equal to 10 mcg/dL in children is a national health objective for 2010. Based on data from the NHANES, there has been a steep decline in the percentage of children ages 1–5 years with blood lead levels this high, 77.8% in 1976–1980 to 4.4% in 1991–1994. Although children in minority populations had comparatively higher levels of blood lead levels, the latest NHANES data collected in 1999–2002 show a continued decrease in blood lead levels for all racial/ethnic populations: the overall prevalence in the U.S. population 1 year of age and older was 0.7%.[32]

Mercury is a neurotoxin. Mercury is a naturally occurring element and can be emitted from power plants and other sources. Mercury can accumulate in soil, streams, and oceans. In time, bacteria can cause chemical changes that transform mercury into methylmercury in soils and water. Like other contaminated soils, soils containing mercury can be a source of mercury poisoning in children as a result of hand-to-mouth activity.[33] Mercury accumulation in soils can be absorbed into plants and later ingested by animals and humans.[34] The most common way people in the United States are exposed to mercury is by eating fish and shellfish (primarily shark, swordfish, king mackerel, or tilefish) that have been contaminated by methylmercury.[35] Dental amalgams contribute very little to human mercury exposure. Exposure to mercury can cause immune, sensory, neurological, motor, and behavior dysfunctions.[36,37]

Mercury exposure in the United States is estimated to occur in approximately 6% to 8% of the 16- to 49-year-old age group, according to data from NHANES.[38] In another study, Asian, Pacific Islander, Native American, and multiracial women had higher prevalence of elevated blood mercury than all other racial/ethnic groups; that is, on the basis of NHANES data, 16.59 +/– 4.0% (mean +/– SE) of adult Asian, Pacific Islander, Native American, and multiracial females had blood mercury levels greater than or equal to 5.8 mcg/L, and 27.26 +/– 4.22% had levels greater than or equal to 3.5 mcg/L. Among other women evaluated, 5.08 +/– 0.90% had blood mercury levels greater than or equal to 5.8 mcg/L, and 10.86 +/– 1.45% had levels greater than or equal to 3.5 mcg/L.[39]

History of Minamata Disease

Minamata disease (also called Chisso-Minamata disease) is a neurologic syndrome resulting from severe mercury poisoning. Symptoms for the disease include ataxia, numbness in hands and feet, general muscle weakness, narrowing of the field of vision, and damage to hearing and speech. Insanity, paralysis, coma, and death may result in extreme cases within weeks of the initial symptoms. The disease may also affect the fetus in the womb.

Minamata disease is named after Minamata city in Kumamoto prefecture, Japan, where the disease was first discovered in 1956. The cause of the disease was methylmercury released in the industrial wastewater from the Chisso Corporation's chemical factory, from 1932 through 1968. On April 21, 1956, a 5-year-old girl presented puzzling symptoms: difficulty walking and speaking and convulsions. A few days later, her younger sister was hospitalized with similar symptoms, and on May 1, the hospital director reported an epidemic of an unknown disease of the central nervous system. Loss of sensation in the hands and feet of patients was also observed, with many unable to grasp small objects or fasten buttons.

It was discovered that victims of the disease were clustered in fishing hamlets around Minamata Bay and that their primary food was fish and shellfish from the bay. Cats and dogs that ate scraps of food from the family table tended to manifest similar symptoms as those found in people. Food poisoning from fish and shellfish was identified as the most likely cause of the illness. On November 4, 1956, Minamata disease was determined to be caused by heavy metal poisoning through consumption of contaminated fish and shellfish.

In February 1959, large quantities of mercury were detected in fish, shellfish, and sludge from Minamata Bay, with the highest concentrations around the Chisso factory wastewater canal in Hyakken Harbour. Thus, the factory was identified as the source of the contamination. Nevertheless, the government and factory did little to prevent the mercury pollution of the bay. Up through March 2001, 2,265 victims of the disease had been officially recognized, with 1,784 having died. Over 10,000 victims have received financial compensation from the Chisso Corporation. Today legal actions continue against Chisso.[40–42]

Fertilizers

Fertilizers are used to add nutrients such as nitrogen, phosphorus, and potassium to soil to enhance the quantity and quality of crop production. Some fertilizers also contain micronutrients such as iron, zinc, and other metals, which are known to enhance plant growth.[43] Like most chemicals, fertilizers are beneficial in moderation but can cause harm if used improperly. For example, nitrogen fertilizers contain nitrates and nitrites that are needed to grow vegetables, but that can also adversely affect health if used excessively: nitrates and nitrites in soil can migrate into drinking-water supplies. Drinking water contaminated with nitrates is known to cause methoglobinemia, a condition in which oxygen is not adequately distributed throughout the body. Because children are especially susceptible to methoglobinemia, it is also known as "blue baby syndrome."[44] Further, after nitrate is converted to nitrite in the body, it may react with amine-containing substances in food that form nitrosamines, which are potent carcinogens.

A positive association has been found in 11 cohorts and 50 case-control studies between nitrite and nitrosamine intake and gastric cancer, but results were inconclusive on the relationship between nitrite and nitrosamine and oesophageal cancer.[45] Some studies have associated nitrates in drinking water with non-Hodgkin's lymphoma.[46] A cohort study conducted in Germany found a significant association between nitrate load in drinking water and the incidence of urothelial cancer in both men and women.[47] A population-based case-control study found no association between long-term water nitrate at levels below 10 mg/L and pancreatic cancer but significant increased risk of pancreatic cancer with increased consumption of dietary nitrate through animal sources.[48] Results from an ecologic study found a significant positive relationship between nitrate levels in drinking water and risk of bladder cancer mortality.[49] However, results of a cohort study conducted in the Netherlands and a case-control study of bladder cancer in Iowa found no association between nitrate exposure and bladder cancer risk.[50,51]

Besides ingestion of contaminated water, fertilizer contaminants can enter the body through direct ingestion of soil, indirect ingestion of contaminated food or meat from animals that were fed contaminated food, inhalation, or absorption through skin. Although poisonings from fertilizers are rare, other health outcomes linked to fertilizers include those outlined in the section on metal contaminants.[52]

Pesticides

Pesticides control or prevent damage to crops by insect infestation. They are known poisons that include insecticides, fungicides, herbicides, bactericides, nematicides, growth regulators, fumigants, and fertilizers. Because pesticides are designed to be toxic, they can also harm humans if used improperly. Most cases of pesticide poisoning occur among agricultural workers. Pesticides enter the workers' bodies primarily through inhalation, absorption through skin, or ingestion. The general population can also suffer pesticide poisoning by ingesting organic contaminants in food that stem primarily from pesticides. It is also possible for pesticide sprayed from an airplane, tractor, or home sprayer to drift or blow onto people who live, work, or go to school near agricultural or related sites. There are three specific forms of pesticide poisoning: organophosphorus poisoning, carbamate poisoning, and chlorinated hydrocarbon poisoning.

Organophosphates and carbamates cause neurological damage by disrupting the enzyme that regulates the neurotransmitter acetylcholine.[53] Other health outcomes of pesticide poisoning include hypertension, bronchospasms and coughing, nausea and vomiting, abdominal cramps, diarrhea, blurred vision, and non-Hodgkin's lymphoma.[46,54] Chlorinated hydrocarbons, a class of synthetic chemicals first produced in the 1930s, are commonly used in pesticides (e.g., DDT). They resist degradation and can be concentrated to poisonous levels in the fatty tissues of animals and humans.

To help protect the more than 2.5 million workers in the United States who handle pesticides, the EPA created the Worker Protection Standard for Agricultural Pesticides (WPS). The WPS restricts the type and quantity of pesticides that can be used; identifies proper safety equipment and clothing; requires all employees who work with or near pesticides to be informed of when and where use occurs; and mandates that all employees who work with or near pesticides receive special training to cover hazards, safety precautions, and emergency procedures. In addition, EPA regulations protect consumers by restricting the type and quantity of pesticides used and requiring all old and new pesticides to be registered with the EPA for analysis.[55]

Food Contaminants

Food contaminants are metals or chemicals (e.g., mercury, pesticides, herbicides, aflatoxins) that make food dangerous for humans if consumed. The previous section focused on chemicals such as lead, cadmium, mercury, sodium, phosphates, nitrites, and nitrates, which affect soil and plants at the growing and processing stage. Food additives and food preparation can also introduce hazardous chemicals into food. In addition, biologic agents such as bacteria and viruses may also negatively affect food.

Food Additives and Chemical Residues

Food additives are substances that are intentionally or unintentionally added to a food product during its processing or production. Intentional food additives have various functions: to enhance flavor, color, aroma, and texture; improve nutritional value; reduce or prevent spoilage; and prevent growth of infectious agents. However, food additives can also have adverse effects. For example, monosodium glutamate, a food seasoning, may cause a burning sensation in the back or neck, forearms, or chest; and tingling, feelings of tightness, flushing, dizziness, headaches, and nausea in sensitive people. Highly sulfited foods or beverages may cause asthma in sensitive individuals. Overfortified or inadequately mixed foods containing nicotinic acid (niacin) can cause flushing, warm sensation, itching, stomach pain, and puffing of face and knees. Excessive nitrification of foods, soils, or water can cause nausea, vomiting, cyanosis, dizziness, weakness, loss of consciousness, and chocolate-brown-colored blood. Some food dyes, such as red 3, have been linked to cancer, noncancerous tumors, and allergies. Certain fat and sugar additives have also been found to be detrimental to health. For example, olestra, a fat substitute, may cause severe diarrhea and abdominal cramps, and stevia, a natural sweetener, may cause cancer.[56]

Some chemicals used in maintaining sanitary food handling (i.e., detergents, cleaning compounds, drain cleaners, polishes, and sanitizers) can contaminate foods if surfaces used for food preparation are improperly rinsed after cleaning. Sodium hydroxide is the most common type of poisoning resulting in foodborne illness. Signs and symptoms of the illness include burning of lips, mouth, and throat; vomiting; abdominal pain; and diarrhea.[57]

Biologic Agents

Biological contaminants are living organisms or their associated toxins. These contaminants include bacteria, viruses, fungi, molds, and house dust. Biological contaminants can be found in water, soil, plants, and animals. They are also common in various occupational settings. Biologic agents may affect food in several ways and affect human health by producing allergic reactions, serious medical conditions, or even death. Table 11.1 presents selected bacteria responsible for foodborne illnesses, along with their connection with habitat and symptoms. In addition, touching food with dirty hands is one way that bacteria and viruses can spread. This is a common form of transmission for enteropathogenic E. coli, salmonellosis, shigellosis (bacillic dysentery), Norwalk virus, amebiasis (amebic dysentery), clostridium perfringens, and typhoid.

TABLE 11.1   Selected Bacteria That Can Exist in Soil or Plants and Affect Human Health

Bacteria	Description	Habitat	Symptoms
Clostridium perfringens	Produces a spore and prefers low-oxygen atmosphere; live cells must be ingested; capable of producing food poisoning	Soil, dust, or feces, held under conditions that permit multiplication of the organism (inadequately cooked or reheated meats)	Cramps and diarrhea within 12 to 24 hours
Clostridium botulinum	Produces a spore and prefers low-oxygen atmosphere; produces a heat-sensitive toxin	Soils, plants, marine sediments, fish	Double vision, blurred vision, drooping eyelids, slurred speech, difficulty swallowing, dry mouth, muscle weakness
Baccillus cereus	Produces a spore and grows in normal oxygen atmosphere	Soil, dust, spices	Mild case of diarrhea and some nausea within 12 to 24 hours
Listeria monocytogenes	Resistant to adverse conditions for long periods of time	Soil, vegetation, water; can survive for long periods in soil and plant materials	Mimics meningitis; immuno-compromised individuals most susceptible

(*continues*)

TABLE 11.1   Selected Bacteria That Can Exist in Soil or Plants and Affect Human Health (continued)

Bacteria	Description	Habitat	Symptoms
Giardiasis	Parasite called Giardia lamblia	Passed in the feces of an infected person or animal; outside the body it is protected by an outer shell; ability to survive in soil, water, food, or surfaces for long periods of time; can become infected by ingesting the parasite	Mild or severe diarrhea, abdominal cramps, bloating, fatigue
Tularemia	Francisella tularensis	Meat, soil, water; can infect humans through mucous membranes, gastrointestinal tract, lungs, skin	Skin ulcers, swollen and painful lymph glands, sore throat, diarrhea or pneumonia, mouth sores, inflamed eyes; inhaling the bacteria can result in abrupt onset of fever, chills, headache, muscle aches, joint pain, dry cough, progressive weakness

(*Source:* Adapted from Wagner, 2006.)[58]

Genetically Modified Food

"Genetic modification" and "biotechnology" are interchangeable terms that refer to a special set of technologies that alter the genetic makeup of living organisms. Recombinant DNA technology refers to the combination of genes from different organisms. The resulting organism is then "genetically modified" or "genetically engineered." In 2003, approximately 167 million acres of genetically modified crops were grown by 7 million farmers in 18 countries. The principal crops were herbicide- and insecticide-resistant soybeans, corn, cotton, and canola. Other crops included virus-resistant sweet potatoes, rice with increased iron and vitamins, and several plants better able to survive extreme weather conditions. In 2003, the countries with about 99% of worldwide genetically modified crops were the United States (63%), Argentina (21%), Canada (6%), Brazil (4%), China (4%), and South Africa (1%). In the future, genetically modified foods are expected to include bananas that produce human vaccines against infectious diseases (e.g., hepatitis B) and fruit and nut trees that yield years earlier. Use of genetically modified foods is expected to plateau in developed countries but increase in developing countries.[59]

Some of the possible benefits of genetically modified food include (1) enhanced taste and quality; (2) reduced maturation time; (3) increased nutrients, yields, and stress tolerance; (4) improved resistance to disease, pests, and herbicides; and (5) improved growing techniques. Environmental benefits include (1) "friendly" bioherbicides and bioinsecticides; (2) conservation of soil, water, and energy; (3) bioprocessing for forestry products; (4) better natural waste management; and (5) more efficient processing. From a societal perspective, we may expect increased food security for growing populations.[59]

There are many controversies that surround genetically modified foods. They may affect human health because of allergens, transfer of antibiotic resistance markers, and for yet unknown reasons. Genetically modified plants may accidentally increase naturally occurring toxins (e.g., solanine). Perhaps a novel toxicity could result, as found with genetically modified potatoes.[60] Genetically modified crops may also harm the ecosystem.[61] Corn engineered to contain the insecticidal toxin from *Bacillus thuringiensis* (Bt) may be associated with death in monarch butterfly caterpillars, [62] although the validity of this study has been questioned.[63] Research has shown that the Bt toxin may leach through plant roots into the soil and there can bind to soil particles, possibly harming soil microorganisms in the short run and causing a disruption to soil ecology.[64,65]

Some possible solutions to these environmental hazards associated with genetically modified crops have been suggested. For example, genes are exchanged between plants via pollen. To ensure that nontarget species will not receive introduced genes from genetically modified plants, a genetically modified plant can be made to be male sterile (i.e., does not produce pollen) or to have pollen that does not contain the introduced gene.[66–68] Creating buffer zones around areas with genetically modified crops has also been suggested.[69,70] However, space restrictions may make this approach infeasible.

Acidic Deposition

An **acid** is a substance that can provide hydrogen ions (H^+) in chemical reactions, whereas bases are substances capable of accepting hydrogen ions in chemical reactions. The **pH scale** is a measure of the acidity of a substance, which ranges from pH 0 (very acidic) to pH 7 (neutral) to pH 14 (basic) (see Figure 11.1). Movement down the scale by 1 unit refers to a tenfold increase in acidity. As pH moves down the scale, the concentration of H^+ ions increases; as the pH moves up the scale, the concentration of H^+ ions decreases.

It is possible for some airborne pollutants produced by smelters, transportation (cars, trucks, and trains), coal-fired electrical power plants, and gas-processing plants to be chemically transformed into acid compounds (see Figure 11.2). The main pollutants producing acidic deposition are sulphur dioxide (SO_2) and oxides of nitrogen (NO_x). In the United States, approximately two-thirds of SO_2 and a quarter of all NO_x come from generating electrical power by burning fossil fuels such as coal. Acid deposition occurs when acidic pollutants in the air are deposited on the ground. **Acid deposition** has two parts: wet and dry. Wet deposition

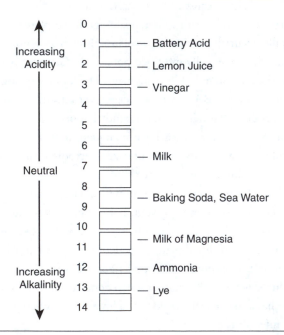

FIGURE 11.1   pH scale. (*Source:* From Environment Canada, 2006.)[71]

falls to earth by mixing with rain or fog, forming mild acids, or by mixing with snow or hail, forming sulfuric and nitric acids as they melt. Sunlight tends to increase the rate of these reactions. Dry deposition refers to particles that form an acid as they mix with water in lakes and rivers and as dry deposition of gases and particles. Prevailing winds can blow the compounds, causing wet and dry acid deposition over hundreds of miles.[72]

Acid deposition has a variety of effects in different areas. In some areas there are natural mechanisms that neutralize acidic deposition (e.g., soils containing limestone that reacts with acidic deposition to neutralize it). "Neutralize" refers to a base being added to an acid until the pH is 7. Acid deposition mixing with rain (**acid rain**) that falls on the leaves of plants interferes with transpiration, and the acid can enter the leaves. Transpiration is the loss of water by evaporation through the stems and leaves of plants. The plant produces food and maintains rigidity through this vital process. Acid deposition can also produce changes in the normal chemistry of soil by leaching important minerals from the soil such as calcium, magnesium, potassium, and sodium. Subsequent reactions of acids with other chemicals in soil can create toxic metals (e.g., aluminum, manganese, mercury, cadmium, and lead),

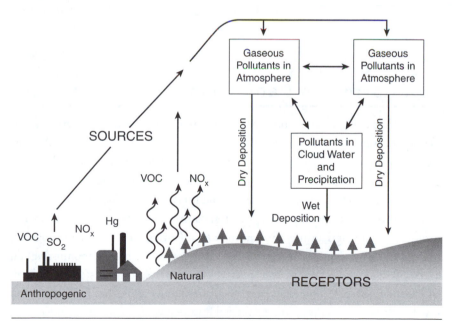

FIGURE 11.2 Acid rain. (*Source:* From EPA, 2006.)[72]

which are more soluble and can be absorbed more readily into plants. Acidic deposition can alter decomposition, limiting important nutrients to plants and damage fish and other living organisms, materials, and human health.

Besides directly affecting crop production, acid rain also affects ecosystems. Most lakes have pH near 8. Lakes possess a natural neutralizing ability to acidic decomposition. Yet long-term exposure to acidic decomposition (e.g., toxic metals like aluminum, mercury, cadmium, and lead) washed into lakes from contaminated soils or from acid rain can lower pH to harmful levels. At pH 7, the carbonates in the water decrease in ability to neutralize acid. At pH 6, microorganisms that play a role in decomposing organic debris on the bottom of the lake die and plankton declines. At pH 5.5 to pH 6, most insect and fish species cannot reproduce and algae mats begin to form along the shoreline. At more extreme pH levels, toxic metals collect in fish and other aquatic life, making them dangerous for human consumption. At pH 4, most fish, frogs, and insects are dead.[73]

Acid rain is measured using the pH scale. Normal rain dissolves some carbon dioxide, resulting in a pH of roughly 5.6. The level of pH in pure water is 7. Acid rain in the range of 4.2 to 5.0 has been recorded in most of the eastern United States and Canada. Examples of pH values in common consumables are carrots (pH is 5.0), bananas (4.6), tomatoes (4.2), apples and soft drinks (3.0), and lemon juice (2.0).[74]

Monitoring Soil and Food

Chemicals in soil can pose serious health risks to children and have become a regulatory focus in the United States. Both the EPA and the Food and Drug Administration (FDA) have jurisdiction over programs to monitor soil and food quality. The EPA operates several programs such as the National Pesticide Information Center, which conducts pesticide research and houses Green Chemistry, a pesticide registry that partners with private chemical companies to mitigate pollution and promote healthy agriculture; the Antimicrobial Pesticide Hotline; and programs on lead and asbestoses. A complete list of EPA programs aimed at monitoring soil and food can be found online at http://www.epa.gov/epahome/pestoxpgram.htm. In addition, the EPA enforces several regulations, including the WPS; the Food Quality Protection Act of 1996; the Federal Insecticide, Fungicide, and Rodenticide Act; and the Federal Food, Drug, and Cosmetic Act. A complete list of EPA laws and regulations can be found online at http://www.epa.gov/epahome/laws.htm. The FDA houses National Food Safety Programs including FoodNet, in which the FDA teams up with the CDC and U.S. Department of Agriculture to track food-borne illnesses; programs to test microbial diseases among vegetables such as sprouts; and reports to the president that track compliance with FDA regulations from "farm to table." A complete list of FDA activities to ensure quality food can be found online at http://www.cfsan.fda.gov/~mow/foodborn.html. Acid rain and its contributing chemicals are monitored by the National Atmospheric Deposition Program, which measures wet deposition, and the Clean Air Status and Trends Network, which measures dry deposition.

Within each EPA and FDA program, epidemiological studies are conducted to assess soil and food quality, test new methods to reduce disease, and affirm compliance with national regulations. Epidemiologic studies assessing soil exposures should take into account peak, average, or cumulative exposures. In turn, this information can assist in determining the association between exposure and disease. Once the exposure is linked to the disease, epidemiologic studies should explore methods of chemical exposure, including metabolic studies of ingested plants, characterization of chemical transformation, and measurement of residues. For example, studies should consider estimates of consumption of contaminated foods and fish. After epidemiologic surveys are conducted, programs should be initiated or altered to incorporate all relevant soil, food, and airborne safety measures.

Key Issues

1. Food contaminants harmful to human health involve two broad groups of metals, fertilizers, pesticides, intentional food additives, other chemical residues, and biologic agents.

2. Abnormally high levels of beneficial chemicals can contaminate food and be harmful to humans. Chemical foodborne illness is called chemical poisoning.

3. Touching food with dirty hands is one way that bacteria and viruses can spread from the intestine. This is a common form of transmission for enteropathogenic E. coli, salmonellosis, shigellosis (bacillic dysentery), Norwalk virus, amebiasis (amebic dysentery), clostridium perfringens, and typhoid.

4. Some common bacteria that can exist in soil or plants and affect human health include clostridium perfringens, clostridium, botulinum, baccillus cereus, listeria monocytogenes, giardiasis, and tularemia.

5. Acidic deposition can alter decomposition, limiting important nutrients to plants and damaging fish and other living things, materials, and human health.

Exercises

Key Terms

Define the following terms.

Acid
Acid deposition
Acid rain
Biological contaminants
Chemical contaminants
Chemical poisoning
Fertilizers
Food additives
Food contaminants
Heavy metals
Pesticides
pH scale

Study Questions

11.1. What are the two broad groups of food contaminants? Provide at least four examples for each group.

11.2. List five metals that pose environmental health hazards. Discuss sources and health outcomes associated with two of those metals.

11.3. How are fertilizers both beneficial and harmful to the environment and one's health?

11.4. Describe the three types of pesticide poisoning.

11.5. What concept is missing from the following statement? "Food additives are substances that are intentionally added to a food product during its processing or production."

11.6. What viruses or bacteria are commonly spread through touching food with dirty hands?

11.7. What is acid deposition?

11.8. What programs and laws have been established to monitor contamination of soil and food in the United States?

References

1. Schutz A, Barregard L, Sallsten G, et al. Blood lead in Uruguayan children and possible sources of exposure. *Environ Res.* 1997;74(1):17–23.
2. Srianujata S. Lead—the toxic metal to stay with human. *J Toxicol Sci.* 1998; 23(supp 2):237–240.
3. Sharpe RT, Livesey CT. Lead poisoning in cattle and its implications for food safety. *Vety Rec.* 2006;159(3):71–74.
4. Kachur AN, Arzhanova VS, Yelpatyevsky PV, von Braun MC, von Lindern IH. Environmental conditions in the Rudnaya River watershed—a compilation of Soviet and post-Soviet era sampling around a lead smelter in the Russian Far East. *Sci Total Environ.* 2003;303(1–2):171–185.
5. Zadnik T. Lead in topsoil, hay, silage and blood of cows from farms near a former lead mine and current smelting plant before and after installation of filters. *Vet Hum Toxicol.* 2004;46(5):287–290.
6. Lanphear BP, Succop P, Roda S, Henningsen G. The effect of soil abatement on blood lead levels in children living near a former smelting and milling operation. *Public Health Rep.* 2003;118(2):83–91.
7. Lynch M, Painter J, Woodruff R, Braden C. Surveillance for foodborne-disease outbreaks—United States, 1998–2002. *MMWR.* 2006;55(10):1–42.
8. Belluck DA, Benjamin SL, Baveye P, Sampson J, Johnson B. Widespread arsenic contamination of soils in residential areas and public spaces: an emerging regulatory or medical crisis? *Int J Toxicol.* 2006;2:109–128.
9. Chou CH, De Rosa CT. Case studies—arsenic. *Int J Hyg Environ Health.* 2003;206(4–5):381–386.
10. Tsuji JS, Benson R, Schoof RA, Hook GC. Health effect levels for risk assessment of childhood exposure to arsenic. *Regul Toxicol Pharmacol.* 2004; 39(2):99–110.
11. International Agency for Research on Cancer. Overall evaluations of carcinogenicity: An updating of IARC monographs (Vols. 1–42, IARC Monographs Supplement 7). Geneva: International Agency for Research on Cancer; 1987.
12. Environmental Protection Agency. Addressing lead at superfund sites. Available at: http://www.epa.gov/superfund/lead/health.htm#Lead. Accessed November 28, 2006.
13. Chowdhury TR, Mandal BK, Samanta G, Basu GK, Chowdhury PP, Chanda CR. Arsenic in groundwater in seven districts of West Bengal, India—the biggest arsenic calamity in the world: the status report up to August 1995. In:

Abernathy CO, Calderon RL, Chappell WR, eds. *Arsenic: Exposure and Health Effects*. New York, NY: Chapman and Hall; 1997.

14. Mandal BK, Chowdhury TR, Samanta G, et al. Chronic arsenic toxicity in West Bengal. *Curr Sci*. 1997;72(2):114–117.

15. British Geological Survey. The groundwater arsenic problem in Bangladesh—background to Phase 2. Available at: http://www.bgs.ac.uk/arsenic/bangladesh/. Accessed June 6, 2007.

16. Environmental Protection Agency. Arsenic in drinking water. Available at: http://www.epa.gov/safewater/arsenic/basicinformation.html. Accessed June 6, 2007.

17. World Health Organization. Arsenic in drinking water. Available at: http://www.who.int/mediacentre/factsheets/fs210/en/. Accessed June 5, 2007.

18. Environmental Protection Agency. Technology transfer network air toxics: antimony compounds 2000. Available at: http://www.epa.gov/ttn/atw/hlthef/antimony.html. Accessed November 28, 2006.

19. Gebel T. Suppression of arsenic-induced chromosome mutagenicity by antimony. *Mutat Res*. 1998;412(3):213–218.

20. U.S. Geological Survey, Mineral Commodity Summaries, January 2007. Available at: http://minerals.usgs.gov/minerals/pubs/commodity/antimony/antimmcs07.pdf. Accessed June 6, 2007.

21. Agency for Toxic Substances and Disease Registry. *Toxicological Profile for Cadmium. Draft for Public Comment*. Atlanta, GA: U.S. Department of Health and Human Services; 1997.

22. Muller M, Anke M. Distribution of cadmium in the food chain (soil-plant-human) of a cadmium exposed area and the health risks of the general population. *Sci Total Environ*. 1994;156(2):151–158.

23. Shute T, Macfie SM. Cadmium and zinc accumulation in soybean: a threat to food safety? *Sci Total Environ*. 2006;371(1–3):63–73.

24. Calíbrese EJ, Kenyon EM. *Air Toxics and Risk Assessment*. Chelsea, MI: Lewis Publishers; 1991.

25. U.S. Department of Health and Human Services (US DHHS). Hazardous Substances Data Bank (HSDB, online database). National Toxicology Information Program, National Library of Medicine, Bethesda, MD; 1993.

26. Hallenbeck WH. Human health effects of exposure to cadmium. *Experientia*. 1984;40(2):136–142.

27. Maclure M. Asbestos and renal adenocarcinoma: a case control study. *Environ Res*. 1987;42:353–361.

28. Dekernion JB, Smith RB. The kidney and adrenal glands. In: Paulson DR, ed. *Genitourinary Surgery*. New York, NY: Churchill Livingstone; 1984.

29. *Stedman's Medical Dictionary for the Health Professions and Nursing*. 5th ed. New York, NY: Lippincott Williams & Wilkins; 2005.

30. Paschal DC, Burt V, Caudill SP, et al. Exposure of the U.S. population aged 6 years and older to cadmium: 1988–1994. *Arch Environ Contam Toxicol*. 2000;38(3):377–383.

31. Stewart WF, Schwartz BS, Davatzikos C, et al. Past adult lead exposure is linked to neurodegeneration measured by brain MRI. *Neurology*. 2006;66(10): 1476–1484.

32. Centers for Disease Control and Prevention. Blood lead levels—United States, 1999–2002. *MMWR*. 2005;54(20):513–516.

33. Maramba NP, Reyes JP, Francisco-Rivera AT, et al. Environmental and human exposure assessment monitoring of communities near an abandoned mercury mine in the Philippines: a toxic legacy. *J Environ Manage*. 2006; 81(2):135–145.

34. Molina JA, Oyarzun R, Esbri JM, Higueras P. Mercury accumulation in soils and plants in the Almaden mining district, Spain: one of the most contaminated sites on Earth. *Environ Geochem Health*. 2006;28(5):487–498.

35. Zhang L, Wong MH. Environmental mercury contamination in China: Sources and impacts. *Environ Int*. 2007;33(1):108–121.

36. Boguszewska A, Pasternak K. Mercury-influence on biochemical processes of the human organism. *Annales Universitatis Mariae Curie-Sk_odowska. Sectio D: Medicina*. 2004;59(2):524–527.

37. Environmental Protection Agency. Mercury. 2006. Available at: http://www .epa.gov/mercury/exposure.htm#3. Accessed November 28, 2006.

38. Mahaffey KR. Mercury exposure: medical and public health issues. *Trans Am Clin Climatol Assoc*. 2005;116:127–153. Discussion 153–154.

39. Hightower JM, O'Hare A, Hernandez GT. Blood mercury reporting in NHANES: identifying Asian, Pacific Islander, Native American, and multiracial groups. *Environ Health Perspect*. 2006;114(2):173–175.

40. Wikipedia: The free encyclopedia. Minamata disease. Available at: http://en .wikipedia.org/wiki/Minamata_disease. Accessed June 6, 2007.

41. Ministry of the Environment, Government of Japan. Minamata disease: the history and measures. Available at: http://www.env.go.jp/en/chemi/hs/minamata 2002/. Accessed June 6, 2007.

42. Harada M. Minamata disease: methylmercury poisoning in Japan caused by environmental pollution. *Crit Rev Toxi*. 1995;25:1–24.

43. Environmental Protection Agency. Nutrient management and fertilizer. Available at: http://www.epa.gov/agriculture/tfer.html. Accessed June 12, 2007.

44. Nitrates in drinking water. Available at: http://www.co.missoula.mt.us/measures/Nitrates.htm. Accessed November 22, 2006.

45. Jakszyn P, Gonzalez CA. Nitrosamine and related food intake and gastric and oesophageal cancer risk: a systematic review of the epidemiological evidence. *World J Gastroenterol*. 2006;12(27):4296–4303.

46. Pearce N, McLean D. Agricultural exposures and non-Hodgkin's lymphoma. Discussion 5-7. *Scand J Work Environ Health*. 2005;31(suppl 1):18–25.

47. Volkmer BG, Ernst B, Simon J, et al. Influence of nitrate levels in drinking water on urological malignancies: a community-based cohort study. *BJU Int*. 2005;95(7):972–976.

48. Coss A, Cantor KP, Reif JS, Lynch CF, Ward MH. Pancreatic cancer and drinking water and dietary sources of nitrate and nitrite. *Am J Epidemiol.* 2004; 159(7):693–701.

49. Chiu HF, Tsai SS, Yang CY. Nitrate in drinking water and risk of death from bladder cancer: an ecological case-control study in Taiwan. *J Toxicol Environ Health A.* 2007;70(12):1000–1004.

50. Zeegers MP, Selen RF, Kleinjans JC, Goldbohm RA, van den Brandt PA. Nitrate intake does not influence bladder cancer risk: the Netherlands cohort study. *Environ Health Perspect.* 2006;114(10):1527–1531.

51. Ward MH, Cantor KP, Riley D, Merkle S, Lynch CF. Nitrate in public water supplies and risk of bladder cancer. *Epidemiology.* 2003;14(2):183–190.

52. Environmental Protection Agency. Estimating risk from contaminants contained in agricultural fertilizers. Available at: http://www.epa.gov/epaoswer/hazwaste/recycle/fertiliz/risk/report.pdf. Accessed November 24, 2006.

53. Environmental Protection Agency. Types of pesticides. Available at: http://www.epa.gov/pesticides/about/types.htm. Accessed November 22, 2006.

54. Joshi S, Biswas B, Malla G. Management of organophosphorus poisoning. 2006. Available at: http://www.nda.ox.ac.uk/wfsa/html/u19/u1913_01.htm. Accessed November 22, 2006.

55. Environmental Protection Agency. Worker protection standard for Agricultural pesticides. Available at: http://www.epa.gov/agriculture/twor.html. Accessed November 22, 2006.

56. Center for Science in the Public Interest. Food safety: food additives. Available at: http://www.cspinet.org/reports/chemcuisine.htm. Accessed November 27, 2006.

57. Tybor PT, Hurst WC, Reynolds E, Schuler GA. Preventing chemical foodborne illness. Available at: http://pubs.caes.uga.edu/caespubs/pubcd/b1042-w.html. Accessed November 28, 2006.

58. Wagner AB. Bacterial food poisoning. Available at: http://aggie-horticulture.tamu.edu/extension/poison.html. Accessed November 28, 2006.

59. Human Genome Project Information. Genetically modified foods and organisms. Available at: http://www.ornl.gov/sci/techresources/Human_Genome/elsi/gmfood.shtml. Accessed June 5, 2007.

60. Ewen SWB, Pusztai A. Effects of diets containing genetically modified potatoes expressing *Galanthus nivalis* lectin on rat small intestine. *Lancet.* 1999; 354:1353–1354.

61. Ferber D. GM crops in the cross hairs. *Science.* 1999;286:1662–1666.

62. Losey JE, Rayor LS, Carter ME. Transgenic pollen harms monarch larvae. *Nature.* 1999;399(6733):214.

63. Niiler E. GM corn poses little threat to monarch. *Nat Biotechnol.* 1999;17: 1154.

64. Saxena D, Flores S, Stotzky G. Insecticidal toxin in root exudates from Bt corn. *Nature.* 1999;402:480.

65. Mulder C, Wouterse M, Raubuch M, Roelofs W, Rutgers M. Can transgenic maize affect soil microbial communities? *PLoS Comput Biol.* 2006;2(9):e128.

66. Daniell H, Datta R, Varma S, Gray S, Lee SB. Containment of herbicide resistance through genetic engineering of the chloroplast genome. *Nat Biotechnol*. 1998;16(4):345–348.

67. Daniell H. New tools for chloroplast genetic engineering. *Nat Biotechnol*. 1999;17(9):855–856.

68. Gressel J. Tandem constructs: preventing the rise of superweeds. *Trends Biotechnol*. 1999;17(9):361–366.

69. Huang F, Buschman LL, Higgins RA, McGaughey WH. Inheritance of resistance to *Bacillus thuringiensis* toxin (DiPel ES) in the European corn borer. *Science*. 1999;284(5416):965–967.

70. Shen FF, Yu YJ, Zhang XK, Bi JJ, Yin CY. Bt gene flow of transgeic cotton. *Yi Chuan Xue Bao*. 2001;28(6):562–567.

71. Environment Canada. Acid rain and the facts. Available at: http://www.ec.gc.ca/acidrain/acidfact.html. Accessed November 28, 2006.

72. Environmental Protection Agency. What is acid rain? Available at: http://www.epa.gov/airmarkets/acidrain/what/index.html. Accessed November 28, 2006.

73. Alberta Environment. Focus on acidic deposition. Alberta, Canada: Crown Copyright; 1993. Available at: http://environment.gov.ab.ca/info/library/Focus_On_Acidic_Deposition.pdf. Accessed December 11, 2006.

74. Elmhurst College. Virtual chembook. Available at: http://www.elmhurst.edu/~chm/vchembook/190acidrain.html. Accessed November 28, 2006.

Water and Health

LEARNING OBJECTIVES

After completing this chapter, you should be able to:

1. Describe the water cycle.
2. Identify selected functions of water in the human body.
3. Identify common diseases associated with water.
4. Define "water pollution" and identify its primary causes.
5. Identify water-monitoring efforts in the United States.

Introduction

The scientific term for **water** is H_2O. It is a clear, odorless, tasteless liquid present in all living things. The smallest possible amount of water consists of a single molecule made up of two hydrogen atoms that attach to a single oxygen atom. The hydrogen atoms have a positive electrical charge, and the oxygen atom has a negative charge. Opposite charges attract such that the charges on the ends of the water molecule attract other water molecules, thereby forming water drops. This is why water sticks together in rivers, oceans, lakes, and your bathtub. Water is the only thing on earth that can take the form of a liquid (rivers, lakes, and ocean), a solid (snow and ice), or a gas (vapor or steam). Water solidifies at 32°F (0°C) and boils at 212°F (100°C) and dissolves more substances than any other liquid.

The surface of the earth consists mostly of water—about 70%. Water is also found underground and in the atmosphere. Of the earth's water, 97% is saltwater, 2% is frozen in ice caps and glaciers, and only 1% is freshwater useful for agriculture, industry, and domestic purposes. Of this small percentage of freshwater, half is below the surface of the earth. It is a limited resource that continually cycles from the earth's surface to the air and then back again to the ground. Water evaporates as heat energy from the sun causes surface water to form into a gas and to rise into the air. When the water cools in the air, it changes into tiny droplets to form clouds. **Condensation** occurs when water changes from a gas to a liquid, resulting in the formation of clouds or steam. Under the right conditions, water eventually falls from clouds in a liquid or solid state (**precipitation**), soaking into the earth's surface or flowing over land in streams, rivers, lakes, and wetlands.

A number of drinking water contaminants have been identified that adversely affect health, including bacteria (coliform bacteria, fecal coliform, E. coli) and parasites (cryptosporidium, giardia); radionuclides (alpha emitters, beta/photon emitters, combined radium 226/228, radon); inorganic contaminants (arsenic, fluoride, lead); synthetic organic contaminants (pesticides and herbicides); volatile organic contaminants; disinfectants (chlorine, choramine, chorine dioxide); and disinfection by-products (total trihalomethanes, haloacetic acids, bromate, chlorite).[1] Water from aquifers (groundwater) is generally microbiologically safe because the water that enters aquifers from the surface is filtered as it passes through several meters of earth. On the other hand, such water is often hard, containing calcium ions, or it may have arsenic, iron, manganese, or other chemicals that may be dangerous to one's health. Surface water in lakes and rivers may not be microbiologically safe because of organic and fecal materials. This is particularly true in farming areas. Surface waters may also be turbid from fine soil particles or colored by natural dyes and acids from decomposing vegetation.[2] In the United States, more than 83 contaminants are monitored. These contaminants are monitored at varying schedules and at different locations throughout the water system.

Water treatment technology and processes are used to address microbiological, chemical, and aesthetic contaminants in raw water. Municipal/public water treatment systems, particularly those that use surface waters as the source water involve a series of steps: (1) removing solids, (2) filtration, (3) disinfection (chlorination/ozonation), and (4) final water treatments (e.g., fluoride, corrosion protection, water softeners).

The purpose of this chapter is to describe the role of water in human health, identify common waterborne diseases, and discuss some of the monitoring efforts used to ensure that safe water standards are met.

Water and Health

All forms of life depend on water. About 70% of human body weight is water. The human brain is 85% water, blood is 82% water, and lungs are 90% water. Dehydration can result in a mere 2% drop in the body's water supply, resulting in fuzzy short-term memory, trouble with basic math, and difficulty focusing on smaller print. Water is vital to cell and organ functions and for healthy living. The U.S. National Research Council recommends that men consume about 3.7 liters of water each day and women about 2.7 liters, in beverages and food.[3]

Some functions of water in the human body follow:

- Water serves as a lubricant.
- Water forms the base for saliva.
- Water forms the fluids that surround the joints.
- Water regulates the body temperature, as the cooling and heating is distributed through perspiration.
- Water helps to alleviate constipation by moving food through the intestinal tract and thereby eliminating waste—the best detox agent.
- Water regulates metabolism.[4]

Health problems can arise by ingesting contaminated water (drinking the water, eating food that has lived in the water) as well as through airborne exposures from materials that can outgas during showering, bathing, swimming, or cooking. It can also be absorbed through the skin. Hence, estimates of exposure from water should take into account airborne exposures related to outgas from water exposure and skin exposure from water. Epidemiologic research has shown that contaminated water can lead to many diseases with multifactorial etiology. It can cause cardiac defects; spontaneous abortions; various cancers; damage to neurological, hepatic, and immunologic functions; and congenital malformations.[5–7]

Waterborne diseases are infectious diseases that are spread primarily through contaminated water. These diseases can be contracted directly or indirectly through exposure to infected vectors, but water is the primary medium for their spreading.

Intestinal (enteric) diseases are generally infectious, transmitted through fecal waste. **Pathogens** are bacteria, viruses, protozoa, or parasitic worms capable of producing diseases. Pathogens are often found in feces of infected persons. Infectious diseases are those where the pathogen is capable of entering, surviving, and multiplying in the host. Such diseases are more common in areas with poor sanitary conditions. Pathogens can travel through water and directly affect persons exposed to the water. Diarrhea, hepatitis, cholera, and typhoid are the more common waterborne diseases, and they occur more frequently in tropical regions of the world.

In addition, several chemicals, both human-made and naturally existing dissolve in water, polluting the water and producing disease among those exposed.

A list of common diseases associated with water is presented in Table 12.1.

TABLE 12.1   Diseases Associated with Water and Their Sources

Disease	Description	Source
Anemia	A condition that occurs when the red blood cells do not carry enough oxygen to the tissues of the body. Several infections related to hygiene, sanitation, safe water, and water management are significant contributors to anemia in addition to iron deficiency. These include malaria, schistosomiasis, and hookworm.	Malnutrition and waterborne or water-related infections; disinfectants in drinking water to kill germs drunk in excess (chloramine, chlorine dioxide)

TABLE 12.1   Diseases Associated with Water and Their Sources (continued)

Disease	Description	Source
Arsenic	Many waters contain some arsenic, and excessive concentrations are known to naturally occur in some areas. Drinking arsenic-rich water over a long period results in various health effects including skin problems (such as color changes on the skin and hard patches on the palms and soles of the feet); skin cancer; cancers of the bladder, kidney, and lung; and diseases of the blood vessels of the legs and feet; and possibly diabetes, high blood pressure, and reproductive disorders.	Arsenic in drinking water. Arsenic contamination in water may also be due to industrial processes such as those involved in mining, metal refining, and timber treatment. Malnutrition may aggravate the effects of arsenic in blood vessels.
Ascariasis	An infection of the small intestine caused by *Ascaris lumbricoides*, a large roundworm. The eggs of the worm are found in soil contaminated by human feces or in uncooked food contaminated by soil containing eggs of the worm. A person becomes infected after accidentally swallowing the eggs.	Eating uncooked food grown in contaminated soil or irrigated with inadequately treated wastewater.
Cancer	Bladder, renal, rectal	Disinfection by-products added to drinking water to kill germs that react with naturally occurring organic matter in water (trihalomethanes, haloacetic acids, bromate)
Campylobacteriosis	Campylobacteriosis is an infection (a bacterium, usually *Campylobacter jejuni* or *C. coli*) of the gastrointestinal tract.	Consumption of contaminated food such as undercooked meats, contaminated water, or raw milk

(continues)

TABLE 12.1 Diseases Associated with Water and Their Sources (continued)

Disease	Description	Source
Cholera	An acute infection of the intestine caused by the bacterium *Vibrio cholerae*	Eating food or drinking water that has been contaminated by the feces of infected persons; raw or undercooked seafood infection in areas where cholera is prevalent and sanitation is poor; vegetables and fruit that have been washed with water contaminated by sewage
Cyanobacterial toxins	Bacteria with symptoms that include skin irritation, stomach cramps, vomiting, nausea, diarrhea, fever, sore throat, headache, muscle and joint pain, blisters of the mouth, and liver damage. Swimmers in water containing cyanobacterial toxins may suffer allergic reactions.	People may be exposed to cyanobacterial toxins by drinking or bathing in contaminated water. The most frequent and serious health effects are caused by drinking water containing the toxins (cyanobacteria), or by ingestion during recreational water contact.
Dengue fever	The clinical features of dengue fever vary according to the age of the patient. Infants and young children may have a feverish illness with rash. Older children and adults may have either a mild feverish illness, or the classical incapacitating disease with abrupt onset and high fever, severe headache, pain behind the eyes, muscle and joint pains, and rash.	Mosquito-borne infection where the mosquitoes find breeding opportunities in small water collections in and around houses: drinking-water containers, discarded car tires, flower vases, and ant traps are well-known breeding places.
Diarrhea	Gastrointestinal infections	Caused by a host of bacterial, viral, and parasitic organisms most of which can be spread by contaminated water (e.g., fecal coliform and *E. coli, cryptosporidium, giardia lamblia*).

TABLE 12.1   Diseases Associated with Water and Their Sources (continued)

Disease	Description	Source
Fluorosis	Ingestion of excess fluoride, most commonly in drinking water, can cause fluorosis, which affects the teeth and bones. Moderate amounts lead to dental effects, but long-term ingestion of large amounts can lead to potentially severe skeletal problems. Severe enamel fluorosis occurs in approximately 10% of children in the United States with water fluoride concentrations at or near 4 mg/L. Paradoxically, low levels of fluoride intake help to prevent dental caries.	The most common cause is contaminated drinking water.
Guinea-worm disease (dracunculiasis)	Guinea-worm disease is a debilitating and painful infection caused by a large nematode (roundworm), *Dracunculus medinensis*.	Infected water
Hepatitis	Broad term for inflammation of the liver	Number of infectious and noninfectious causes. Two of the viruses that cause hepatitis (hepatitis A and E) can be transmitted through water and food; hygiene is therefore important in their control.
Japanese encephalitis	Viral disease that infects animals and humans causing inflammation of the membranes around the brain	Mosquito-borne infection where the mosquitoes find breeding opportunities in small water collections in and around houses: drinking-water containers, discarded car tires, flower vases, and ant traps are well-known breeding places.

(continues)

TABLE 12.1   Diseases Associated with Water and Their Sources (continued)

Disease	Description	Source
Lead poisoning	Too much lead can damage various systems of the body including the nervous and reproductive systems and the kidneys, and it can cause high blood pressure and anemia. Lead accumulates in the bones and lead poisoning may be diagnosed from a blue line around the gums. Lead is especially harmful to the developing brains of fetuses and young children and to pregnant women. Lead interferes with the metabolism of calcium and Vitamin D.	Exposure to lead through water is generally low in comparison with exposure through air or food. The main source of lead in drinking water is (old) lead piping and lead solders.
Leptospirosis	Bacterial disease	Human infection occurs through direct contact with the urine of infected animals or by contact with a urine-contaminated environment, such as surface water, soil, and plants.
Malaria	World's most common parasitic infectious disease	Transmitted by mosquitoes that breed in fresh or occasionally brackish water.
Malnutrition	Characterized by inadequate or excess intake of protein, energy, and micronutrients such as vitamins, and the frequent infections and disorders that result	Water supply, sanitation and hygiene, given their direct impact on infectious disease, especially diarrhea, are important for preventing malnutrition.
Methaemoglobinaemia	Decreased ability of blood to carry vital oxygen around the body	The most common cause is high levels of nitrates in drinking water.
Onchocerciasis or river blindness	Parasitic disease caused by *Onchocerca volvulus*, a thin parasitic worm that can live for up to 14 years in the human body. The disease is transmitted from one person to another through the bite of a blackfly (*Simulium*).	The blackfly lays its eggs in the water of fast-flowing rivers.

TABLE 12.1   Diseases Associated with Water and Their Sources (continued)

Disease	Description	Source
Ringworm or tinea	Typically mild disease of the skin, scalp, or nails caused by a fungus	The link with water is via poor personal domestic hygiene and shortage of water for cleaning and washing.
Scabies	A contagious skin infection that spreads rapidly in crowded conditions and is found worldwide.	Personal hygiene is an important preventive measure, and access to adequate water supply is important in control.
Schistosomiasis	A water-based disease that is considered the second most important parasitic infection after malaria in terms of public health and economic impact. The signs following infection are rashes or itchy skin.	Infection occurs when free-swimming larvae penetrate human skin.
Trachoma	An infection of the eyes that may result in blindness after repeated re-infections	Primary interventions advocated for preventing trachoma infection include improved sanitation, reduction of fly-breeding sites, and increased facial cleanliness (with clean water) among children at risk of disease.
Typhoid and paratyphoid fevers	Infections caused by bacteria that are transmitted from feces to ingestion. Caused by the bacteria *Salmonella typhi* and *Salmonella paratyphi*, respectively. Typhoid and paratyphoid germs are passed in the feces and urine of infected people.	Clean water, hygiene, and good sanitation prevent the spread of typhoid and paratyphoid. Contaminated water is one of the pathways of transmission of the disease.

(*Source:* Modified from EPA, 2006; WHO, 2006.)[1,8]

To further illustrate, let's consider the connection between drinking arsenic-rich water over a long period and cancer. An older study conducted among residents in an endemic area of chronic arsenic exposure on the southwest coast of Taiwan found a dose–response relationship between arsenic levels in drinking water and mortality from lung cancer, bladder cancer, and kidney cancer.[9] Studies in the United States and Argentina have found a synergistic effect between smoking and high levels of arsenic exposure in water and the risk of bladder cancer.[10,11] In another study involving arsenic in drinking-water wells in Finland, bladder cancer was associated with arsenic concentrations and daily dose during the third to ninth years preceding the cancer diagnosis.[12] Futher, a study conducted in Cordoba, Argentina, found evidence that arsenic ingestion increases the risk of lung and kidney cancers.[13]

Arsenic in drinking water has also been associated with skin cancer. In a study conducted by the Wisconsin Division of Public Health in 19 rural townships, a high percentage of private drinking-water wells contained traces of arsenic. There were 2,233 household wells tested, with 6,669 residents providing information on water consumption and health. Median arsenic level was 2.0 microg/L, with 80% of the wells below the federal drinking-water standard of 10 mcg/L, but 11% had an arsenic level of above 20 mcg/L. Residents at least 35 years of age who had consumed arsenic-contaminated water for at least 10 years were significantly more likely to have a history of skin cancer than others. Tobacco use, which was also associated with increased risk of skin cancer, had a synergistic effect with arsenic producing an even higher risk of skin cancer.[14]

Among waterborne diseases, diarrhea has the largest impact on the world's health. The largest waterborne disease outbreak in the United States in which diarrhea was a primary symptom occurred in Milwaukee in 1993. An estimated 403,000 became ill from March 23 through April 8. The cause of the illness was a significant distribution of *Crypotosporidium* from sewage that found its way into the filtration system of a drinking-water plant.[15] Each year about 4 billion cases of diarrhea occur and 1.8 million deaths occur, mostly in children younger than 5. In addition, about 1 in 10 people in the developing world have intestinal worms that can cause infections resulting in cognitive impairment, massive dysentery, or anemia; about 6 million people are visually impaired because of trachoma; and about 200 million people are infected by schistosomiasis.[16]

Although an adequate supply of fresh and clean drinking water is necessary to sustain life, 1.1 billion people are without access to quality water and 2.6 billion are without basic sanitation. Without adequate clean water and sanitation facilities, disease rates increase, poverty increases, and economic and social productivity fall.[16]

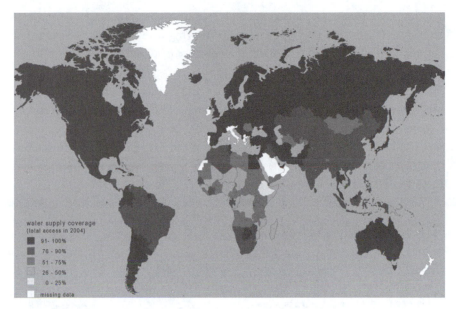

FIGURE 12.1   Drinking water coverage per country, total access in 2004. (*Source:* From WHO, 2006.)[17]

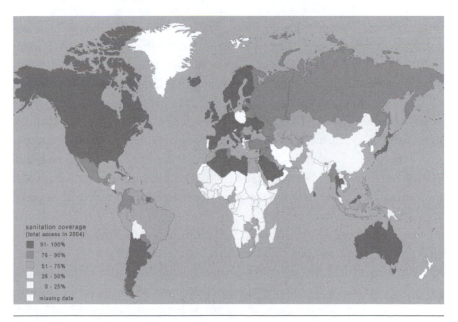

FIGURE 12.2   Sanitation coverage per country, total access in 2004. (*Source:* From WHO, 2006.)[17]

The World Health Organization (WHO) Joint Monitoring Program for Water Supply and Sanitation provides area maps showing drinking water coverage per country (see Figure 12.1) and sanitation coverage per country (see Figure 12.2). The percentage with improved water supply coverage throughout the world in 2004 was 83% (95% urban and 73% rural). This percentage is up from 78% (95% urban and 64% rural) in 1990. As evident, the increase in improved water supply coverage was primarily in rural areas. The global percentage with access to sanitation facilities was 59% (80% urban and 39% rural) in 2004. In 1990 corresponding percentages were 49% (79% urban and 26% rural). Again, the improvement in sanitation coverage was primarily in rural areas.[17]

Yet despite progress being made, considerably more work is needed to ensure improved water quality and sanitation facilities, primarily in developing rural areas of the world.

Water Pollution

Water pollution, produced by human activities, has adverse effects upon bodies of water (lakes, rivers, oceans, groundwater), making them unsafe for drinking, fishing, swimming, and other activities. Natural phenomena that may change water quality and the ecological status of water (e.g., storms, earthquakes, etc.) are not considered to be pollution. Water pollution can come from a number of different sources. If it originates from a single source, such as a factory, it is called **point-source pollution**. If it comes from many sources it is **nonpoint-source pollution**.

Water pollutants include a spectrum of chemicals, pathogens, and changes to the water's physical chemistry (acidity, conductivity, temperature, excess nutrient loading). Naturally occurring or human-made industrial waste (e.g., fluoride, arsenic, lead, petrochemicals, selenium, other heavy metals) in water can have serious health effects. Pathogens include disease-causing organisms such as bacteria, viruses, and protozoans. They enter water through untreated sewage, storm drains, septic tanks, and runoff water from farms.

There are several sources of water pollution: industrial discharging of toxic chemicals, mercury, solvents, polychlorinated biphenyls (PCBs), and sulfur dioxide; untreated sewage; surface runoff containing pesticides; slash and burn farming practices; surface runoff containing spilled petroleum products; excess nutrients added to water runoff containing detergents or fertilizers; and leakage of underground storage tanks into aquifers. Organic water pollutants include insecticides and herbicides, pathogens, tree and brush debris from logging operations, and volatile organic compounds coming from improper storage. Inorganic water pollutants include heavy metals, sulfur dioxide from power plants, radioactive waste, chemical waste, fertilizers (including nitrates and phosphates), acidity in mine drainage, and silt in surface runoff. Sewage and farm waste lead to oxygen depletion in water, potentially damaging ecosystems.[18]

To summarize, the main source of freshwater pollution is untreated waste, chemical discharges, and runoff from agricultural fields. Industrial growth, urbanization, and greater use of synthetic organic substances are largely to blame for water pollution. Freshwater for agriculture represents about 69% of total annual use of freshwater worldwide, followed by industrial (23%) and domestic use (8%). More developed countries tend to use a smaller percentage of their freshwater for agriculture and more for industry and for personal use compared with developing countries.[19–21] Developed countries suffer more from chemical discharges into water, mainly groundwater (95% of freshwater in the United States is groundwater), than developing countries.[22] On the other hand, water pollution in developing countries is mainly attributed to agricultural runoff in water sources.

According to the Second United Nations World Water Development Report, more than a billion people lack safe drinking water. Highlights from the report follow:

- An estimated 1.1 billion people do not have access to an adequate supply of drinking water and 2.6 billion fail to have access to basic sanitation. Over half live in China and India.
- An estimated 1.6 million lives could be saved every year by providing access to safe drinking water, sanitation, and hygiene.
- The quality of water is declining in most regions because the diversity of freshwater species and ecosystems is deteriorating rapidly. The hydrological cycle needs a healthy environment to function properly.
- Ninety percent of natural disasters are related to water events. These events are on the increase (see Chapter 14).
- Fifty-five percent more food will be required to feed the earth's population by 2030. Already, 70% of all freshwater used by humans is for crops.
- Half of humanity currently lives in towns and cities. This is estimated to increase to two-thirds by 2030, requiring more water in urban areas. Approximately 2 billion of these people are estimated to be living in slums and squatter settlements.

- Water is an important resource for generating energy, which translates to economic development.
- Wasteful water use through leakages in pipes and canals and illegal connections is widespread.[23]

Per capital household water consumption is highest in developed regions of the world (see Figure 12.3), yielding better hygiene and sanitation in those places and, therefore, better health. The United States has the highest per capita consumers of water (see Figure 12.4). It is estimated that by 2025 the United States will be responsible for more than 10% of global per capita household water consumption.[24]

Consider that the daily per capita water use in a typical single-family U.S. home is 69.3 gallons, most of which is used in the bathroom. Installation of more efficient water fixtures and checking for leaks can reduce daily per capita water use by about 35%.[25]

Use	Gallons per capita	Percentage of total
Showers	11.6	16.8%
Clothes washers	15.0	21.7%
Dishwashers	1.0	1.4%
Toilets	18.5	26.7%
Baths	1.2	1.7%
Leaks	9.5	13.7%
Faucets	10.9	15.7%
Other domestic use	1.6	2.2%

Monitoring Water

In the United States, water is monitored by federal, state, and local agencies, universities, dischargers, and volunteers. The federal **Clean Water Act** is a law that provides standards for regulating pollution discharges in ambient water. State regulations and guidelines further evaluate levels of contaminants according to type of water body (e.g., surface, recreation, marine). Data on water quality are used to characterize waters, identify emerging problems, assess whether water pollution control programs are effective, direct pollution control efforts, and respond to emergencies (e.g., oil spills, flooding). The Environmental Protection Agency (EPA) has various programs that provide data for monitoring water standards.

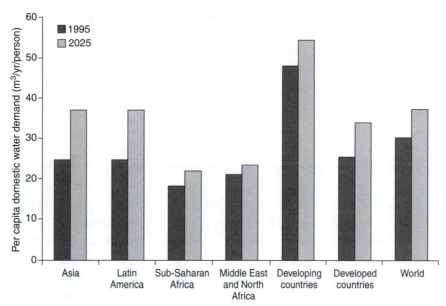

FIGURE 12.3 Per capita household water consumption by region. (*Source:* From IFPRI, 1998.)[26]

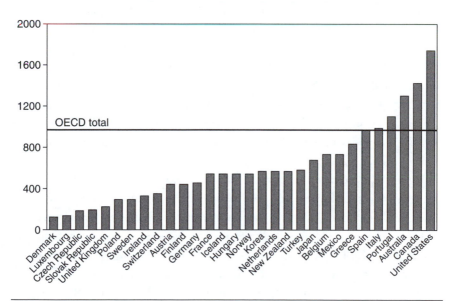

FIGURE 12.4 Water abstractions: m³ per capita, 2002 or latest available year. (*Source:* From OECD Factbook, 2005.)[27]

As public awareness and concern increased over water pollution, the Federal Water Pollution Control Act Amendments of 1972 were enacted. They were amended in 1977, becoming the Clean Water Act. The act gave the EPA authority to set control standards for all contaminants in surface waters. The act requires a permit to discharge any pollutant from a point source into waters, and it provided a grant program for funding the construction of sewage treatment plants. It also identifies the need for planning to address nonpoint-source pollutants. Many changes have been made to the original Clean Water Act.[28]

Initially the Clean Water Act focused on chemical pollutants. However, since the 1990s it has given more attention to physical and biological pollutants. In addition, regulation initially focused on discharges from point-source facilities. Little attention was given to runoff from streets, farms, construction sites, and so on. However, since the late 1980s, much more attention has been given to polluted runoff. A shift in focus has also been toward a more holistic watershed-based approach. Similar emphasis is placed on protecting healthy waters and restoring contaminated waters. Many issues are considered, not just those under regulatory authority.[29]

As authorized by the Clean Water Act in 1972, the National Pollutant Discharge Elimination System (NPDES) allows for programs to control water pollution through regulating point sources (e.g., pipes or human-made ditches) of discharged water pollutants. If a home is connected to a municipal system, uses a septic system, or does not have a surface discharge, it does not require an NPDES permit. However, a permit is necessary for an industrial, municipal, and other facility if its discharge goes directly to surface waters. Authorized states generally administer the NPDES permit program. State program status is available at http://cfpub.epa.gov/npdes/statestats.cfm. Information on NPDES regulations is available at http://cfpub.epa.gov/npdes/regs.cfm?program_id=0. The NPDES permit program is responsible for notable improvements to the United States' water quality.

Figure 12.5 presents a map of the Wasatch Front in northern Utah, available through the EPA's Envirofacts Data Warehouse at http://www.epa.gov/enviro/index.html. The map shows regulated water discharge sites and impaired water bodies and streams. The site allows you to map regulated water discharge sites, as well as regulated sites of hazardous waste, air emissions, toxic releases, and Superfund sites for any area in the United States.

Indicators used in monitoring programs also include proportion of marine and freshwater recreational waters failing to meet water quality regulations; proportion of treated recreational waters failing to meet state and local standards; number

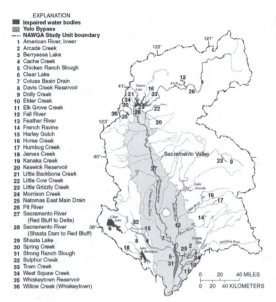

EXPLANATION
- Impaired water bodies
- Yolo Bypass
- NAWQA Study Unit boundary

1 American River, lower
2 Arcade Creek
3 Berryessa Lake
4 Cache Creek
5 Chicken Ranch Slough
6 Clear Lake
7 Colusa Basin Drain
8 Davis Creek Reservoir
9 Dolly Creek
10 Elder Creek
11 Elk Grove Creek
12 Fall River
13 Feather River
14 French Ravine
15 Harley Gulch
16 Horse Creek
17 Humbug Creek
18 James Creek
19 Kanaka Creek
20 Keswick Reservoir
21 Little Backbone Creek
22 Little Cow Creek
23 Little Grizzly Creek
24 Morrison Creek
25 Natomas East Main Drain
26 Pit River
27 Sacramento River
    (Red Bluff to Delta)
28 Sacramento River
    (Shasta Dam to Red Bluff)
29 Shasta Lake
30 Spring Creek
31 Strong Ranch Slough
32 Sulphur Creek
33 Town Creek
34 West Squaw Creek
35 Whiskeytown Reservoir
36 Willow Creek (Whiskeytown)

FIGURE 12.5   EPA-regulated water discharge sites, impaired water bodies and streams in Sacramento River Basin. (*Source:* Courtesy of USGS.)

of health-related closure days for water recreation areas; volume of point-source discharges according to type of contaminant, such as permitted sanitary waste disposal, sewage, and intentional spills and discharges; levels of fecal coliform and mercury in shellfish beds; and levels of mercury, dioxin, and PCBs in fish.

The **Safe Drinking Water Act** of 1974 sets quality standards for drinking water and oversees the states and localities that implement those standards. Hundreds of organizations around the United States conduct some form of water-quality monitoring. These include federal agencies, the EPA, and the U.S. Geological Survey. The primary indicator used to monitor drinking water is the number and proportion of drinking-water systems failing to meet water-quality regulations and guidelines by specific type of water supply. Other indicators may be the number of citations for noncompliance with standards for free chlorine levels, number of point-source discharges into drinking-water aquifers, and levels of naturally occurring toxicants.

The EPA's civil enforcement program takes legal action to see that polluters come into compliance with the federal environmental laws. The efforts of this program have prevented the release of millions of tons of illegal pollution into water, have fostered the cleanup of contamination, and have halted the reoccurrence of pollution. Enforcement activities are conducted through 10 regional offices, with headquarters in Washington, D.C. Environmental laws are administered and environmental improvements achieved through collaboration with state, local, and tribal governments, as well as with the Department of Justice.[30]

Adverse health effects may also be used as indicators for monitoring ambient water and drinking water. In the case of ambient water, outbreaks by source (fish, shellfish) and etiologic agent (biologic, toxic, and other) may be used. For drinking water, cases of methemoglobinemia or outbreaks attributed to drinking water (including bottled water) may be considered. More information on indicators for ambient water or drinking water is provided in Appendix I.

The **United Nations Global Environment Monitoring System** (GEMS) Water Program, established in 1978, is the primary source for global water quality data. Key activities include monitoring, assessment, and capacity building throughout the world. The state and trends of regional and global water quality are provided through GEMS. The United Nations Environmental Program's (UNEP's) GEMS/Water Program involves participating government entities that monitor and assess water quality. A GEMStat Web site at http:gemstat.org has surface and groundwater quality data sets collected by the GEMS/Water Global Network. Currently there are 2,800 stations, 2 million records, and over 100 parameters in the network (see Figure 12.5). During 2005 through 2007, coverage has doubled, but monitoring stations are still greatly needed in areas of Africa, small islands, and west Asia.

In 2002, more than 83% of the world had received improved drinking-water sources. In addition, global sanitation coverage rose from 49% in 1990 to 58% in

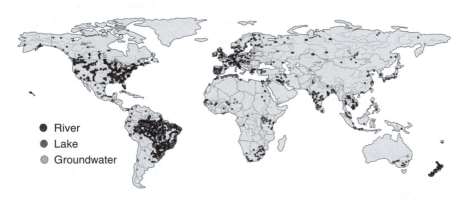

FIGURE 12.6   UNEP GEMS/Water Global Network worldwide distribution of over 2,800 monitoring stations. (*Source:* ©United Nations Environment Programme Global Environment Monitoring System/Water Programme, 2007.)[31]

2002. These statistics demonstrate the positive efforts of many agencies throughout the world to improve water quality and subsequent quality of life for millions of people.

Many obstacles remain in achieving improved drinking-water sources for all human beings. One of the most difficult factors to overcome is outpacing the world's population growth. To illustrate, for Peru to maintain its 1990 level it would have had to ensure drinking-water services to more than 350,000 people per year. Between 1990 and 2002 they have actually surpassed that monumental mark and have provided improved drinking-water sources to more than 480,000 people per year, which means that Peru raised the coverage from 74% to 81% in that time span.[32]

Key Issues

1. Health problems can arise by ingesting contaminated water as well as through airborne exposures from materials that can outgas during showering, bathing, swimming, or cooking. Contaminated water can also be absorbed through the skin.

2. Waterborne diseases are infectious diseases that are spread primarily through contaminated water. Whether these diseases are contracted directly or indirectly through exposure to infected vectors, water is the primary medium for spread of these diseases.

3. Several chemicals, both human-made and naturally existing, dissolve in water, polluting the water and producing disease among those exposed.

4. Each year about 4 billion cases of diarrhea and 1.8 million deaths occur, mostly in children younger than 5. In addition, about 1 in 10 people in the developing world have intestinal worms that can cause infections resulting in cognitive impairment, massive dysentery, or anemia; about 6 million people are visually impaired because of trachoma; and about 160 million people are infected by schistosomiasis.

5. The percentage with improved water supply coverage throughout the world in 2004 was 83% (95% urban and 73% rural). This percentage is up from 78% (95% urban and 64% rural) in 1990.

6. The main source of freshwater pollution is untreated waste, chemical discharges, and runoff from agricultural fields. Industrial growth, urbanization, and greater use of synthetic organic substances are largely responsible for water pollution.

Exercises

Key Terms

Define the following terms.

Clean Water Act
Condensation
H_2O
Nonpoint-source pollution
Pathogens
Point-source pollution
Precipitation
Safe Drinking Water Act
United Nations Global Environment Monitoring System
Water
Water pollution
Waterborn diseases

Study Questions

12.1. Describe common waterborne diseases, including sources of water contamination and health outcomes associated with contaminated water.

12.2. Define "water pollution" and describe its common sources.

12.3. Contrast water use in developed and developing nations.

12.4. What is the Clean Water Act and how has it expanded in recent years?

12.5. Access the EPA site http://www.epa.gov/enviro/index.html and identify regulated water-discharge sites and impaired water bodies and streams.

References

1. Environmental Protection Agency. Drinking water contaminants. Available at: http://www.epa.gov/safewater/hfacts.html. Accessed June 4, 2007.
2. Water Legislation and Substance/Quality Database. Canadian Water and Wastewater Association. Municipal Drinking Water Services. Available at: http://www.cwwa.ca/legislation/faqs/MunicipalWater.htm. Accessed June 4, 2007.
3. Food and Nutrition Board. *Dietary Reference Intakes: Water, Potassium, Sodium, Chloride, and Sulfate.* Washington, DC: The National Academies Press; 2004. Available at: http://www.iom.edu/?id=18495&redirect=0. Accessed December 6, 2006.

4. Advanced Purification Engineering Corporation. Water education. Available at: http://www.freedrinkingwater.com/water-education/water-health.htm. Accessed December 6, 2006.

5. Bove F, Shim Y, Zeitz P. Drinking water contaminants and adverse pregnancy outcomes: a review. *Environ Health Perspect.* 2002;110:61–74.

6. Morris RD. Drinking water and cancer. *Environ Health Perspect.* 1995; 103(S8):225–231.

7. Reif JS, Hatch MC, Bracken M, Holmes LB, Schwetz BA, Singer PC. Reproductive and developmental effects of disinfection by-products in drinking water. *Environ Health Perspect.* 1996;104(10):1056–1061.

8. World Health Organization. Water sanitation and health. Available at: http://www.who.int/water_sanitation_health/diseases/diseasefact/en/index.html. Accessed December 6, 2006.

9. Chen CJ, Chen CW, Wu MM, Kuo TL. Cancer potential in liver, lung, bladder and kidney due to ingested inorganic arsenic in drinking water. *Br J Cancer.* 1992;66(5):888–892.

10. Steinmaus C, Yuan Y, Bates MN, Smith AH. Case-control study of bladder cancer and drinking water arsenic in the western United States. *Am J Epidemiol.* 2003;158(12):1193–1201.

11. Bates MN, Rey OA, Biggs ML, et al. Case-control study of bladder cancer and exposure to arsenic in Argentina. *Am J Epidemiol.* 2004;159(4):381–389.

12. Kurttio P, Pukkala E, Kahelin H, Auvinen A, Pekkanen J. Arsenic concentrations in well water and risk of bladder and kidney cancer in Finland. *Environ Health Perspect.* 1999;107(9):705–710.

13. Hopenhayn-Rich C, Biggs ML, Smith AH. Lung and kidney cancer mortality associated with arsenic in drinking water in Cordoba, Argentina. *Int J Epidemiol.* 1998;27(4):561–569.

14. Knobeloch LM, Zierold KM, Anderson HA. Association of arsenic-contaminated drinking-water with prevalence of skin cancer in Wisconsin's Fox River Valley. *J Health Popul Nutr.* 2006;24(2):206–213.

15. Mac Kenzie WR, Hoxie NJ, Proctor ME, et al. A massive outbreak in Milwaukee of cryptosporidium infection transmitted through the public water supply. *N Engl J Med.* 1994;331(3):161–167.

16. World Health Organization. The Joint Monitoring Programme for Water Supply and Sanitation: The health aspects of water supply and sanitation. Available at: http://www.wssinfo.org/en/141_wshIntro.html. Accessed December 6, 2006.

17. World Health Organization. The Joint Monitoring Programme for Water Supply and Sanitation: Water supply data at global level. Available at: http://www.wssinfo.org/en/22_wat_global.html. Accessed December 6, 2006.

18. Wikipedia: The free encyclopedia. Water pollution. Available at: http://en.wikipedia.org/wiki/Water_pollution. Accessed December 6, 2006.

19. Engelman R, LeRoy P. *Sustaining water: Population and the Future of Renewable Water Supplies.* Washington, DC: Population Action International; 1993.

20. European Schoolbooks (ES). *The Battle for Water: Earth's Most Precious Resource*. Cheltenham, UK: ES; 1994.

21. United Nations, Department for Policy Coordination and Sustainable Development. *Critical trends—Global Change and Sustainable Development*. New York, NY: United Nations; 1997.

22. Wikipedia: The free encyclopedia. Water. Available at: http://wikipedia.org/wiki/Water. Accessed December 6, 2006.

23. United Nations. United Nations World Report 2, Water, A Shared Responsibility. Available at: http://environment.about.com/gi/dynamic/offsite.htm?zi=1/XJ&sdn=environment&zu=http%3A%2F%2Fportal.unesco.org%2Fen%2Fev.php-URL_ID%3D32057%26URL_DO%3DDO_TOPIC%26amp%3BURL_SECTION%3D201.html. Accessed December 6, 2006.

24. Rosegrant MW, Cai X, Cline SA. *Global Water Outlook to 2025: Averting an Impending Crisis*. International Food Policy Research Institute (IFPRI) and the International Water Management Institute (IWMI); 2002.

25. Vickers A. *Handbook of Water Use and Conservation*. Amherst, MA: WaterPlow; 2001.

26. International Food Policy Research Institute. Graphs on water. Available at: http://www.ifpri.org/media/water_graphs.htm#usage. Accessed December 6, 2006.

27. Organization for Economic Co-Operation and Development. Water consumption. Available at: http://www.oecd.org/dataoecd/42/27/34416097.pdf. Accessed December 6, 2006.

28. Environmental Protection Agency. Clean Water Act. Available at: http://www.epa.gov/r5water/cwa.htm. Accessed December 6, 2006.

29. Environmental Protection Agency. Introduction to the Clean Water Act. Available at: http://www.epa.gov/watertrain/cwa/. Accessed December 7, 2006.

30. Environmental Protection Agency. Civil enforcement. Available at: http://epa.gov/compliance/civil/programs/sdwa/index.html. Accessed June 5, 2007.

31. UNEP GEMS/Water Programme. Water quality outlook. Available at: http://www.gemswater.org/common/pdfs/water_quality_outlook.pdf. Accessed June 4, 2007.

32. World Health Organization. Drinking water coverage. Available at: http://www.who.int/water_sanitation_health/monitoring/jmp04_3.pdf. Accessed December 6, 2006.

Radiation and Health

LEARNING OBJECTIVES

After completing this chapter, you should be able to:

1. Describe the electromagnetic spectrum.

2. Describe pathways by which people are exposed to radiation.

3. Identify common health problems associated with radiation exposure.

4. Discuss some of the difficulties faced by epidemiologic radiation studies.

5. Describe radiation monitoring programs.

Introduction

All humans are regularly exposed to radiation; it is present in the air, water, soil, and food. Natural sources of radiation include the earth's crust (e.g., uranium, radium, plutonium) and the cosmos (originating from outer space and the sun). Natural radiation varies considerably by location. Radiation increases with altitude and increased radioactive materials in the earth. For example, people in Colorado are exposed to higher levels of radiation than people in most other areas of the United States because of the comparatively high altitude and the high levels of uranium deposits in the Colorado plateau. Artificial sources of radiation include:

- Industrial uses of radiation: nuclear power plants, nuclear weapons, industrial particle accelerators
- Radioactive waste produced by industrial processes that use radioactive materials: coal-fired power plant emissions, "orphan" radioactive sources in scrap metal, by-products from oil and gas drilling
- Medical radiation: diagnostic nuclear medicine, mammography, medical X-rays, radiation therapy
- Radioactive materials in consumer products: luminous clocks and watches, glazed and tinted products, tobacco products
- Transportation and storage: treatment of spent fuel
- Misuse of radioactive substances
- In the United States, radon gas accounts for the majority of annual radiation exposure, and cosmic, terrestrial, internal radiation, and human-made sources account for the remaining exposure (see Figure 13.1).

Because we are constantly exposed to natural and artificial sources of radiation, and given the epidemiologic evidence linking radiation with disease, monitoring and controlling radioactive exposures in the workplace and the ambient environment are important to public health. The purpose of this chapter is to describe the electromagnetic spectrum, the pathways by which people are exposed to radiation, common health problems associated with radiation exposure, challenges associated with epidemiologic radiation studies, and radiation monitoring programs.

Radiation

Radiation is energy emitted as either a particle or a wave, spreading out as it travels. Low-energy (long wavelength) radiation is produced by radars, radios, and elec-

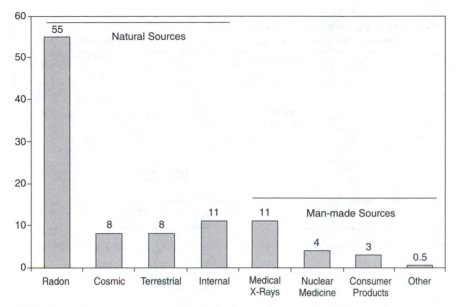

FIGURE 13.1   Sources of radiation exposure, United States. (*Source:* From NCRP, 1987.)[1]

tric and magnetic fields from high-voltage electric power lines, microwave ovens, desktop computers, and television sets. Each of these sources of radiation improves our standard of living in various ways. Sources of high-energy (short wavelength) radiation also contribute to our quality of life; they include nuclear power, which reduces the stresses to the environment from producing power with fossil fuels; X-rays to improve diagnosis and monitoring of disease; and radiation to control insects and preserve food. High-energy radiation is also responsible for generating stratospheric ozone. However, the potential harmful effects of high-energy radiation on human health are well understood. There is also evidence that long-term exposure to low-energy radiation can negatively affect health.[2]

Electromagnetic Spectrum

The different forms of electromagnetic radiation are distinguished by their wavelength (see Figure 13.2). Wavelength refers to the distance between two adjacent wave crests. The size of the wavelength is associated with frequency (the number of wave peaks that occur in a given time): longer wavelengths are associated with

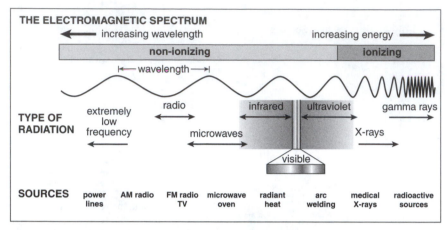

FIGURE 13.2   Types and sources of radiation. (*Source:* From ARPNSA, 2006.)[3]

---

lower frequency, and shorter wavelengths are associated with higher frequency. Wavelengths and frequency are measured on a continuous scale. It has been useful to divide the electromagnetic spectrum into **nonionizing** (radiation with longer wavelengths or lower frequency) and **ionizing radiation** (radiation with shorter wavelengths or higher frequency). Ionizing radiation has enough energy to remove electrons from atoms or molecules (groups of atoms), with the high potential of damaging living tissue.

The sun produces **ultraviolet (UV) radiation**, which has wavelengths shorter than visible light. UV is commonly divided into three bands on the electromagnetic spectrum: **UVA** (wavelengths 320–400 nanometers); **UVB** (wavelengths 280–320 nm); and **UVC** (wavelengths shorter than 280 nm). Note that a nanometer, a common unit to describe wavelengths of electromagnetic radiation, is a distance of one billionth of a meter. The UVA band of radiation has wavelengths that are just shorter than visible violet light. It is not absorbed by stratospheric ozone. Although most UVB is absorbed by stratospheric ozone, that which does contact the earth (or received from sun lamps) has various harmful effects such as damaging DNA, crops, and marine organisms. In humans it is a risk factor for melanoma of the skin and other types of skin cancer. Protecting oneself from UVB radiation is very important, particularly as ozone depletion continues. Although extremely dangerous, UVC is entirely absorbed by stratospheric ozone and normal oxygen. UVC is responsible for generating ozone.

Nonionizing and Ionizing Radiation

Nonionizing radiation, from shortest to longest wavelength, includes visible light (also lasers), infrared, microwaves, radar waves, television, radio waves, and electric and magnetic fields (e.g., high-voltage electric power lines). Such radiation does not interact strongly enough with electrons to ionize atoms. Nonionizing radiation below levels that cause heating is thought to be harmless. However, there continues to be debate over the health effects of long-term exposure.

Ionizing radiation is harmful to human health because it can damage living tissues. It consists of either particle radiation or electromagnetic radiation. Ionizing particle radiation (e.g., electrons, neutrons, atomic ions) carries enough energy to ionize an atom or molecule by removing an electron from its orbit. **Electromagnetic radiation** is a stream of photons (particles with zero mass) traveling in a wave-like pattern at the speed of light. Each photon contains a certain amount of energy: those with the highest energy have the shortest wavelengths. Electromagnetic radiation can ionize an atom (remove an electron from its orbit) if the energy per photon is high enough (i.e., wavelength short enough). Ionizing radiation, from shortest to longest wavelength, consists of cosmic rays, gamma rays, X-rays, and UV light (excluding UVA).

Ionizing radiation can penetrate human cells, depositing energy among atoms that creates changes leading to biologic damage. Ionizing radiation is dangerous to the human body because of direct exposure, but most damage occurs when radioactive material is emitted inside the body. For example, as radioactive iodine in the body is used by the thyroid, its accumulation often results in cancer of the thyroid. If radioactive isotopes are present in air, water, soil, plants, or animals, it may be taken into the body. If the dose is sufficient, radiation poisoning can occur because ionizing radiation interferes with cell division. Ionizing radiation can cause burns, cancer, and genetic mutations.[4]

Pathways by Which People Are Exposed to Radiation

Signs and symptoms of radiation sickness as well as the severity of health effects from radiation exposure depend on the amount of radiation received and the exposure pathway. The three basic pathways are inhalation (breathing radioactive materials into the lungs), ingestion (swallowing radioactive material), and direct (external) exposure. These pathways need to be considered when calculating exposure or estimating exposure effects. Ionizing radiation exposure may be external or internal to the body. Injury resulting from external radiation will depend on (1) total dose, (2) dose rate, and (3) percentage and region of the body exposed. Greater potential for human harm is associated with increases in a combination of these factors. The probability that an adverse health effect will occur is associated with the size of the dose.

Certain compounds such as potassium, uranium, and thorium are radioactive and can emit radiation when the nucleus breaks down or disintegrates. Radon-222 is produced by decaying radium-226, which can be found in almost all rock and soil. Typically, very low concentration levels of radon are found in the air, but concentrations indoors may accumulate and be much higher. The half-life of radon-222 is 3.8 days.[5] Uranium-238 is radioactive as well as very toxic; that is, a sample that contains enough atoms to pose a radiation hazard also poses a chemical hazard. The Environmental Protection Agency (EPA) regulates uranium-238 as both a radiation hazard and a chemical hazard.[6] The decay chains for uranium-238 and radon-222 are shown in Figure 13.3. As shown, uranium-238 decays to eventually become a stable form of lead.

Three types of ionizing radiation produced by radioactive material or other sources are (1) **alpha particles,** (2) **beta particles,** (3) and **gamma rays.** Direct, external exposure is of limited concern if it involves alpha particles because they cannot penetrate the outer layer of skin (see Figure 13.4). Beta particles are a concern because they can burn the skin and damage eyes. Gamma radiation is of greatest concern because radionuclides emitted from gamma rays can travel long distances and penetrate the body.[8]

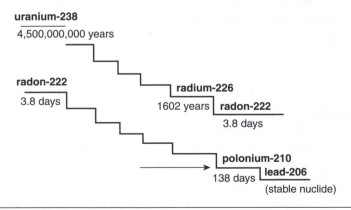

FIGURE 13.3   Uranium-238 decay chain. (*Source:* From EPA, 2006.)[7]

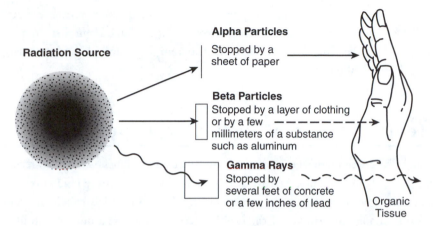

FIGURE 13.4 Sources of radiation: The penetrating powers of alpha and beta particles, and gamma rays. (*Source:* From EPA, 2006.)[9]

Exposure to radiation through inhalation is primarily through contaminated dust, smoke, or gaseous radionuclides (e.g., radon). Radioactive particles entering the lungs can remain there for some time. **Radionuclides** slowly decay, emitting high-energy particles as the atom breaks down. Exposure continues as long as decay continues. When radionuclides emit alpha or beta particles, large amounts of energy are transferred to surrounding tissue, damaging DNA or other cellular material.

Ingested radioactive exposure to alpha- and beta-emitting radionuclides is of most concern because they can expose the entire digestive system, kidneys, other organs, and bones to harmful radiation. Radionuclides rapidly cleared from the body are of less concern.

Measuring Radiation

Ionizing radiation can be measured by the rate of radioactive emissions coming from the body (radioactivity) or by the amount of energy absorbed by material such as the body. **Becquerel** (Bq) is the international standard for radioactivity (i.e., rate at which radioactive materials decay). One Bq refers to the amount of radioactive material required to have disintegration in one second. Health studies are typically concerned with absorption of radiation into the human body. The most common dose units include **rad**, **rem**, **gray** (Gy), and **sievert** (Sv). Dose is a measure of energy that is absorbed in matter. Rad (U.S.) and Gy (international) are unit measures of absorbed dose, with 1 Gy = 100 rad. *Dose equivalent* relates to the energy deposited and the effectiveness of that dose in human tissue to produce biological cell damage. The basic units are rem (U.S.) and Sv (international), with 1 Sv = 100 rem.[10]

Health Effects of Radiation Exposure

The link between radioactive materials and uncommon illnesses has been recognized for about a century. As early as 1910, an association between radiation and skin cancer was observed. A number of epidemiologic studies have made this connection. Long-term studies of the health effects of Japanese atomic bomb blast survivors, populations exposed to nuclear-testing fallout, and uranium miners are among the best known.[6]

Radiation exposure may be chronic or acute. **Chronic exposure** is long-term continuous or frequent recurrence at low doses over an extended period of time. The effects of chronic radiation exposure occur some time after the initial exposure. Chronic exposure has been associated with benign tumors, precancerous lesions, cancer (leukemia, breast, bladder, colon, liver, lung, esophagus, ovarian, multiple myeloma, and stomach), cataracts, skin changes, and chromosomal aberrations. Ionizing radiation is a potent carcinogen because of its ability to break chemical bonds in atoms and molecules. Cancer is the primary health effect resulting from radiation exposure. Cancer occurs when genes that regulate cell duplication, apoptosis (cell suicide), or DNA repair are injured or damaged. **Acute exposure**, on the other hand, is characterized by a large, single dose or series of doses of radiation in a short time period, and adverse health outcomes manifest themselves relatively quickly.[11]

Cancer risk from radiation compared with cancer risk in general has been estimated by health physicists. If persons in a group of 10,000 were each exposed to 1 rem of ionizing radiation over their lifetime, five or six more deaths from cancer would be expected. About 2,000 deaths from cancer would be expected from nonradiation causes. Hence, exposure to 1 rem of radiation over time would increase this number of cancer deaths to 2,005 or 2,006.[6] The normal rate of exposure for most people is about 0.3 rem (or 300 millirem) every year from natural background sources of radiation, mostly radon. Another 60 millirem of exposure occurs every year, on average, from human-caused radiation such as from medical, commercial, and industrial activities. The yearly limit of all sources of human-caused radiation among nonradiation workers set by the Nuclear Regulatory Commission (NRC) is 100 mrem (=l msv). The yearly limit for radiation workers set by the NRC is 5 rem.

Individual cells attempt to repair the damage resulting from radiation, but if the damage is too extensive, or mistakes occur in the natural repair process, adverse health effects result. High doses of radiation may kill cells and damage tissues and organs immediately. Signs and symptoms of acute radiation often include nausea and vomiting, diarrhea, skin burns, loss of appetite, fainting, fatigue, weakness, dehydration, inflammation of tissues, anemia, and hair loss. A range of health effects associated with various levels of radiation exposure is shown in Table 13.1.

Children are more sensitive to radiation exposure than adults because they are growing more rapidly, and cells are dividing more rapidly. There is a greater chance that radiation exposure and DNA damage can cause more significant health problems during this developmental time. Hence, radiation standards set by the EPA consider variability in sensitivity attributed to age and gender.[6]

TABLE 13.1 Health Effects of Radiation According to Dose

Exposure (rem)	Health Effect	Time to Onset
< 5	Radiation burns; more severe as exposure increases	
5–10	Changes in blood chemistry	
50	Nausea	hours
55	Fatigue	
70	Vomiting	
75	Hair loss	2–3 weeks
90	Diarrhea	
100	Hemorrhage	
400	Death from fatal doses	within 2 months
1,000	Destruction of intestinal lining	
	Internal bleeding	
	Death	1–2 weeks
2,000	Damage to central nervous system	
	Loss of consciousness	minutes
	Death	hours to days

Source: From EPA, 2006.[6]

Beyond cancer, the next most common health effects of radiation are teratogenic and genetic mutations. "Teratogenic" refers to mutations in the embryo or fetus that result from abnormal maternal homeostasis or direct exposure of the fetus in utero to radiation. Fetuses are most sensitive from 8 to 15 weeks after conception. Consequences of radiation exposure can include reduced head or brain size, slowed growth, and mental retardation. Scientists estimate that 4 per 1,000 fetuses between 8 and 15 weeks old exposed to 1 rem would become mentally retarded. Genetic mutation is when the parent passes on a genetic error to his or her child. It is estimated that these occur in about 50 children per million live births when both parents were exposed to 1 rem.[6]

The types of adverse health effects that can be associated with radiation exposure prior to conception include:[12]

- early fetus loss
- childhood cancer
- chromosomal anomalies
- other congenital anomalies
- late fetus loss
- neonatal death
- sex ratio

Although ionizing radiation represents a possible teratogen for the fetus, this is dependent on the dosage and the gestational age of the fetus. Maternal thyroid exposure to diagnostic radiation is associated with a slight reduction in birth weight.[13] Embryo exposure to radio frequency—an extremely low frequency—and intermediate frequency electromagnetic fields has not shown an adverse affect on childhood development.[14]

While the epidemiologic evidence has established the health effects of high-dose exposure, focus in epidemiologic research is now on the health effects of low-dose exposure. There is controversy in this area of research, as well as many challenges for studying this particular topic. A case–control study of radiological technicians, those consistently exposed to low-grade radiation as part of their job taking X-rays, determined there was no association between exposure and lung cancer.[15] However, another study on female radiological technicians found increased breast cancer rates among those who had been practicing technicians before 1940 when radiation restrictions were less stringent and among those women who began working before age 17.[16] A study of Canadians exposed to low-dose radiation at work showed that those with preexisting cancer were more likely to develop malignant cancer, but not develop new cancers. The response was significantly dose-dependent.[17] Some experts feel that epidemiological studies cannot adequately determine the health hazards of very low dosages of radiation, so a linear extrapolation from studies of higher doses (but still low) is the best estimate. Others argue that a linear relationship does not adequately model the effects of very low dosages.[18] Research in the area is often inconsistent due to several factors. It is difficult to measure low-grade radiation status consistently, especially over time. In addition, with the relatively consistent exposure to environmental radiation in almost all parts of the world, several sources of confounding are possible.

Radiation is a common form of cancer treatment. Ionizing radiation is used to kill cancer cells and shrink tumors. In the United States, roughly half of all cancer patients undergo radiation therapy, either alone or in combination with surgery and/or other cancer treatments. Radiation therapy is classified as external or internal. External radiation is most common and comes from a machine outside the body. Internal radiation is implanted into or near the tumor in small capsules or some other type of containers. The type of radiation used depends on the type of cancer. Treatment planning and simulation are actions taken first to improve the precision and effectiveness of the treatment and then to minimize damage to healthy tissues.[19]

Deaths from Leukemia Example

The intense study of radiation-induced leukemia of atomic bomb survivors in Japan has been unparalleled. This is made possible by the Atomic Bomb Casualty Commission and the Radiation Effects Research Foundation in Hiroshima and Nagasaki, which have monitored the occurrence of leukemia in atomic bomb survivors. Research has added a great deal to our understanding of the natural history of radiation-induced leukemia, from the latency period and the shape of the dose–response curve, to the clinical symptoms and survival times associated with the disease.

To illustrate the relationship between radiation exposure and leukemia, consider the following data involving leukemia- and nonleukemia-related deaths for the areas including Hiroshima and Nagasaki, Japan (see also Table 13.2). These data were collected from 1950 to 1970, the two decades following the atomic bombing of World War II.

TABLE 13.2 Deaths from Leukemia Observed by the Atomic Bomb Casualty Commission (1950–1970)

Age	Cause of death	Dose (rad) Not in City	0–9	10–49	50–99	100–199	200+
0–9	Leukemia	0	7	3	1	4	11
	Other	5015	10752	2989	694	418	387
10–19	Leukemia	5	4	6	1	3	6
	Other	5973	11811	2620	771	792	820
20–34	Leukemia	2	8	3	1	3	7
	Other	5669	10828	2798	797	596	624
35–49	Leukemia	3	19	4	2	1	10
	Other	6158	12645	3566	972	694	608
50+	Leukemia	3	7	3	2	2	6
	Other	3695	9053	2415	655	393	289

Source: From Sugiura and Otake, 1974.[20]

The death rate from leukemia was 130 per 100,000. Age-group specific death rates were not significantly different [Mantel-Haenszel chi-square (1) = 0.88, p = 0.3489]. The rate of death from leukemia follows a strong dose–response relationship (see Figure 13.5), which is statistically significant [Mantel-Haenszel chi-square (1) = 245.05, p < 0.0001]. The result from this statistic is similar to the Mantel-Haenszel trend test (i.e., 251.06, p < 0.0001).

Monitoring Radiation

The EPA is the primary federal entity for regulating and monitoring radiation exposure. The EPA has several responsibilities to maintain surveillance programs and develop guidelines. Its Office of Air and Radiation develops programs and regulations to reduce radiation exposure and air pollution. Scientists at the EPA determine areas of high exposure risk such as mines, nuclear reactors and other industrial operations, nuclear waste storage facilities, and so on. The EPA also sets certain limits on radiation exposure; these limits are implemented or adapted by other national or local commercial and governmental agencies to protect the public and employees from excessive and potentially harmful exposure. These regulations can apply to many different situations, including acceptable levels of

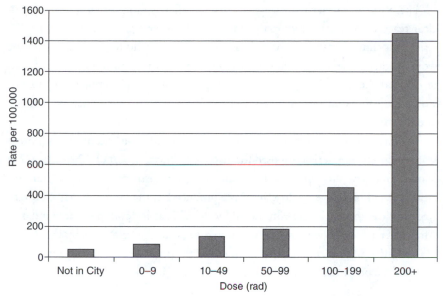

FIGURE 13.5 Leukemia death rate according to dose in Japan (1950–1970)

radiation in drinking water and safe levels of exposure in uranium mines and nuclear reactors.[21]

UV light is one form of radiation exposure the EPA monitors. Monitoring indicators of UV light are presented in Appendix I. These indicators include the number of days that the UV light index exceeds a safe threshold. Incidence and mortality are also useful measures of UV light exposure, as are injuries attributed to UV light, such as the number of corneal burns, incidence of cataracts, and number of other eye injuries. Public health education about UV light may be measured by determining the proportion of adults who follow protective measures to prevent melanoma, skin cancer, and eye problems.

Radon is also monitored by the EPA. The Indoor Radon Abatement Act of 1988, Sections 307 and 309, directed the EPA to identify areas in the country with potentially elevated indoor radon levels. Thus, the EPA has developed a map of radon zones throughout the country to show radon potential, based on indoor radon measurements, geology, aerial radioactivity, soil permeability, and foundation type.

The NRC is another federal agency that specifically monitors and regulates nuclear reactors, materials (radioactive metals and minerals), and wastes. It has set strict guidelines for the use of radioactive materials including limiting the time workers can handle them; requiring labeling and warning signs on radioactive materials and the areas in which they are kept; requiring the reporting of lost or stolen radioactive materials; and specifying how nuclear waste must be handled and disposed of.[22]

The EPA sets the standards that will protect public health and the environment from radioactive material proposed for disposal at Yucca Mountain, Nevada. Yucca Mountain is a facility intended to become the final disposal site for all spent nuclear fuel and high-level radioactive waste produced in the United States. Substantive public comments were considered by the EPA as it developed the standards. After interagency review, the EPA expected to issue the standards by the end of 2007. Different government agency roles in the approval, monitoring, and operation of the potential Yucca Mountain Repository follow:

- National Academy of Sciences (NAS): provided technical recommendations the EPA must use while developing develop public health and environmental standards
- EPA: provided standards for protection of public health and the environment (consistent with NAS recommendations)
- NRC: determines whether the proposed facility can meet the EPA standards, thereby influencing whether construction authorization and a license for operations are granted or not; if approved and built, will inspect and monitor the facility
- U.S. Department of Energy: submits license application to the NRC; upon approval, designs, constructs, and operates the facility; also manages the shipping of waste
- Congress and the president: approved the development of a Yucca Mountain site as a nuclear waste facility; passed legislation for the EPA to provide standards for a Yucca Mountain facility
- U.S. Department of Transportation: regulates transportation of waste now stored at 126 locations across the United States to the Yucca Mountain facility; enforces requirements on shipping contracts, routes, and vehicles[23]

The Occupational Safety and Health Administration (OSHA) enforces limits set on radiation exposure in the workplace. It requires that employers keep their workplaces free of health hazards and provide adequate protection to employees who work with hazardous materials. OSHA has set standards in many aspects of industry, such as requiring the safe disposal of hazardous waste; requiring those operating X-ray devices and other radiation-emitting materials to be trained and capable; limiting the amount of time employees can be exposed to sources of radiation; and limiting exposure of radioactivity in people younger than 18.[24]

There are several other organizations, national and international, governmental and nongovernmental, that promote radiation safety through numerous means. They include:

- The International Radiation Protection Association is an organization committed to increasing protection from radiation throughout the world. It holds international conferences, encourages the development of local radiation-protection societies, and encourages international research.[25]
- The National Council on Radiation Protection and Measurements (NCRP) is a national organization whose primary mission is to communicate to the public the scientific findings concerning radiation hazards and protection practices. The NCRP works with several other organizations to establish a uniform and informed approach to regulating and monitoring radiation levels around the country.[25]
- The International Commission on Radiological Protection is an organization that also seeks to encourage radiation-protective measures. It provides recommendations on safe exposure levels to governments and agencies worldwide.[26]

Key Issues

1. The electromagnetic spectrum represents a kind of radiation where electric and magnetic fields vary simultaneously, from power lines to visible light to gamma rays.
2. Nonionizing radiation, from shortest to longest wavelength, is visible light (also lasers), infrared, microwaves, radar, television, radio waves, and electric and magnetic fields (e.g., high-voltage electric power lines). Such radiation does not interact strongly enough with electrons to ionize atoms.
3. Nonionizing radiation below levels that cause heating is thought to be harmless. However, debate continues on the health effects of long-term exposure.

4. Ionizing radiation is dangerous to human health. It can damage any living tissue in the human body. It is sufficiently energetic to break the bonds that hold molecules together to form ions.

5. While the epidemiologic evidence has established the health effects of high-dose exposure, focus in research is now on the health effects of low-dose exposure.

6. The EPA is the primary federal body for regulating and monitoring radiation exposure. The EPA maintains surveillance programs and develops guidelines.

7. The Nuclear Regulatory Commission (NRC) is a federal agency that specifically monitors and regulates nuclear reactors, materials, and waste.

8. The Occupational Safety and Health Administration (OSHA) enforces limits set on radiation exposure in the workplace.

Exercises

Key Terms

Define the following terms.

Acute exposure
Alpha particles
Becquerel
Beta particles
Chronic exposure
Electromagnetic radiation
Gamma ray
Gray
Ionizing radiation
Nonionizing radiation
Rad
Radiation
Radionuclides
Rem
Sievert
Teratogenic
Ultraviolet radiation

UVA
UVB
UVC

Study Questions

13.1. List several sources of both natural and human-made radiation. Which are most likely to affect the area where you live?

13.2. Describe the different classifications of radiation and give examples of each: low-energy (long wavelength) vs. high-energy (short wavelength); ionizing vs. nonionizing.

13.3. What forms of UV light are most dangerous to human health? To which types are humans most at risk of being exposed?

13.4. What factors influence the severity of damage to a person exposed to radiation?

13.5. What are the three major pathways of radiation exposure? Give examples of each.

13.6. List some common adverse health effects associated with radiation exposure.

13.7. Why are children and developing fetuses more susceptible to radiation-associated health problems than adults?

13.8. What are the challenges of studying the effects of low-dose radiation on health?

13.9. Why are radiation-monitoring agencies and institutions necessary? Describe the duties of the EPA, NRC, and OSHA in monitoring and regulating radiation exposure.

References

1. National Council on Radiation Protection and Measurements. *Ionizing radiation exposure of the population of the United States, NCRP Report No. 93*. Washington, DC: National Council on Radiation Protection and Measurements; 1987.

2. Environmental Protection Agency. Understanding radiation. Available at: http://www.epa.gov/radiation/understand/index.html. Accessed December 6, 2006.

3. Australian Radiation Protection and Nuclear Safety Agency. Ionizing and non-ionizing radiation. Available at: http://www.arpansa.gov.au/basics/ion_nonion.htm. Accessed December 6, 2006.

4. Wikipedia: The free encyclopedia. Ionizing radiation. Available at: http://en.wikipedia.org/wiki/Ionizing_radiation. Accessed December 6, 2006.

5. Environmental Protection Agency. Radon. Available at: http://www.epa.gov/radiation/radionuclides/radon.htm. Accessed June 7, 2007.

6. Environmental Protection Agency. Health effects. Available at: http://www.epa.gov/radiation/understand/health_effects.htm. Accessed December 6, 2006.

7. Environmental Protection Agency. Decay chains. Available at: http://www.epa.gov/radiation/understand/chain.htm. Accessed June 7, 2007.

8. Environmental Protection Agency. Exposure pathways. Available at: http://www.epa.gov/radiation/understand/pathways.htm. Accessed December 6, 2006.

9. Environmental Protection Agency. Ionizing radiation fact sheet series. Available at: http://www.epa.gov/radiation/docs/ionize/402-f-98-009.htm. Accessed December 6, 2006.

10. Centers for Disease Control and Prevention. Radiation measurement. 2006. Available at: http://www.bt.cdc.gov/radiation/measurement.asp. Accessed December 6, 2006.

11. Environmental Protection Agency. Ionizing radiation fact sheets series: No. 2. 2006. Available at: http://www.epa.gov/radiation/docs/ionize/402-f-98-010.htm. Accessed December 6, 2006.

12. Wilkinson P, ed. *Environmental Epidemiology*. New York, NY: Open University Press; 2006.

13. De Santis M, Di Gianantonio E, Straface G, et al. Ionizing radiations in pregnancy and teratogenesis: a review of literature. *Reprod Toxicol*. 2005;20(3): 323–329.

14. Juutilainen J. Developmental effects of electromagnetic fields. *Bioelectromagnetics*. 2005;7:S107–S115.

15. Rajaraman P, Sigurdson AJ, Doody MM, et al. Lung cancer risk among US radiologic technologists, 1983–1998. *Int J Cancer*. 2006;119:2481–2486.

16. Doody MM, Freedman DM, Alexander BH, et al. Breast cancer incidence in US radiologic technologists. *Cancer*. 2006;106:2707–2715.

17. Hazelton WD, Moolgavkar SH, Curtis SB, et al. Biologically based analysis of lung cancer incidence in a large Canadian occupational cohort with low-dose ionizing radiation exposure, and comparison with Japanese atomic bomb survivors. *J Toxicol Environ Health A*. 2006;69(11):1013–1038.

18. Brenner DJ, Sachs RK. Estimating radiation-induced cancer risks at very low doses: rationale for using a linear no-threshold approach. *Radiat Environ Biophys*. 2006;44(4):253–256.

19. National Cancer Institute. Radiation therapy for cancer: Questions and answers. 2004. Available at: http://www.cancer.gov/cancertopics/factsheet/Therapy/radiation. Accessed June 7, 2007.

20. Sugiura N, Otake M. An extension of the Mantel-Haenszel procedure to K 2 x C contingency tables and the relation to the logit model. *Comm Stat.* 1974; 3:829–842.

21. Environmental Protection Agency. About EPA's radiation protection program. 2006. Available at: http://www.epa.gov/radiation/about/index.html. Accessed December 6, 2006.

22. U.S. Nuclear Regulatory Commission. What we do. Available at: http://www .nrc.gov/what-we-do.html. Accessed December 6, 2006.

23. Environmental Protection Agency. EPA Yucca Mountain fact sheet #4. Available at: http://www.epa.gov/radiation/docs/yucca/402-f-05-028.pdf. Accessed May 7, 2007.

24. U.S. Department of Labor, Occupational Safety & Health Administration. Ionizing radiation standards. Available at: http://www.osha.gov/SLTC/ radiationionizing/standards.html. Accessed December 6, 2006.

25. International Radiation Protection Association. Available at: http://www.irpa .net/index.php?option=com_content&task=blogcategory&id=94&Itemid=60. Accessed December 6, 2006.

26. International Commission on Radiological Protection. Some more information about ICRP. Available at: http://www.icrp.org/about.asp. Accessed December 6, 2006.

Climate Change and Health

LEARNING OBJECTIVES

After completing this chapter, you should be able to:

1. Define and distinguish between "climate" and "weather."

2. Indicate why epidemiologic studies generally assess the relation between weather and health and not climate and health.

3. Define "global warming," "greenhouse gases," and "greenhouse effect."

4. Identify natural sources of global warming and discuss the impact these sources have on climate change.

5. Identify human activities that lead to global warming and discuss the impact these causes have on climate change.

6. Identify human causes of deforestation.

7. Identify human causes of stratospheric ozone depletion.

8. Discuss current policies and technologies aimed at mitigating the impacts of global warming.

9. Identify selected environmental and health effects associated with global warming.

10. Be familiar with why climate change has the potential to alter the distribution of vectors.

11. Identify ways deforestation directly and indirectly affects human health.

12. Discuss the relationship between climate change and frequency of natural disasters.

13. Identify selected health effects associated with ozone depletion.

Introduction

Changes in the earth's climate have been naturally occurring since the creation of the planet. Yet a growing body of evidence is attributing some climate changes to human-made environmental pollutants. Global warming and ozone depletion are environmental events influenced by human activity. The World Health Organization (WHO) has provided a summary of direct and indirect health effects associated with climate change (see Figure 14.1). Climate change can directly affect health through extreme temperatures, increased floods and severe storms, droughts, increased frequency of waterborne and foodborne diseases, and a change pattern in vector- and rodent-borne diseases. Climate change can indirectly affect health by disrupting modern-day methods of food production and by hurting economic productivity.

Climate is how temperature, precipitation, and wind characteristically prevail in a region over many years. **Weather**, on the other hand, is the state of the atmosphere (temperature, moisture, wind velocity, barometric pressure) at a specific time and place. Climate change involves statistically significant changes in the mean state of the climate (temperature or amount of precipitation) or in its variability that persist over periods of time on the order of decades or longer; in other words, climate change is the long-term change in the average weather condition for a particular area.

Epidemiologic studies do not generally evaluate health according to climate change, but rather assess the association between health and weather. This is because health is typically associated with something that is more immediate—weather conditions at a point and place in time that vary from day to day. Time–series studies

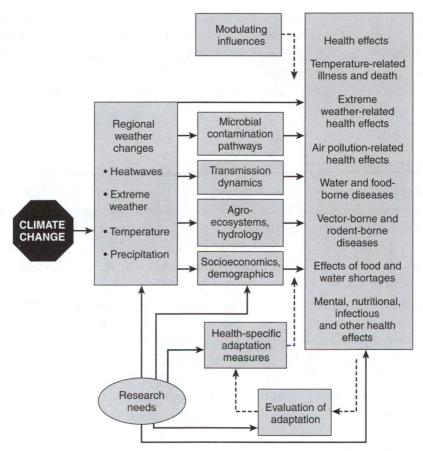

FIGURE 14.1   Climate change and human health. (*Source:* From WHO, 2006.)[1]

are generally used to evaluate the relationship between short-term changes in health and changes in temperature and precipitation measured at similar temporal resolutions. To study the relation between health and climate is much more complex because the association between long-term health experiences and exposure to different time-averaged climate conditions is likely to be confounded by factors such as people adapting to living in a warmer climate. Adaptation may include alteration of behaviors and/or structural changes.[2]

Although epidemiologic studies cannot effectively investigate climate and health, they can effectively assess the relationship between weather and health, thereby providing an indirect measure of the impact of climate on health and evidence supporting the need to reduce environmental pollutants. Epidemiologic research can also identify how to limit adverse health effects associated with climate change. The purpose of this chapter is to present evidence of a changing climate due to human activity. Epidemiologic evidence of the health effects associated with weather changes and ozone depletion will also be discussed.

Global Warming

Global warming refers to an average increase in the earth's temperature, which in turn causes changes in climate. An increase in the earth's temperature is the result of both natural causes and human activities, including greenhouse gases, ozone depletion, deforestation, and volcanoes, to name a few. The total force of such causes has led to a 0.6 to 0.8°C increase in the earth's temperature over the past 100 years, with half of the temperature increase occurring in the last 25 to 30 years.[3] Climate modeling indicates that during this century the approximate average temperature could increase another 1.5 to 5.8°C.[4] A time–series analysis shows the combined global land and marine surface temperature record for the years 1850 to 2005. The year 1998 was the warmest on record, followed by 2005. The temperature increase in the past has been associated with an increased incidence of natural disasters such as hurricanes, heat waves, droughts, forest fires, and melting of glaciers. Extreme weather anomalies will likely increase in the future.

Greenhouse Gases and the Greenhouse Effect

To understand major natural and human-made causes of global warming, an understanding of greenhouse gases and the greenhouse effect is needed. **Greenhouse gases,** gases that absorb infrared radiation in the atmosphere, include water vapor (H_2O), carbon dioxide (CO_2), methane (CH_4), nitrous oxide (N_2O), chlorofluorocarbons (CFCs), ozone (O_3), phosphofluorocarbons (PFCs), hydrofluorocarbons (HFCs), and hydrochlorofluorocarbons (HCFCs). The **greenhouse effect** refers to the "trapping" of infrared radiation from the earth by greenhouse gases in the atmosphere. The effects of greenhouse gases are illustrated in Figure 14.3. The greenhouse effect begins with absorption of ultraviolet (UV) radiation from the sun by the earth's surface. After absorption of UV radiation, the earth emits excess heat in the form of infrared radiation. Under "normal" circumstances, infrared radiation passes through the earth's atmosphere because it is primarily composed of argon

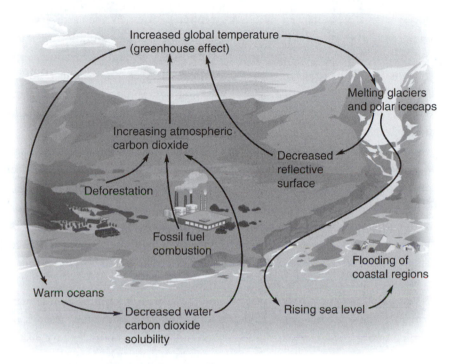

FIGURE 14.3 The Greenhouse Effect. (*Source:* © Jones and Bartlett Publishers.)

and diatomic molecules such as oxygen (O_2) and nitrogen (N_2). When molecules absorb energy such as infrared radiation, their bonds rotate, vibrate, and stretch. However, diatomic molecules, such as O_2 and N_2, have relatively strong, stable bonds and therefore do not react greatly with infrared radiation. Greenhouse gases, on the other hand, have more flexible bonds, which allow infrared radiation to cause significant movement in greenhouse gases. This interaction is what "traps" infrared radiation when greenhouse gases are prevalent in the earth's atmosphere. The net result of this reaction is the warming of the earth's surface.[6]

Natural Sources of Global Warming

Water vapor is the most abundant greenhouse gas in the earth's atmosphere and has been increasing in the earth's atmosphere by about 3% each year since the 1970s.[8] Although increases in water vapor occur chiefly by natural causes, this process is greatly influenced by other greenhouse gases. As the earth's average temperature rises, the melting of glaciers and increased evaporation of water from oceans lead to more water vapor in the atmosphere and more cloud coverage. Not only do increases in water vapor enhance the greenhouse effect, but increased cloud coverage adds to global warming by trapping heat in the earth's lower atmosphere. Sixty percent of expected global warming is due to feedbacks such as water vapor.[9]

Other factors that naturally contribute to global warming include solar rays and volcanoes. Many argue that large increases in UV radiation (or solar irradiance) could explain global warming. While indirect measures have shown an increase in solar irradiance over the past few decades, the contribution of solar rays to global warming appears to be small when compared with the impact of greenhouse gases. Solar irradiance accounts for about 0.3 W/m^2 forcing power on climate change, while CO_2 alone contributes 1.4 W/m^2 forcing power.[9] **Climate forcing power** is a measure of imposed perturbation to the earth's energy balance.

Volcanoes also contribute about 0.2 to 0.5 W/m^2 forcing power on climate change. When volcanoes erupt, large amounts of dust, gas, and other aerosols are expelled into the stratosphere. Although volcanic eruptions initially have a large impact on climate, typically causing a short period of cooler climate, the aerosols ejected remain in the atmosphere only for one to two years. Therefore, unless large volcanic eruptions occur frequently over a long period of time, volcanic eruptions do not greatly contribute to climate change or global warming.[9]

The Year Without a Summer

History tells about weather aberrations influenced by volcanic eruptions involving unusually low temperatures, dark clouds, little sunlight and darkness during the day, crop failures, and flooding in typically dry places. In 1815, for example, Mount Tamora erupted on the island of Sumbawa, Indonesia. This added to ashes and dust already in the atmosphere from earlier volcanic eruptions in La Soufriere on Saint Vincent in the Caribbean in 1812 and Mayon in the Philippines in 1814. Temperatures fell throughout the world because less sunlight was able to pass through the atmosphere. The greatest changes in the climate resulted in New England, the Canadian Maritimes, Newfoundland, and northern Europe. "In May of 1816, frost killed off most of the crops that had been planted, and in June two large snowstorms in eastern Canada and New England resulted in many human deaths. Nearly a foot of snow was observed in Quebec City in early June. In July and August, lake and river ice were observed as far south as Pennsylvania. Rapid, dramatic temperature swings were common, with temperatures sometimes reverting from normal or above-normal summer temperatures as high as 95°F (35°C) to near-freezing within hours. Even though farmers south of New England did succeed in bringing some crops to maturity, maize (corn) and other grain prices rose dramatically. Oats, for example, rose from 12¢ a bushel the previous year to 92¢ a bushel."[10]

Human Activities That Contribute to Global Warming

The largest human-related contributors to global warming are greenhouse gases. **Greenhouse gases** contribute to global warming not only through the greenhouse effect, but by depleting the stratospheric ozone layer. Specifically, CO_2, CH_4, N_2O, HFCs, and PFCs create the greenhouse effect, while CFCs and HCFCs deplete the ozone layer.[11] Among greenhouse gases, CO_2 and CFCs are considered the most hazardous gases because each is the greatest human-caused contributor to the greenhouse effect and ozone depletion, respectively (see Table 14.1).

Since 1850, about 18% of atmospheric CO_2 can be attributed to human activities, primarily fossil fuel production and use, cement production, and changes in land use.[13] Table 14.2 provides information from the Intergovernmental Panel on Climate Change (IPCC) on which human processes produce CO_2 and the level of CO_2 emissions associated with those processes. In the year 2000, emissions of CO_2 from fossil fuels totaled about 23.5 Gt of CO_2 per year.[4] Because of this rapid increase in CO_2 emissions, CO_2 levels in the atmosphere have increased from around 280 ppmv to 370 ppmv since the Industrial Revolution. If this trend continues, researchers predict that by the twenty-second century, CO_2 levels will range from 490 to 1260 ppmv.[3]

Although methane (CH_4) and nitrous oxide (N_2O) are not as prevalent as carbon dioxide, they too contribute to the greenhouse effect. CH_4 is about 21 times more powerful at warming the earth's atmosphere than carbon dioxide.[14] As shown in Figure 14.4, levels of methane and nitrous oxide have increased in the United States and worldwide in recent years. Levels of methane are influenced by rice

TABLE 14.1   Greenhouse Gases Influenced by Human Activities[a]

Variable	CO_2	CH_4	N_2O	CFC-11	HCFC-22	CF_4
Pre-industrial concentration	280 ppmv	700 ppbv	275 ppbv	0	0	0
Concentration in 1994	358 ppmv	1720 ppbv	312 ppbv[b]	268 pptv[b]	110 pptv	72 pptv[b]
Annual rate of increase in concentration	1.5 ppmv (0.4%)	10 ppbv (0.6%)	0.8 ppbv (0.25%)	0 pptv (0%)	5 pptv (5%)	1.2 pptv (2%)
Atmospheric lifetime, yr.[b]	50–200[d]	12[e]	120	50	12	50,000

[a]The rates for CO_2, CH_4, and N_2O are based on data for the decade beginning 1984; the rates for the other gases are based on data for recent years (1990s).

[b]Average time spent by a gas in the atmosphere after it is emitted.

[c]Estimated from 1992–1993 data.

[d]No single lifetime for CO_2 can be defined because of the different rates of uptake from different sink processes. Sinks are systems such as forests and oceans that can uptake greenhouse gases.

[e]Adjusted to take into account the indirect effect of methane on its own lifetime. CFCs also deplete ozone in the stratosphere and are now controlled by the Montreal Protocol. HCFCs have been temporarily permitted as substitutes for CFCs but are also potent greenhouse gases.

Source: From Haines et al., 2006, as adapted from Houghton, JT et al.[12]

TABLE 14.2 CO_2 Emission Sources and Amounts

Process	Number of Sources	Emissions ($MtCO_2$ yr^{-1})
Fossil fuels		
Power	4,942	10,539
Cement production	1,175	932
Refineries	638	798
Iron and steel industry	269	646
Petrochemical industry	470	379
Oil and gas processing	N/A	50
Other sources	90	33
Biomass		
Bioethanol and bioenergy	303	91
Total	7,887	13,468

Source: From IPCC, 2005.[4]

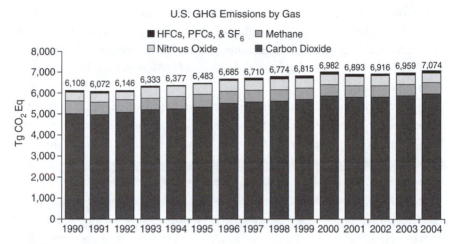

FIGURE 14.4 U.S. greenhouse gas emission by gas. (*Source:* From EPA, 2004.)[15]

cultivation, biomass burning, and cattle and sheep ranching, but are also the result of decaying material in landfills, coal mining, oil drilling, and other power-producing processes. An estimated 60% of global methane emissions are associated with human activities. Natural sources include wetlands (76%), termites (11%), oceans (8%), and emissions from global hydrates.[14] The estimated climate forcing power of methane is 0.7 W/m^2.[9] The principal sources of nitrous oxide are energy use (42%), agriculture (33%), and industry (25%). Nitrous oxide is largely the product of both agricultural and industrial activities such as combustion of waste and power production. The estimated climate forcing power of nitrous oxide is 0.15 W/m^2.[9] Globally, greenhouse gas emissions are expected to continue to increase through 2030 and beyond, with the level of greenhouse gas emissions in developing countries expected to surpass those of developed countries by 2015.[16]

Halocarbon substances are greenhouse gases that contain carbon and halogens (i.e., chlorine, fluorine, or bromine) and are known to degrade the ozone. The most notorious halocarbons are CFCs. Because CFCs remain in the atmosphere for 50 to 100 years, and in some cases up to 300 years, they contribute greatly to climate change.[11] Between 1950 and 2000, the production of halocarbon gases increased in the United States at an alarming rate. In 1950, the global atmospheric mixing ratio of CFCs was around 0 ppt. By 2000, the global atmospheric mixing ratio of CFCs ranged from about 100 to 550 ppt, depending on the specific CFC (see Figure 14.5). Because of the rapid increase of halocarbons emitted into the atmosphere, the Montreal Protocol was created in 2000 to mitigate halocarbon production by establishing policies on the amount of halocarbons industries could produce. After this time, levels of halocarbons in the atmosphere dropped dramatically.

However, during the time of high halocarbon gas production, the amount of stratospheric ozone decreased by 3% worldwide. Decreases in stratospheric ozone have been especially great for the Antarctic region of the earth, which at times has been 40–50% below pre-1950 ozone levels. As shown in Figure 14.6, column ozone over the Antarctic region has decreased by about 150 Dobson units (DUs) in the past four decades. Although the amount of stratospheric ozone varies depending on season, such a significant drop could be explained by the increased presence of halocarbons in the atmosphere.[11] Because ozone strongly absorbs UV-radiation from the sun, depletions in ozone can lead to global warming. The direct climate forcing of CFCs is about 0.35 W/m^2.[9]

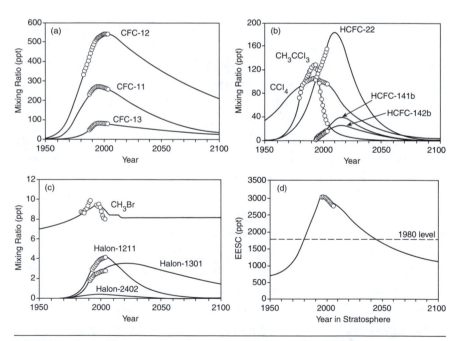

FIGURE 14.5 Global atmospheric mixing ratios for select halocarbon gases from the year 1950 to 2000. (*Source:* From IPCC, 2005, p. 95.)[11]

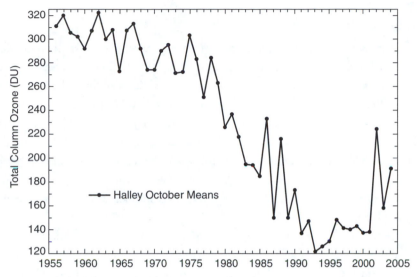

FIGURE 14.6 The total column ozone for the years 1950 to 2000. (*Source:* From IPCC, 2005, p. 94.)[11]

Besides greenhouse gases, another major human-related factor in global warming is land-coverage variability, which includes agriculture and forestation. Because crop production is a vital food source and forests are a vital source of lumber and fuel, these resources are constantly fluctuating. Because plants need CO_2 to flourish, many argue that increases in CO_2 would help maximize agriculture. However, this argument is true only for a short period of time. Although increased levels of CO_2 can initially enhance forest and crop growths, the effect soon wears thin as global temperatures increase because of elevated levels of CO_2 and deforestation. Eventually this can lead to constantly declining crop production.[9]

In addition, because crops and forests require many resources to thrive, including money, land, and labor, they can actually strain societies and ecosystems. As a result of stressed resources, crop production can slow, leading to increased CO_2 in the atmosphere. Also, plants not only take in CO_2, but they also give it off. Therefore there is a fine balance between maximizing CO_2 intake and minimizing CO_2 release from vegetation. It is estimated that the climate forcing from deforestation is -0.2 W/m^2.[9]

Deforestation

Over the last two decades, tropical regions have experienced deforestation rates that exceed 12 million hectares (unit of area equal to 10,000 square meters) per year. Forests have virtually disappeared in 25 countries, while an additional 29 countries have suffered forest cover losses of more than 90%.[17] Globally, each year an estimated 16 million hectares of forest are cut, bulldozed, or burned; this is comparable to losing an area of forest the size of Montana (U.S.) every year.[18] Based on the current rates of cutting and replanting, the World Bank calculates that forests will entirely disappear within the next 60 years.[19] These estimates are especially worrisome considering the vital roles that forests play in maintaining the well-being of populations.

The causes of deforestation are many and varied. Much deforestation has been fueled by a rising demand for forest services such as food, water, wood, paper products, and fuel. Between 1960 and 2000, wood harvests for paper products tripled because of increased demand.[17] Increased consumption of these forest products has been coupled with an increase in the production of other services that have required the clearing of forests. Such practices include farming and cattle herding. Demand for the combination of wood and food products has led to increased land area for services like agriculture and herding, and decreased area for forests. Thus, the expansion of some services has come at the expense of another service.[17]

Agriculture uses more than half of the habitable land on the planet, and the very practice of agriculture destroys more than 250,000 square kilometers of forests each year.[20] In the 30 years between 1950 and 1980, more land was converted to cropland than in the 150-year span between 1700 and 1850.[17] One of the driving forces of land conversion is economic pressure. In order to survive economically, farmers have to respond to consumer demand. The need to export more product forces farmers to expand their farming area at the expense of forests. Although most people think that these practices will positively contribute to gross national product, when the depletion of natural resources and damage from carbon emissions are considered, net national savings decrease by 5%.[17] Many studies have shown that benefits for sustainable management of forests exceed the benefits of converting the forest land.

Another leading cause of deforestation is cattle herding. The international demand for beef has necessitated the expansion of cattle herding lands. Forests and critical habitats have been cleared to make room for cattle herding.[21] Brazil, one of the most critically deforested regions, has suffered from the expansion of cattle herding. The lucrative beef business has been estimated to contribute to between 38% and 73% of the deforestation in Brazil. Over just an 18-month period, Brazil expected to lose a forest area the size of Denmark to cattle herding.[21] Some of this expansion for herding and farming may be justified, because as the global population expands, more food and forest products are necessary. However, the presence of forests is also essential, and a balance between expansion and maintenance of forests should be sought.

Forests benefit the globe by regulating climate and absorbing carbon dioxide. Because forests absorb carbon dioxide, they are vital in regulating the supply and control of fresh air.[19] Since 1750, the atmospheric concentration of carbon dioxide has increased 32%, primarily because of forest loss.[17] In addition, when forests are destroyed, rain washes phosphates away, causing the ground to become unproductive. Further, forests have other life-sustaining benefits. Half a billion people are dependent on forests either for the entirety or for a portion of their daily diets.[18] An additional 4.6 billion people depend on water supplies from forest systems.[17] Forests provide timber and wood for energy fuel to about 1 billion people.[19] Forest systems are also essential because they regulate 57% of total water runoff, and by doing so, help to control flooding and protect against soil erosion.[17] In addition, they provide the largest natural habitat for wildlife (50–90%). If forests disappear, these wildlife habitats would be destroyed. The environment provided by forest ecosystems is also necessary for the growth of certain medicinal plants.

The Carbon Cycle

Carbon is the fourth most common element in our universe, after hydrogen, helium, and oxygen, and serves as the building block of life. The geological carbon cycle moves carbon between rocks and minerals, seawater, and the atmosphere. Carbon cycling also occurs biologically. Through the process called photosynthesis, green plants absorb sunlight and take up CO_2 through small openings in leaves to create fuel for building plant structures. The carbon is incorporated into the biomass of trees and plants, with some being released as CO_2 through respiration. Oxygen is also produced during photosynthesis. Approximately half of biomass is carbon, which can make its way into the soil when the trees and plants decay. Carbon can return to the atmosphere as CO_2 if the soil is stirred up or if the biomass is burned.[22]

Oceans can absorb and release carbon dioxide. The exchange is largely influenced by the surface water temperature and currents, and by photosynthesis and respiration of sea plants. Cold temperatures take up CO_2 whereas warmer temperatures release CO_2. Upward and downward currents in the ocean are influenced by temperature. Hence, upward moving currents such as those found in the tropics carry carbon dioxide to the surface where it is released into the atmosphere. Finally, the carbon cycle involving algae (e.g., phytoplankton) in the sea is much quicker than for trees and plants on land where carbon is stored in the biomass and in soil.[22]

Although there are natural fluxes in the carbon cycle, human activities (primarily fossil fuel burning and deforestation) are causing atmospheric CO_2 levels to increase. Consequently, CO_2 levels are higher now than they have been for over the last half-million years.[23] The global carbon cycle is presented in Figure 14.7. Thus, scientists estimate that fossil fuel burning contributes 5.5 gigatons of carbon into the atmosphere each year. Deforestation contributes another 1.6 gigatons of carbon into the atmosphere each year. Measures of atmospheric CO_2 since 1957, when regular measuring began, indicate that of the 7.1 gigatons released into the atmosphere each year by human activity, 3.2 gigatons remain there, resulting in

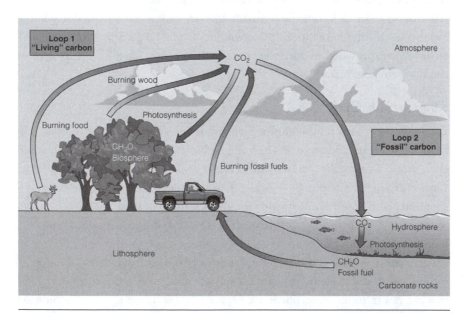

FIGURE 14.7   The global carbon cycle. (*Source:* © Jones and Bartlett Publishers.)

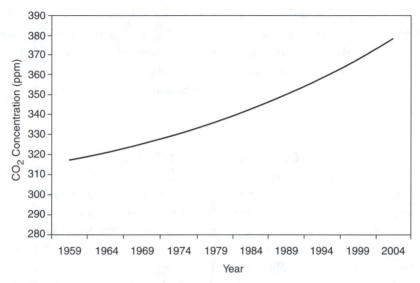

FIGURE 14.8 Atmospheric carbon dioxide concentration

an increase in atmospheric CO_2 (see Figure 14.8). In contrast to the CO_2 concentrations shown in the figure, from 9000 BC to about 1900, CO_2 levels ranged from 260 ppm to 280 ppm.

The Nitrogen Cycle

Nitrogen is essential to life, making up approximately 78% of air (by weight), and is the second most common element found in the human body.[24] Although it is a nutrient to human life and naturally cycles through the air, water, and land, it is a hazardous pollutant if it becomes overabundant.

Environmental problems have resulted from humans interfering with the nitrogen cycle. Fuel combustion releases various compounds into the atmosphere, including nitrogen oxides (NO_x). Nitrogen oxides react with oxygen in the air, resulting in nitrous oxide gas (N_2O), which is a greenhouse gas. If levels of N_2O are too high in the air, the earth's temperature will rise. Further, N_2O can interact with stratospheric ozone to break down the ozone layer. As already discussed, the ozone layer protects life from UV radiation, which can cause serious sunburns and skin cancer in animals and humans (see Chapter 13).

Nitrogen dioxide can also react with hydrogen to form nitric acid (HNO_3). Nitric acid causes acid deposition (acid rain). Trees, plants, and marine ecosystems can be damaged because of increased acidic levels in soil and water (see Chapter 11). High nitrogen concentrations in estuaries and other coastal waters can result in low oxygen levels and possibly no oxygen in bottom waters because of stimulated blooms of algae (e.g., phytoplankton).

Human Causes of Stratospheric Ozone Depletion

Ozone (O_3) is an odorless gas composed of three atoms of oxygen. It is harmful to breathe. About 90% of ozone is in the earth's stratosphere, the atmospheric region at an altitude of 10 to 15 kilometers. This region and the region that is 15 to 40 kilometers (10–25 miles) about the surface of the earth are known as the ozone layer (see Figure 14.9). Because the stratosphere absorbs UV radiation, warmer air is in the upper stratosphere and cooler air is in the lower stratosphere. Commercial airplanes travel in the lower stratosphere. Ozone completely absorbs UVC and most of UVB, which are harmful to living things. Below the strastosphere and extending down to the surface of the earth is the atmospheric region known as the

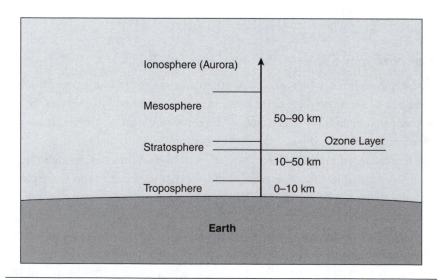

FIGURE 14.9   Layers of the earth's atmosphere

troposphere. This is where almost all weather occurs, with temperatures decreasing with higher altitude. Convection, the process of warm air rising, cooling, and then falling back to earth, produces wind currents and weather patterns. To provide perspective on the elevation of atmospheric regions, the world's highest mountain, Mt. Everest, which is 8.8 kilometers high, can be used as a reference.[16]

Ozone depletion describes a slow, steady decline in the total amount of ozone in the earth's stratosphere below normal levels after accounting for seasonal cycles and location (about 3% per decade over the past 20 years) and a decrease in stratospheric ozone over the polar regions of the earth (see Figures 14.10 and 14.11). The ozone hole on September 9, 2006, was the largest ever observed, at 11.4 million square miles. The general decreasing trend and monthly variability in average total ozone are shown in Figure 14.12.

Ozone levels can be described in various ways. The most common measure of ozone levels is the DU, which measures how much ozone is in a column of air. One hundred DUs of ozone brought to the earth's surface is equivalent to 1 millimeter thick. Ozone levels tend to vary from 250 to 300 DUs throughout the year. Seasonal variation in ozone levels is more extreme in temperate regions. There are several ozone-depleting substances: CFCs, HCFCs, halons, methyl bromide, carbon tetrachloride, and methyl chloroform. Although these ozone-depleting substances are generally stable in the troposphere, intense UV in the stratosphere can cause these substances to break down, releasing atomic chlorine and bromine that deplete ozone. While chemical destruction and creation of ozone occurs naturally, these ozone-depleting substances adversely influence this balance, causing lower ozone levels than normal.

CFCs are chemical compounds that consist of chlorine, fluorine, and carbon atoms. They have been widely used as refrigerants, industrial solvents, blowing agents in manufacturing foam products, and propellants for aerosol sprays. Once released in the air, CFCs rise slowly into the stratosphere and can remain there for several years. UV radiation destroys CFC molecules, producing chlorine atoms that react with ozone, converting ozone to normal oxygen. One chlorine atom can destroy 100,000 molecules of ozone. HCFCs are a class of chemicals that have been used to replace CFCs. HCFC is a compound consisting of hydrogen, chlorine, fluorine, and carbon. Like CFCs, the chlorine in HCFCs depletes stratospheric ozone, but at a much lower level than CFCs. Production of HCFCs will eventually be stopped.

Other ozone-depleting substances include halons, methyl bromide, carbon tetrachloride, methyl chloroform, and hydrobromofluorocarbon (HBFC). Halons are

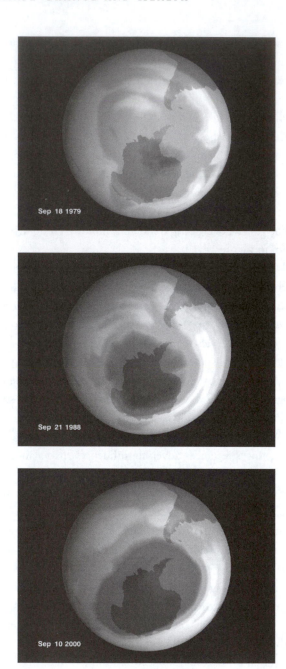

FIGURE 14.10   Images of ozone concentrations over Antarctica in September 1979, 1988, and 2000. (*Source:* Courtesy of NASA/Goddard Space Flight Center/Scientific Visualization Studio)

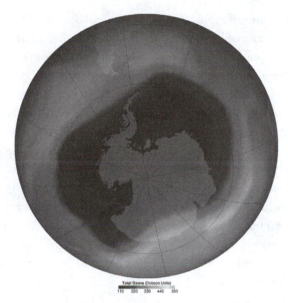

FIGURE 14.11   Image of Antarctic ozone hole in September 2006. (*Source:* Courtesy of NASA)

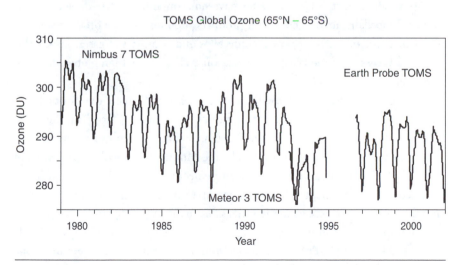

FIGURE 14.12   Trends in stratospheric global ozone. (*Source:* From Wikipedia, 2006.)[27]

compounds consisting of bromine, fluorine, and carbon. Fire-extinguishing agents are the primary source of halons. Because bromine, the compound in halons that causes ozone depletion, is much more damaging to the ozone layer than chlorine, these substances have not been produced in the United States since the end of 1993. Methyl bromide is a compound consisting of carbon, hydrogen, and bromine. Because it too contains bromine, it depletes stratospheric ozone. Although it is an effective pesticide for fumigating soil and various agricultural products, U.S. production ended at the end of 2000. Carbon tetrachloride, a compound consisting of one carbon atom and four chlorine atoms, is used in various industrial processes, such as production of CFCs. It had previously been used as a solvent until it was found to be carcinogenic. Methyl chloroform is a compound used as an industrial solvent and consists of carbon, hydrogen, and chlorine. HBFC is a compound consisting of hydrogen, bromine, fluorine, and carbon. Although not regulated in the original Clean Air Act (CCA), it has been added as a regulated substance.

Potential replacements for ozone-depleting substances are hydrocarbon (HC), compounds consisting of carbon and hydrogen, and HFC, compounds consisting of hydrogen, fluorine, and carbon. HCs include the highly flammable substances methane, ethane, propane, cyclopropane, butane, and cyclopentane. HCs are relatively inexpensive to produce, do not cause ozone depletion, have little global warming potential, and have low toxicity. Since the late 1970s, consumer aerosol products in the United States have not contained ozone-depleting substances. Propellants used in consumer products and most aerosol products that do not deplete the ozone layer now include HCs and compressed gases. HFCs also do not deplete the ozone layer. However, some HFCs have high global warming potential.

In 1987, the **Montreal Protocol** on Substances that Deplete the Ozone Layer was signed as an international treaty to protect the ozone by stopping the emission of halocarbon gases and other substances that deplete the ozone layer.[28] Ozone-depleting substances controlled by the Montreal Protocol are presented in Table 14.3. The protocol requires that future decisions by parties of the protocol be based on current scientific, environmental, technical, and economic information from worldwide experts in these areas. Since the 1987 Montreal Protocol, assessment of advances in understanding on these topics was made in 1989, 1991, 1994, 1998, and 2002. Primary findings from the Scientific Assessment of Ozone Depletion (2002) are presented in Table 14.4.

TABLE 14.3   Ozone-Depleting Substances Controlled by the Montreal Protocol Including Atmospheric Lifetimes and Relative Contributions to Ozone Depletion

Ozone-Depleting Substance	Atmospheric Lifetime, yrs.	Global Warming Potential for 100-yr. Horizon[*]
Chlorofluorocarbons (CFCs)		
CFC-11	45	4680
CFC-12	100	10720
CFC-113	85	6030
CFC-114	200	9880
CFC-115	1700	7250
Hydrochlorofluorocarbons (HCFCs)		
HCFC-22	12	1780
HCFC-123	1.3	76
HCFC-124	5.8	599
HCFC-141b	9.3	713
HCFC-142b	17.9	2270
HCFC-22ca	1.9	120
HCFC-22cb	5.8	586
Halons		
Halon-1211	16	1860
Halon-1301	65	7030
Halon-2402	20	1620
Methyl bromide	0.7	5
Carbon tetrachloride	26	1380
Methyl chloroform	5	144

*Values adopted under the United Nations Framework Convention on Climate Change for the national inventories.

Source: Data from IPCC, 2005.[11]

TABLE 14.4   Primary Findings from the Scientific Assessment of Ozone Depletion, 2002

Changes in Ozone-Depleting Compounds

- In the troposphere, total combined ozone-depleting compounds are declining slowly from their peak in 1992–1994 (total chlorine is declining whereas bromine is increasing, but at a slower rate).
- Nonindustrial sources of CFCs, halons, and major chlorocarbons trapped in snow since the late 19th century were insignificant.
- HCFCs in the lower atmosphere are still increasing.
- In the stratosphere, total chlorine abundance is at or near its peak, whereas bromine abundance is likely still increasing.
- Very short-lived organic chlorine-, bromine-, and iodine-containing source gases can deplete ozone, but it is more difficult to estimate their potentials than longer-lived substances like CFCs.

Changes in the Ozone Layer over the Poles and Globally

- Large depletion of springtime Antarctic ozone due to halogens over the past decade has occurred (with daily total column values reaching 60–70% less than prior to ozone-hole conditions).
- Maximum total column ozone due to halogens has been reduced by as much as 30% in the winters during the last decade.
- Ozone remains depleted in midlatitudes of both hemispheres. Compared with the pre-ozone period of 1980, 1997–2001 losses in total column ozone were about 4% at northern midlatitudes in winter–spring; about 2% at northern midlatitudes in summer–fall; and about 6% at southern midlatitudes on a year-round basis.
- Models predict that springtime Antarctic ozone levels will start increasing by 2010, based on projected decreases of halogens.
- A future arctic polar ozone hole similar to that in the Antarctic is unlikely.
- Global ozone layer recovery is linked mainly to decreasing chlorine and bromine, although other contributing factors are likely.

Changes in Ultraviolet Radiation

- Enhanced values of UV radiation are observed under the Antarctic ozone hole.
- Decreases in ozone column amounts results in increases in UV radiation in mid- to high latitudes.

The Ozone Layer and Climate Change

- A global and annual mean cooling of the stratosphere has occurred over the last two decades, with the cooling greater in the upper stratosphere.
- There is an increase in stratospheric water vapor, which contributes to cooling the lower stratosphere and depleting ozone through chemical interactions.

TABLE 14.4   (continued)

Implications for Policy Formulation

- The Montreal Protocol is effective, with ozone-layer depletion expected to begin to ameliorate within the next decade and the Antarctic ozone hole predicted to disappear by 2050.

- Ozone-depleting substances in the atmosphere are currently at or near their highest. Full compliance will not substantially alter the ozone layer for at least a decade.

- Approaches to accelerate recovery of the ozone layer are limited.

- Failure to comply with the Montreal Protocol would prevent recovery of the ozone layer (e.g., continued production of ozone-depleting substances at the 1999 level would extend recovery to well beyond 2100).

- New approaches are needed to effectively estimate the impacts of very short-lived ozone-depleting substances.

- Ozone depletion and climate change are interconnected. For example, as CFCs decline because of the Montreal Protocol's provision, their contribution to global warming declines. However, substitute compounds for CFCs (e.g., HFCs and HCFCs) can contribute to global warming.

Source: United Nations Environment Programme, 2002.[29]

Policy to Curb Global Warming

In 1992, delegates from 154 nations met in Rio de Janeiro, Brazil, to discuss global warming at the United Nations Conference on Environment and Development.[30] From this conference came a treaty known as the **United Nations Framework Convention on Climate Change** (UNFCCC). UNFCCC recognizes that climate change is influenced by each country of the world and in turn affects each country of the world. Therefore, UNFCCC challenges countries to "gather and share information on greenhouse gas emissions, national policies and best practices; launch national strategies for addressing greenhouse gas emissions and adapting to expected impacts, including the provision of financial and technological support to developing countries; and cooperate in preparing for adaptation to the impacts of climate change."[32] There were 189 UNFCCC members.

On December 11, 1997, delegates from the United Nations met in Kyoto, Japan, to once again discuss global warming. During this conference, the **Kyoto Protocol** was established to strengthen UNFCCC by setting standards for greenhouse gas emissions among countries that ratified the protocol. On November 12,

1998, the Clinton administration signed the Kyoto treaty, despite unanimous resolution by the U.S. Senate not to ratify it. The protocol came into force February 16, 2005. Such standards include drastically decreasing the production of halocarbon gases and decreasing other greenhouse gas emissions by a certain percentage depending on a given country's current emissions levels. Today, 165 nations have ratified the Kyoto Protocol UNFCCC.[32] The United States, the largest producer of greenhouse gases, withdrew its support in 2001. One of George W. Bush's first acts as president was to pull the United States out of the Kyoto accords. His rationale was that the protocol was too costly and that the science behind global warming was questionable.

On February 14, 2002, President Bush announced global climate change initiatives. He said, "Today, I'm announcing a new environmental approach that will clean our skies, bring greater health to our citizens, and encourage environmentally responsible development in America and around the world."[33] The Bush administration's Clear Skies initiative was submitted to Congress in February 2003 as a proposal to amend the CAA. The CAA (see Chapter 10) is the primary federal law that governs air quality in the United States. However, the Clear Skies legislation would weaken and delay health protections that are already required by the CAA. Specifically, according to the Natural Resources Defense Council, "The Clear Skies legislation sets new targets for emissions of sulfur dioxide, mercury, and nitrogen oxides from U.S. power plants. But these targets are *weaker* than those that would be put in place if the Bush administration simply implemented and enforced the existing law! Compared to current law, the Clear Skies plan would allow three times more toxic mercury emissions, 50 percent more sulfur emissions, and hundreds of thousands more tons of smog-forming nitrogen oxides. It would also delay cleaning up this pollution by up to a decade compared to current law and force residents of heavily polluted areas to wait years longer for clean air compared to the existing Clean Air Act."[34] The new Clear Air Act failed to make it out of committee in 2005 and is unlikely to be considered again in the U.S. Congress in the near future.

To further decrease greenhouse emissions, researchers are developing technologies to capture CO_2 for further use or sequestration. Examples of such innovations include polymer-metallic membranes used to separate out and capture CO_2 from industrial gas by-products; liquid absorbents or solid sorbents that trap CO_2 from mixed-gas streams and then release CO_2 into a separate gas stream; and refrigeration or liquefying separations that require cooling of gases to liquid followed by distillation.[4]

Besides the United Nation's efforts to monitor greenhouse gas emissions, several organizations are in place to monitor and provide data useful for conducting epidemiologic studies of the association between climate change and health. These are listed in Appendix II and include Environmental Protection Agency (EPA) Flood Hazard Mapping; EPA National Environmental Satellite; Data and Information Service; National Weather Service; National Severe Storms Laboratory; Occupational Safety and Health Administration; Housing and Urban Development; and Statistics and Data. Some useful indicators for monitoring associations between global warming, disasters, and health include the proportion of residents that have homes in a floodplain, number of days where the temperature exceeds safe thresholds, amount of excessive rainfall, number of safety violations at nuclear power plants, and proportion of population living in damaged or destroyed homes (see Appendix I).

Global Warming and Health: An Overview of Select Examples

Epidemiologic studies have associated health events with climate conditions like global warming and ozone depletion. Global warming can adversely affect health by causing a disruption in food production and economic performance. It may also increase the occurrence of illness, injury, and death because of more extreme temperatures, increased floods and severe storms, droughts, increased frequency of and changing patterns in waterborne, foodborne, vector-borne, and rodent-borne diseases. Ozone depletion leads to higher levels of UVB radiation reaching the earth's surface, which is associated with skin cancer, skin damage, cataracts, suppression of the body's immune system, and interference with the physiological and developmental process of plants.

Earlier in this chapter we discussed how greenhouse gases and other natural and human factors contribute to global warming. In turn, global warming leads to changes in the environment. Environmental changes associated with global warming include melting of arctic glaciers; increases in floods, hurricanes, heat waves, and forest fires; changes in ecosystems such as coral reefs; extinctions of some amphibian species; and increases in the spread of infectious diseases among human populations.

Over the past several decades, the earth's atmosphere and ocean surfaces have warmed, leading to increased glacier melting and evaporation from oceans. Glacier melting has been especially prevalent in the arctic regions where temperatures have increased by almost twice the rate of the rest of the earth. If this rate remains constant, scientists project that arctic temperatures could increase by 4°C to 7°C in the next 100 years. Because of increasing temperatures in this region, arctic sea ice has decreased distinctly and ocean levels have risen (see Figure 14.13).[35] In turn, rising ocean levels and increased evaporation cause air to become saturated with moisture, and storms are more likely to form and lead to heavier rain and snow as the air moves from oceans to land. In one study, researchers compared 51 simulated tropical storms under current conditions with 51 simulated storms under high atmospheric CO_2 conditions. The study concluded that CO_2-induced warming led to more intense hurricanes.[36]

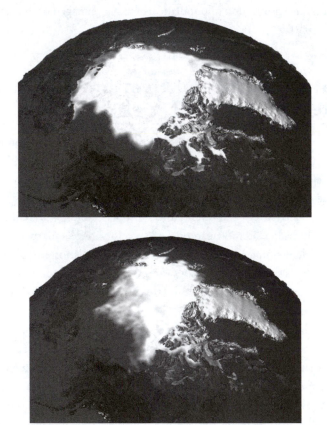

FIGURE 14.13   Patterns of Arctic sea ice in the years 1979 and 2003. (*Source:* Courtesy of NASA/Goddard Space Flight Center/Scientific Visualization Studio)

In addition to changing weather patterns, global warming has the potential to change ecosystems. One dramatic example of this is occurring in the Seychelles, a small island country with one of the largest coral reefs in the Indian Ocean. Over the past several years, Seychelles has experienced an increase in extreme weather conditions characterized by much wetter wet seasons and much drier dry seasons. As a result of increased temperatures and extreme weather, the Seychelles coral reef has begun to be bleached, causing death of the coral. Depending on the depth of the coral and other factors, some areas of the coral reef have been bleached upwards of 74% to 100%. Because coral reefs are home to hundreds of species and two of the main industries in Seychelles are fishing and tourism, coral reef bleaching will not only have a drastic effect on this ecosystem, but on this country's economy.[38]

Another outcome of global warming that is especially worrisome is the increased spread of infectious diseases. Due to increased precipitation in wet months and excessive heat in dry months, many officials fear that the incidence of infectious diseases will increase due to weather conditions optimal for the spread of disease. While causal relationships between global warming and increases in disease transmission are hard to establish, some researchers are beginning to find evidence for this connection among animal populations. In one study, researchers found that 67% of 110 species of harlequin frogs have become extinct in Central and South America over the past two decades with 78–83% of extinctions occurring during years with unusually warm weather. Specifically, researchers asserted that because temperatures in the tropical Americas have increased over the past several years, nighttime temperatures are now at the optimal temperature for the transmission of *B. dendrobatidi*, a bacterium known to kill harlequin frogs.[39]

Evidence of increased infectious diseases due to climate change is also starting to surface among human populations. During 1998, the hottest year of the past century, storms associated with **El Niño** (warming of the ocean surface off the western coast of South America) and hurricanes were abnormally frequent and intense, causing massive deforestation, forest fires, and flooding. As a result, Indonesia and Brazil experienced an epidemic of respiratory illness and Central America experienced increases in water- and insect-borne diseases such as cholera and malaria.[12]

However, data from all over the world indicate that changes in climate affect health in more ways than just promoting the spread of infectious diseases. Impacts of climate change on global health also include malnutrition from changes in crops, heat-related illnesses from excessive heat exposure, injury and death from natural disasters, vector-borne illnesses from changes in migrating animals, asthma and allergies from air pollutions, and many more.[12] The remainder of this chapter will specifically explore the association between global warming and health in terms of vector-borne disease, deforestation, natural disasters, and ozone depletion.

Global Warming and Vector-borne Disease

A **vector** is an invertebrate animal (e.g., tick, mite, mosquito, bloodsucking fly) capable of transmitting an infectious agent among vertebrates.[24] A vector can spread an infectious agent from an infected animal or human to other susceptible animals or humans through its waste products, bite, body fluids, or indirectly through food contamination. Vector-borne diseases kill millions of people each year (see Figure 14.14). Malaria is the leading vector-related cause of death. In 2002, an estimated 1,272,000 people died from this disease worldwide.[40] Vectors do not regulate their internal body temperature. Hence, they are sensitive to temperature (see Figure 14.15). In addition, because mosquitoes primarily use shallow pools of rainwater for breeding, a time lag between rainfall and diseases associated with mosquitoes is well established.[41,42]

Consequently, climate change has the potential to alter the distribution of vectors by altering the weather conditions that influence their breeding places (water, vegetation, or host). Temperature can also influence rates of reproduction and mat-

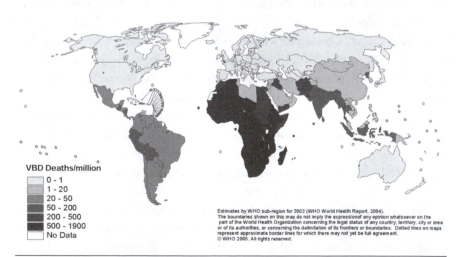

VBD Deaths/million

- 0 - 1
- 1 - 20
- 20 - 50
- 50 - 200
- 200 - 500
- 500 - 1900
- No Data

Estimates by WHO sub-region for 2002 (WHO World Health Report, 2004).
The boundaries shown on this map do not imply the expressionof any opinion whatsoever on the part of the World Health Organization concerning the legal status of any country, territory, city or area or of its authorities, or concerning the delimitation of its frontiers or boundaries. Dotted lines on maps represent approximate border lines for which there may not yet be full agreement.
© WHO 2005. All rights reserved.

FIGURE 14.14   Death from vector-borne disease. (*Source:* ©WHO 2005. All rights reserved.)

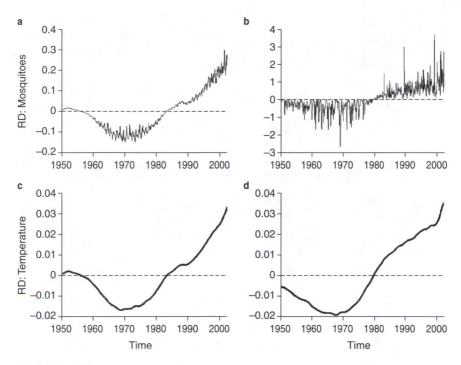

RD: Relative difference

FIGURE 14.15 Mosquito abundances (a and b) and temperature (c and d) for two sites in East African highlands: Kericho (a and c) and Kabale (b and d). (*Source:* Pascual et al., 2006.)[45]

uration of the infectious agent in the vector organism and the survivability of the organism. Disease transmission requires the vector and the pathogen to be present in the same place and at the same time in adequate number.[43] Common vector-borne diseases are presented in Table 14.5, along with their climate-epidemic link.

The potential global warming has on humidity, altered rainfall, and sea levels has been discussed. These factors, combined with temperature, demographic, and societal factors, influence the risk of disease transmission through vector organisms.[47] Some of the many factors that combine with temperature, relative humidity, and precipitation patterns that influence vector-borne disease transmission include land use and irrigation systems, sewage and waste management systems, housing type and location, availability of screens and air conditioning, and human population density. For example, climate change may introduce vector-borne disease into new areas or decrease the distribution of vectors in others because of factors

TABLE 14.5 Common Vector-Borne Diseases According to Population at Risk and Climatic Epidemic Link

Disease	Vector	Population at Risk	Global Burden (DALYs)	Distribution	Evidence for Interannual Variability	Climate Epidemic Link	Strength of Temporal Climate Sensitivity
Malaria	Female *Anopheles* mosquitoes	2,400 million (40% of world's population)	46,486,000	Endemic in > 100 countries throughout the tropics and subtropics and some temperate areas	*****	Change in temperature and rainfall associated epidemics; other locally relevant factors also important, including vector characteristics, immunity, population movements, drug resistance, and environmental changes	+++++
Schistosomiasis	Water snail	500–600 million	1,702,000	Africa, East Asia, South America	*	Increases in temperature and rainfall affect seasonal transmission and geographical distribution	+

Disease	Vector	Population at risk	Number infected	Distribution		Climate sensitivity	
Lymphatic filariasis	Female *Culex*, Anopheles, *Aedes* and *Mansonia* mosquitoes	1 billion	5,777,000	Africa, India, South America, South Asia, and Pacific Islands	-	Temperature and rainfall determine the geographical distribution of vectors and disease	++
African trypanosomiasis	Male or female tsetse flies	55 million	1,525,000	Sub-Saharan Africa	***	Changes in temperature and rainfall; cattle density and vegetation patterns also relevant	++
Leishmaniasis	Female *Phlebotomine* sand flies	350 million	2,090,000	Africa, Central Asia, Europe, India, South America	**	Increases in temperature and rainfall associated with epidemics	+++
Onchocerciasis	Female *Simulid* black flies	120 million	484,000	Africa, Southwest Asia, South America	*	Evidence for climate effects on spatial distribution and seasonal vector biting rates, but not temporal variation in disease	-

(*continues*)

TABLE 14.5 (continued)

Disease	Vector	Population at Risk	Global Burden (DALYs)	Distribution	Evidence for Interannual Variability	Climate Epidemic Link	Strength of Temporal Climate Sensitivity
American typanosomiasis (Chagas disease)	Blood-feeding male or female *Reduviid* bugs	100 million	667,000	South and Central America	*	Presence of bugs associated with high temperatures, low humidity, and specific vegetation types	+
Dengue	Female *Aedes* mosquitoes	3,000 million	616,000	Africa, Europe, South America, Southeast Asia, Western Pacific	****	High temperatures, humidity, and rainfall associated with epidemics in some areas; nonclimatic factors also important	+++
Japanese encephalitis	Female *Culex* and *Aedes* mosquitoes	300 million	709,000	Southeast Asia	***	High temperatures and heavy rains associated with epidemics	+++

Disease	Vector		Burden	Distribution		Climate sensitivity	
St Louis encephalitis	Female *Culex* and *Aedes* mosquitoes	NA	Not quantified	North and South America	***	High temperatures and heavy precipitation associated with epidemics	+++
Yellow fever	Female *Aedes* and *Haemagogus* mosquitoes	468 million in Africa	Not quantified	Africa, South and Central America	****	High temperatures and heavy rains associated with epidemic	++
West Nile virus	Female *Culicine* mosquitoes	NA	Not quantified	Africa, Central Asia, Southwest Asia, Europe, North America	***	High temperatures and heavy precipitation associated with onset of epidemic; Nonclimatic factors may have more important impact	++
Ross River virus	Female *Culicine* mosquitoes	NA	Not quantified	Australia and Pacific Islands	**	High temperatures and heavy precipitation associated with epidemic	+++

(continues)

TABLE 14.5 (continued)

Disease	Vector	Population at Risk	Global Burden (DALYs)	Distribution	Evidence for Interannual Variability	Climate Epidemic Link	Strength of Temporal Climate Sensitivity
Murray Valley fever	Female *Culex* mosquitoes	NA	Not quantified	Australia	**	Heavy rains and below average atmospheric pressure associated with epidemics	+++
Lyme disease	Ixodid ticks	NA	Not quantified	Asia, Europe, and North America	*	Temperature and vegetation patterns associated with distribution of vectors and disease	+

Source: Adapted from WHO, 2004; WHO, 2005.[1,46]

*very weak variability; **some variability; ***moderate variability; ****strong variability; *****very strong variability.

+climate link is very weak; ++climate plays a moderate role; +++climate plays a significant role; ++++climate is an important factor; +++++climate is the primary factor in determining at least some epidemics, based on published quantitative (statistical) data.

like droughts. Although climate change in the future may play a significant role in infectious diseases, to date there is little evidence that recent resurgence in infectious diseases is attributed to climate change. Rather, population growth, urbanization, deforestation, changes in land use, changes in agricultural practices, commerce, international travel, microbial adaptation and change, and other factors have been primarily responsible for epidemic transmission occurrence.[48–50]

Investigating the influence of climate change on the frequency and pattern of vector-borne disease may involve laboratory data or epidemiologic data collected in the field. Laboratory studies allow researchers to investigate under tightly controlled conditions the effects of temperature and humidity on breeding and feeding activities of vectors. However, it may be difficult to fully generalize the laboratory results to the field given other factors that influence vector behavior and survival (e.g., land use, urbanization, and spraying). On the other hand, disease and vector monitoring systems in multiple areas can allow researchers to compare vector-borne disease across several climate conditions.

Deforestation and Health

Deforestation has the potential to directly and indirectly affect human health. Increased emission of greenhouse gases caused by loss of forest cover can propagate a vicious cycle because deforestation leads to a decrease in rainfall, which then signifies increased deforestation. Deforestation can also lead to increased floods, which can lead to an increase in disease such as cholera. Two examples illustrate the damaging effects deforestation can have on a society. In 1997–1998 when Indonesia burned 10 million hectares of forest, it cost $9.3 billion in increased health care costs, lost production, and lost tourism revenues, and affected 20 million people. When China cleared its coastal mangroves, it experienced increased susceptibility to tropical storms and increased downstream flooding of the Yangtze River.[17] These outcomes are examples of indirect influences on health status through impoverishment and loss of resources or livelihoods. Deforestation can also act as a direct cause of health problems.

Changes in ecosystems like forests can affect the amount and spread of pathogens. For example, deforestation leads to a decrease in medicinal plants and species, which leads to ecological imbalances, which in turn lead to the emergence and spread of infectious diseases.[18] Because forests are effective at managing disease, deforestation can lead to increased incidence of infectious diseases like malaria, dengue fever, schistosomiasis, lymphatic filariasis, Japanese encephalitis, Chagas disease, cholera, Lyme disease, meningitis, and West Nile virus.[17] Deforestation also causes loss of habitat; without specific habitats, certain predators disappear. This interruption of the food chain creates an increase in the amount of disease-carrying prey. Small animals can carry diseases such as the Marburg virus, HIV-1, Junin virus, and Lyme disease.[19]

Thus, deforestation affects health in both indirect and direct ways. Deforestation is especially harmful to population health when the definition of health is all-inclusive (emotional, physical, social, and spiritual). Loss of forests can negatively affect people in each of these aspects. Expansion of farming and herding lands, in addition to extensive use of forest products, should be limited to mitigate the negative health outcomes that deforestation can produce.

Climate Change and Frequency of Natural Disaster

On August 25, 2005, Hurricane Katrina swept ashore on the southern Louisiana coast, knocking out power and submerging parts of New Orleans. Katrina was responsible for 1,836 deaths and an estimated $81.2 billion (2005 U.S. dollars) in damage.[51] Reaction to the storm by federal, state, and local governments was highly criticized, resulting in investigations by the U.S. Congress and the resignation of the director of the Federal Emergency Management Agency (FEMA). A cartoon depicting arks lined up like houses with the heading "More realistic FEMA guidelines for rebuilding New Orleans" is reflective of this criticism, with the postscript: "A complete description of materials and how to build it are available in Genesis, Chapter 6:14–16."

Environmental conditions following natural disasters such as Hurricane Katrina increase the risk for infectious disease. (See Table 14.6.) This may be caused by a lack of functioning toilets and potable water, an increase of exposure to water-borne agents and vectors like mosquitoes, wound injuries, and crowding and unsanitary conditions in evacuation centers.[52,53] These are ideal conditions for the spread of common bacteria that cause diarrhea, such as *shigella*, rotoviruses, Norwalk virus, and enteropathic *Escherichia coli*.

In recent decades the total number of reported natural disasters increased from about 80 in 1974 to over 400 in 2002 (see Figure 14.16). Between 1974 and 2003 there were 6,367 natural disasters, not including epidemics. As a result of

TABLE 14.6 Cases of Selected Diseases and Conditions after Hurricane Katrina, August–September 2005

Disease/Condition[*]	No. of Cases	States Reporting	Population
Dermatologic Infectious Conditions			
Methicillin-resistant *Staphylococcus aureus* infections	30 (3 confirmed)	Texas	Evacuees
Vibrio vulnificus and *V. parahaemolyticus* wound infections Oklahoma, Texas	24 (6 deaths)	Arkansas, Arizona, Georgia, Louisiana, Mississippi	Evacuees
Tinea corporis	17	Mississippi	Rescue workers
Noninfectious			
Arthropod bites (likely mite)	97	Louisiana	Rescue workers
Diarrheal disease			
Acute gastroenteritis, some attributed to norovirus	Approximately 1,000	Louisiana, Mississippi, Tennessee, Texas	Evacuees
Nontoxigenic *V. cholerae* O1	6	Arizona, Georgia, Mississippi, Oklahoma, Tennessee	Evacuees
Nontyphoidal *Salmonella*	1	Mississippi	Evacuees
Respiratory disease			
Pertussis	1	Tennessee	Evacuees
Respiratory syncytial virus	1	Texas	Evacuees
Streptococcal pharyngitis	1	Texas	Evacuees
Tuberculosis	1	Pennsylvania	Evacuees
Other conditions			
Presumed viral conjunctivitis	Approximately 200	Louisiana	Evacuees

[*]Other diseases and conditions, for which the number of cases was unknown, included scabies; circumferential lesions at waist; contact dermatitis; erythematous, popular, pustular rash consistent with folliculitis; immersion foot; prickly heat; influenza-like illness and upper respiratory infections; and head lice.

Source: From CDC, 2005.[53]

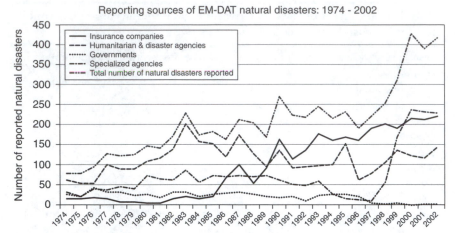

FIGURE 14.16   Reporting sources of EM-DAT natural disasters: 1974–2002. (*Source:* Guha-Sapir et al., 2004.)[54]

these disasters 5.1 billion people were cumulatively affected, 182 million persons were made homeless, more than 2 million deaths were reported, and damages were estimated at $1.38 trillion. Over the last century the total number of natural disasters increased sharply (see Figure 14.17). The largest increasing trends in disasters reflect floods and windstorms. Epidemics have also shown an increase in trend.

Although these data are compelling, changes in reporting may have caused some of the increase; although these data are suggestive of an association between global warming and an increase in natural disasters, they do not confirm a causal association. Nevertheless, some researchers believe that the observed increase in natural disasters in recent years is real, particularly because of El Niño, which is especially associated with droughts and floods.[56]

In 2006, there were 214 episodes of flooding worldwide, along with 6,921 deaths, almost 18 million people displaced from their homes, and almost $10 billion in damage. Clustering of flood events is seen primarily along the equator and tropical latitudes. In 2005, there were 156 episodes of flooding worldwide, almost 8,000 deaths, over 18 million people displaced from their homes, and almost $82 billion in damage.

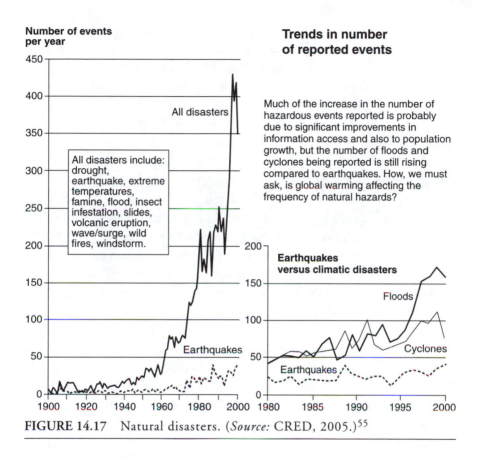

FIGURE 14.17   Natural disasters. (*Source:* CRED, 2005.)[55]

Ozone Depletion and Health

Epidemiologic studies have shown that greater exposure to **UVB radiation** (that portion of the electromagnetic spectrum capable of damaging organisms; wavelength 290–320 nanometers) due to ozone depletion is associated with skin cancer, skin problems, cataracts, and immune system suppression. In the United States, skin cancer incidence is at epidemic levels. One in every five Americans will develop skin cancer during his or her lifetime. The most serious form of skin cancer is melanoma, which is one of the fastest growing types of cancer in the United States. In the past decade the incidence of melanoma has doubled. The primary risk factor for melanoma is blistering sunburn during childhood. Nonmelanoma skin cancers (basal cell carcinoma and squamous cell carcinoma) are less deadly but threaten disfigurement and more serious health problems. Other skin damage that is related to **ultraviolet radiation** includes **actinic keratoses** (skin growths on sun-exposed body areas) and premature aging of the skin. UV radiation is also associated with increased risk of cataracts, which are characterized by a loss of transparency in the lens of the eye and thereby clouds vision. Finally, overexposure to UV radiation may result in suppression of the functioning of the body's immune system, as well as the skin's natural defenses. The health consequences might be impaired response to immunizations, increased sensitivity to sun exposure, and adverse reactions to selected medications.[57]

Human health is also indirectly affected by ozone depletion and corresponding increases in UVB radiation because it affects plants, marine ecosystems, and biogeochemical cycles. Physiological and developmental processes of plants can be adversely affected by UVB radiation. Increasing UVB radiation may also disrupt plant competitive balance, herbivory, plant diseases, and biogeochemical cycles. In addition, UVB radiation has been shown to reduce survival rates of phytoplankton and to cause damage to early developmental stages of fish, shrimp, crab, amphibians, and other animals. There are serious implications of decreased reproductive capacity and impaired larval development on the population of animals that eat these smaller creatures. Increases in solar UV radiation adversely affect terrestrial and aquatic biogeochemical cycles, thereby altering sources and sinks of greenhouse and chemically important trace gases and contributing to the atmospheric buildup of greenhouse gases.[58]

Key Issues

1. Epidemiologic studies rarely evaluate health according to climate change, but rather assess the association between health and weather. This is because health is typically associated with something that is more immediate—weather conditions at a point and place in time that vary from day to day.

2. Global warming refers to an average increase in the earth's temperature, which in turn causes changes in climate. Increases in the earth's temperature are the result of both natural causes and human activities.

3. Greenhouse gases are those that absorb infrared radiation in the atmosphere. The greenhouse effect refers to the "trapping" of infrared radiation from the earth by greenhouse gases in the atmosphere.

4. Natural factors that contribute to global warming include water vapor, cloud coverage, solar rays, and volcanoes.

5. Human activities that contribute to global warming include greenhouse gases, which cause the greenhouse effect and ozone depletion, and land variability.

6. Consequences of climate change, such as global warming, include melting of arctic glaciers; increases in flood, hurricanes, heat waves, and forest fires; changes in ecosystems such as coral reefs; extinctions of species such as frogs; and increases in the spread of infectious diseases among human populations.

7. Deforestation is influenced by factors such as rising demand for land for farming, cattle herding, wood, paper products, and fuel.

8. Ozone depletion describes a slow, steady decline in the total amount of ozone in the earth's stratosphere below normal levels after accounting for seasonal cycles and location (about 3% per decade over the past 20 years), and a decrease in stratospheric ozone over the polar regions of the earth.

9. The Montreal Protocol has been effective at eliminating environmental contaminants associated with stratospheric ozone-layer depletion.

10. The Montreal Protocol, UNFCCC, Kyoto Protocol, and carbon dioxide capture technologies all seek to alleviate global warming impacts.

11. The impact natural disasters have on human health is an epidemiologic question.

12. Global warming is associated with an increase in infectious disease, malnutrition from changes in crops, heat-related illnesses from excessive heat exposure, injury and death from natural disasters, vector-borne illnesses from changes in migrating animals, asthma and allergies from air pollutions, and many more.

13. Changing weather conditions influence rates of reproduction and maturation of the infectious agent in the vector organism and the survivability of the organism. Disease transmission requires the vector and the pathogen to be present in the same place and at the same time in adequate number.

14. Epidemiologic studies have shown that greater exposure to UVB radiation because of ozone depletion is associated with skin cancer, skin problems, cataracts, and immune system suppression.

15. The mounting epidemiologic evidence associating global warming and ozone depletion with adverse health events has provided support for protocols and technologies to reduce global warming and stratospheric ozone depletion.

Exercises

Key Terms

Define the following terms.

Actinic keratoses
Climate
Climate forcing power
El Niño
Global warming
Greenhouse effect
Greenhouse gases
Halocarbon substances
Kyoto Protocol
Montreal Protocol
Ozone
Ozone depletion
Ultraviolet radiation
United Nations Framework Convention on Climate Change
UVB radiation
Vector
Weather

Study Questions

14.1. What is the difference between weather and climate? Why is weather more useful to epidemiologists?

14.2. What are greenhouse gases and the greenhouse effect? Why can an increase in greenhouse gases lead to global warming?

14.3. Give at least two examples each of natural and human factors influencing global warming. Discuss how these factors contribute to global warming.

14.4. There are two major ways to increase global warming: increasing greenhouse gases (the greenhouse effect) or depleting the ozone layer. Discuss the effects of both, and the two combined.

14.5. Explain the role of both the stratosphere and troposphere in protecting the earth from warming. What changes occur in these atmospheric layers to contribute to global warming?

14.6.   Matching:

___Water vapor   a) Gas in the atmosphere that absorbs harmful
___Carbon dioxide   UV light
___Halocarbons   b) Most common greenhouse gas; affected by
___Ozone   deforestation
                        c) Increased amounts can lead to increased hur-
                           ricanes, storms, and other weather changes
                        d) Industrial chemicals that can deplete the ozone
                           layer

14.7.   What are three consequences of increasing temperatures in the arctic regions?

14.8.   Explain three ways that global warming leads to increased spread of infectious diseases.

14.9.   If increased temperatures and humidity led a dry, mosquito-free area to become more humid with more standing water, how could the prevalence of vector-borne diseases in this area change?

14.10.   Global warming can influence human health through which of the following factors (choose all that apply).
         a. Increased natural disasters
         b. Economic changes and strain
         c. Exposure to more extreme temperatures
         d. Increase in infectious disease rates

14.11.   What are ways that deforestation can *directly* lead to adverse health outcomes?

14.12.   How would changes in reporting lead to a perceived increase in natural disasters?

14.13.   What are some of the serious complications associated with a depleting ozone layer and increased UV exposure for humans, plant, and animal species?

References

1. World Health Organization. Climate change and health. Available at: http://www.who.int/globalchange/climate/en/. Accessed November 25, 2006.
2. Wilkinson P, ed. *Environmental Epidemiology*. New York: Open University Press; 2006.
3. U.S. Department of Commerce: National Climatic Data Center. Available at: http://lwf.ncdc.noaa.gov. Accessed October 10, 2006.

4. International Panel on Climate Change. Carbon dioxide capture and storage. 2005:22–23, 109–110. Available at: http://arch.rivm.nl/env/int/ipcc/pages_media/SRCCS-final/SRCCS_TechnicalSummary.pdf. Accessed November 16, 2006.

5. Brohan P, Kennedy JJ, Harris I, Tett SB, Jones PD. Uncertainty estimates in regional and global observed temperature changes: a new dataset from 1850. *J Geophys Res.* 2006;111:D12106.

6. Environmental Protection Agency. Climate change. Available at: http://www.epa.gov/climatechange/kids/greenhouse.html. Accessed October 10, 2006.

7. Wikipedia: The free encyclopedia. Greenhouse effect. Available at: http://en.wikipedia.org/wiki/Greenhouse_effect. Accessed November 30, 2006.

8. Dai A. Recent climatology, variability, and trends in global surface humidity. *Journal of Climate.* 2006;19:3589–3606.

9. National Academy of Sciences. *Climate Change Science: An Analysis of Some Key Questions.* Washington, DC: National Academy Press; 2001.

10. Wikipedia: The free encyclopedia. Year without a summer. Available at: http://en.wikipedia.org/wiki/Year_Without_a_Summer. Accessed June 8, 2007.

11. International Panel on Climate Change. Safeguarding the ozone layer and the global climate system: issues related to hydrofluorocarbons and perfluorocarbons. 2005. Available at: http://arch.rivm.nl/env/int/ipcc/pages_media/SROC-final/SROC01.pdf. Accessed November 14, 2006.

12. Haines A, McMichael A, Epstein P. Environment and health: global climate change and health. *J Canadian Med Assoc.* 2006;163:729–734.

13. Oak Ridge National Laboratory. Carbon Dioxide Information Analysis Center: Frequently asked global change questions. Available at: http://cdiac.ornl.gov/pns/faq.html. Accessed October 11, 2006.

14. Environmental Protection Agency. Methane. Available at: http://www.epa.gov/methane/scientific.html. Accessed June 15, 2006.

15. Environmental Protection Agency. The U.S. inventory of greenhouse gas emission and sinks: fast facts. 2004. Available at: http://www.epa.gov/climatechange/emissions/downloads06/06FastFacts.pdf. Accessed November 14, 2006.

16. Environmental Protection Agency. Global greenhouse gas data. Available at: http://www.epa.gov/climatechange/emissions/globalghg.html. Accessed June 8, 2007.

17. Millennium Ecosystem Assessment. *Ecosystems and Human Well-being: A Framework for Assessment.* Washington, DC: Island Press; 2005.

18. Frumkin H. *Environmental Health: from Global to Local.* San Francisco, CA: John Wiley & Sons, Inc.; 2005.

19. Vajpeyi DK, ed. *Deforestation, Environment, and Sustainable Development: Comparative Analysis.* Westport, CT: Greenwood Publishing Group; 2001.

20. Berriman M, Fraser R. News from near and far. *New Vegetarian and Natural Health.* Spring 2004.

21. Errey S. *The True Cost of a Burger: News from the World Vegetarian Congress in Brazil.* Florianopolis, Brazil: World Vegetarian Congress; 2004.

22. National Aeronautics and Space Administration. The carbon cycle. Available at: http://earthobservatory.nasa.gov/Library/CarbonCycle/carbon_cycle.html. Accessed June 8, 2007.

23. Lorius CJ, Jouzel C, Ritz L, et al. A 150,000-year climatic record from Antarctic ice. *Nature.* 1995;316:591–596.

24. *Stedman's Medical Dictionary for the Health Professions and Nursing.* 5th ed. New York, NY: Lippincott, Williams & Wilkins; 2005.

25. National Aeronautics and Space Administration. Goddard Space Flight Center. Unusually small Antarctic ozone hole this year attributed to exceptionally strong stratospheric weather systems. 2002. Available at: www.gsfc.nasa.gov/topstory/20020926ozonehole.html. Accessed November 24, 2006.

26. National Aeronautics and Space Administration. NASA and NOAA announce ozone hole is a double record breaker. Available at: http://www.nasa.gov/vision/earth/lookingatearth/ozone_record.html. Accessed November 24, 2006.

27. Wikipedia: The free encyclopedia. Ozone depletion. Available at: http://en.wikipedia.org/wiki/Ozone_depletion. Accessed November 24, 2006.

28. *Alternative fluorocarbons environmental acceptability study.* Available at: http://www.afeas.org/montreal_protocol.html. Accessed October 17, 2006.

29. United Nations Environment Programme. *Scientific assessment of ozone depletion: executive summary.* Available at: http://ozone.unep.org/pdfs/Scientific_assess_depletion/05-ExecutiveSummary.pdf. Accessed November 25, 2006.

30. Wikipedia: The free encyclopedia. *UNFCCC.* 2006. Available at: http://en.wikipedia.org/wiki/United_Nations_Framework_Convention_on_Climate_Change. Accessed October 17, 2006.

31. United Nations Framework Convention on Climate Change. *The United Nations Framework Convention on Climate Change: Essential Background.* 2006. Available at: http://unfccc.int/essential_background/convention /items/ 2627.php. Accessed October 17, 2006.

32. United Nations Framework Convention on Climate Change. *Kyoto Protocol.* 2006. Available at: http://unfccc.int/kyoto_protocol/background/items/3145 .php. Accessed November 25, 2006.

33. The White House. President announces clear skies & global climate change initiatives. Available at: http://www.whitehouse.gov/news/releases/2002/02/ 20020214-5.html. Accessed June 9, 2007.

34. Natural Resources Defense Council. Dirty skies: The Bush administration's air pollution plan. Available at: http://www.nrdc.org/air/pollution/qbushplan .asp. Accessed June 9, 2007.

35. Watson RT. International Panel on Climate Change Core Writing Team, eds. *Climate Change 2001: Synthesis Report. A Contribution of Working Groups I, II, and III to the Third Assessment Report of the Intergovernmental Panel on Climate Change.* Cambridge, UK: Cambridge University Press; 2001.

36. Knutson T, Tuleya R, Kurihara Y. Simulated increase of hurricane intensities in a CO_2-warmed climate. *Science.* 1998;279:1017–1020.

37. National Aeronautics and Space Administration. NASA watches arctic ice. Available at: http://www.nasa.gov/centers/goddard/news/topstory/2005/arctic ice_decline.html. Accessed June 12, 2007.

38. Payet R, Agricole W. Climate change in the Seychelles: implications for water and coral reefs. *Ambio.* 2006;35:182–189.

39. Blaustein A, Dobson A. A message from the frogs. *Nature.* 2006;439: 143–144.

40. World Health Organization. The World Health Report 2004. Available at: http://www.who.int/whr/2004/en/report04_en.pdf. Accessed November 30, 2006.

41. Kilian AD, Langi P, Talisuna A, Kabagambe G. Rainfall pattern, El Niño and malaria in Uganda. *Trans R Soc Trop Med Hyg.* 1999;93:22–23.

42. Odongo-Aginya E, Ssegwanyi G, Kategere P, Vuzi PC. Relationship between malaria infection intensity and rainfall pattern in Entebbe peninsula, Uganda. *Afr Health Sci.* 2005;5(3):238–245.

43. McCarthy JJ, Canziani OF, Leary NA, Dokken DJ, White KS, eds. Contribution of working group II to the third assessment report of the intergovernmental panel on climate change (chap. 9). In: *Climate Change 2001: Impacts, Adaptation, and Vulnerability.* Available at: http://www.grida.no/climate/ipcc_tar/wg2/index.htm. Accessed November 30, 2006.

44. World Health Organization. The Health and Environment Linkages Initiative. 2006. Available at: http://www.who.int/heli/risks/vectors/vector/en/. Accessed November 30, 2006.

45. Pascual M, Ahumada JA, Chaves LF, Rodo X, Bouma M. Malaria resurgence in the East Adrican highlands: temperature trends revisited. *Proc Natl Acad Sci U S A.* 2006;103:5829–5834. Available at: http://www.pnas.org/cgi/content/full/103/15/5829. Accessed November 30, 2006.

46. World Health Organization. Using climate to predict infectious disease epidemics. Available at: http://www.who.int/globalchange/publications/infect diseases.pdf. Accessed November 30, 2006.

47. Gubler DJ. Dengue and dengue hemorrhagic fever. *Clin Microbiol Rev.* 1998; 11:480–496.

48. Lederberg J, Oates SC, Shope RE. *Emerging Infections: Microbial Threats to Health in the United States.* Washington, DC: Institute of Medicine, National Academy Press; 1992.

49. Gubler DJ. Aedes aegypti and Aedes aegypti-borne disease control in the 1990s: top down and bottom up. *Am J Trop Med Hyg.* 1989;40:571–578.

50. Gubler DJ. Resurgent vector borne diseases as a global health problem. *Emerg Infect Dis.* 1998;4:442–450.

51. Wikipedia: The free encyclopedia. Hurricane Katrina. Available at: http://en.wikipedia.org/wiki/Hurricane_Katrina. Accessed November 25, 2006.

52. Centers for Disease Control and Prevention. Tropical storm Allison rapid needs assessment—Houston, Texas, June 2001. *MMWR.* 2002;51:365–368.

53. Centers for Disease Control and Prevention. Infectious disease and dermatologic conditions in evacuees and rescue workers after Hurricane Katrina—multiple states, August–September, 2005. *MMWR.* 2005;54:1–4.

54. Guha-Sapir D, Hargitt D, Hoyois P. Thirty years of natural disasters 1974–2003: the numbers. Centre for Research on the Epidemiology of Dis-

aster & Universitaires De Louvain: UCL Presses. Available at: http://www.em-dat.net/documents/Publication/publication_2004_emdat.pdf. Accessed November 25, 2006.

55. Centre for Research on the Epidemiology of Disasters. Available at: http://maps .grida.no/go/graphic/trends_in_natural_disasters. Accessed November 25, 2006.

56. Kovats R, Bouma M, Hajat S, Worrall E, Haines A. El Niño and health. *Lancet.* 2003;362:1481–1489.

57. Environmental Protection Agency. SunWise Program: Health effects of over-exposure to the sun. Available at: http://www.epa.gov/sunwise/uvandhealth .html#iss. Accessed November 25, 2006.

58. Environmental Protection Agency. Ozone depletion: The effects of ozone depletion. Available at: http://www.epa.gov/ozone/science/effects.html. Accessed November 25, 2006.

Measures and Data Sources for Environmental Public Health Indicators

Source: Environmental Public Health Indicators Project; NCEH, EHHE; January 2006.

Air, Ambient (Outdoor)

Indicator	Suggested Measure	Potential Data Source
Hazards		
Criteria pollutants in ambient air *(core)*	1) Annual high levels of criteria pollutants: carbon monoxide (CO), lead (Pb), nitrogen dioxide (NO$_2$), ozone (O$_3$), PM$_{10}$, sulfur dioxide (SO$_2$) *(core)* 2) Tons of criteria pollutants released in ambient air *(core)*	**EPA:** National Air Quality and Emissions Trends Report; NMMAPS; NEI; Urban Air Toxics Program; TRI/EPCRA; AIRS **States or local jurisdictions:** environmental protection agencies, especially those with indicator projects; Urban Air Toxics Programs
Hazardous or toxic substances in ambient air *(core)*	1) Tons of one or more hazardous or toxic substances released in ambient air *(core)* 2) Number of reports of noncompliance for emissions releases *(developmental)*	**ATSDR:** HSEES **EPA:** National Air Quality and Emissions Trends Report; NMMAPS; NEI; TRI/EPCRA; AIRS **NOAA (NWS)** **States or local jurisdictions:** environmental protection agencies, especially those with indicator projects; Urban Air Toxics Programs
Motor vehicle emissions *(core)*	1) Vehicle miles driven per capita *(core)* 2) Average fuel efficiency of registered motor vehicles *(optional)*	**CB:** census data **DOE (EIA)** **DOT, FHA:** NPTS
Residence in nonattainment areas *(core)*	1) Percentage of human population residing in nonattainment areas (for criteria air pollutants) *(core)*	**CB:** census data **EPA:** National Air Quality and Emissions Trends Report, NMMAPS
Exposures		
(None identified)		
Health Effects		
Unusual pattern of asthma events *(core)*	1) Number of asthma-related deaths *(core)* 2) Incidence of asthma *(core)* 3) Rates of hospitalization and emergency department visits for acute asthma events *(core)*	**CDC:** NHAMCS, NHDS, NVSS **States or local jurisdictions:** CDI surveillance; ME/Cs; vital statistics

Air, Ambient (Outdoor) Continued

Indicator	Suggested Measure	Potential Data Source
Health Effects Continued	4) Number of work days missed because of asthma *(optional)*	
	5) Number of school days missed because of asthma *(optional)*	
	6) Proportion of population filling prescriptions for asthma medication *(developmental)*	
Unusual pattern of cardiovascular or respiratory events *(core)*	1) Incidence of cardiovascular and respiratory events *(core)*	**CDC:** NHAMCS, NHDS, NVSS **States or local jurisdictions:** CDI surveillance; vital statistics
	2) Rates of hospitalization and emergency department visits for acute cardiovascular and respiratory events *(core)*	
Interventions		
Programs that address motor vehicle emissions *(core)*	1) Proportion of population residing in jurisdictions that have vehicle emissions mandates *(core)*	**CB:** census data **DOT (FHA):** NPTS **States or local jurisdictions:** environmental protection and transportation agencies, especially those with indicator projects
	2) Number of public education messages to encourage the use of personal transportation alternatives (e.g., "ozone action day") *(optional)*	
Alternate fuel use in registered motor vehicles *(core)*	1) Proportion of registered vehicles powered by alternative fuel *(core)*	**DOE (EIA)** **States or local jurisdictions:** transportation agencies
Availability of mass transit *(core)*	1) Proportion of population for whom mass transit is available *(core)*	**CB:** census data **CDC:** BRFSS; NHIS **DOT (FHA):** National Bicycle and Walking Study; NPTS
	2) Proportion of population who chose personal transportation alternatives (e.g., walking, bicycling) *(optional)*	**States or local jurisdictions:** CDI surveillance; transportation agencies

(continues)

Air, Ambient (Outdoor) Continued

Indicator	Suggested Measure	Potential Data Source
Interventions Continued		
Programs that address hazardous or toxic substances in ambient air *(optional)*	1) Number of jurisdictions that have air toxics monitoring programs *(optional)*	**EPA** **States or local jurisdictions:** environmental protection agencies
	2) Number of operating permits for releases of hazardous air pollutants *(optional)*	
	3) Number of fines for hazardous releases violations *(optional)*	

Air, Indoor

Indicator	Suggested Measure	Potential Data Source
Hazards		
Tobacco smoke in homes with children *(core)*	1) Proportion of children residing in households with adult smokers *(core)*	**CB:** census data **CDC:** BRFSS; NHIS; YRBSS **EPA** **American Legacy Foundation** **States or local jurisdictions:** CDI surveillance; environmental protection agencies, especially those with indicator projects
	2) Proportion of households with adult smokers *(core)*	
	3) Proportion of children who smoke *(optional)*	
Hazardous or toxic substances in indoor air *(optional)*	1) Proportion of houses with group I dust mite in beds *(optional)*	**CDC** **HUD:** National Survey of Lead and Allergens in Housing **NIEHS**
	2) Proportion of houses with > 0.1 unit/g German cockroach dust in beds *(optional)*	
	3) Proportion of schools with indoor air hazards *(developmental)*	
Exposures (None identified)		

Air, Indoor Continued

Indicator	Suggested Measure	Potential Data Source
Health Effects		
CO poisoning (not fire-related) *(core)*	1) Number of deaths from CO poisoning *(core)* 2) Number of hospitalizations and emergency department visits attributed to CO exposure *(core)*	**CDC:** NHAMCS; NHDS; NVSS **States or local jurisdictions:** injury and CDI surveillance; hospital discharge data; ME/Cs; vital statistics
Unusual pattern of respiratory events *(optional)*	1) Number of emergency department visits in which an airborne agent is suspected *(optional)* 2) Number of deaths in which an airborne agent is suspected *(optional)*	**CDC:** NHAMCS; NHDS; NVSS **States or local jurisdictions:** CDI surveillance; ME/Cs; vital statistics
Interventions		
Policies that address indoor air hazards in schools *(core)*	1) Proportion of schools with indoor air policies *(core)* 2) Proportion of schools with smoke-free and tobacco-free policies *(core)*	**CDC:** NHIS; SHPPS; YRBSS **EPA** **States or local jurisdictions:** CDI surveillance; STATE
Laws pertaining to smoke-free indoor air *(core)*	1) Number of jurisdictions with laws on smoke-free indoor air *(core)* 2) Proportion of resident population in jurisdictions with laws pertaining to smoke-free indoor air *(core)*	**CB:** census data **CDC, NIOSH** **States or local jurisdictions:** STATE; health agencies, occupational safety and health divisions
Indoor air inspections *(core)*	1) Number of complaint-related indoor air inspections *(core)*	**CDC (NIOSH)** **OSHA**
Use of best practices for protecting indoor air *(optional)*	1) Number of local jurisdictions with ordinances requiring CO detectors in apartment buildings *(optional)* 2) Proportion of non-manufacturing work force that occupies office buildings for which indoor air quality management practices address human health *(optional)*	**CDC:** NHIS, NIOSH surveillance systems **EPA** **OSHA:** health agencies, occupational safety and health divisions **States or local jurisdictions:** health agencies, occupational safety and health divisions; local OSHA; STATE

(continues)

Air, Indoor Continued

Indicator	Suggested Measure	Potential Data Source
Health Effects Continued	3) Proportion of resident population for which programs are available for testing radon in high-risk homes *(optional)*	

Water, Ambient

Indicators	Suggested Measures	Potential Data Sources
Hazards		
Monitored contaminants in ambient water *(core)*	1) Levels of contaminants monitored under CWA and state regulations and guidelines by type of water body (e.g., surface, recreational, marine) *(core)*	**EPA:** BEACH Program; CWA compliance data **USDA** **USGS (NAWQA)** **States or local jurisdictions:** public drinking water utilities; environmental protection and natural resources agencies; pool inspection program
	2) Proportion of marine and freshwater recreational waters that fail to meet water quality regulations and guidelines *(core)*	
	3) Proportion of treated recreational waters that fail to meet state and local standards for free chlorine levels by type of recreational water (swimming pools, water parks, play fountains) *(core)*	
	4) Number of health-related closure days for marine and freshwater recreational areas *(optional)*	
	5) Land-use patterns *(developmental)*	
Point-source discharges into ambient water *(core)*	1) Volume of point-source discharges by type of contaminant (permitted sanitary waste disposal, sewage overflows, unintentional discharges and spills) *(core)*	**EPA:** BEACH program **FDA**

Water, Ambient Continued

Indicator	Suggested Measure	Potential Data Source
Health Effects Continued	2) Levels of mercury, dioxin, PCB, other in recreational (fishing) water bodies *(developmental)*	
Contaminants in shellfish and sport and commercial fish *(core)*	1) Levels of fecal coliform and mercury in shellfish beds *(core)* 2) Levels of mercury, dioxin, and PCB in sport and commercial fish *(core)*	**FDA** **States or local jurisdictions:** shellfish and food safety programs in health and natural resources agencies
Exposures		
(None identified)		
Health Effects		
Outbreaks attributed to fish and shellfish consumption *(core)*	1) Number of outbreaks by source (fish, shellfish) and etiologic agent (biologic, toxic, other) *(core)*	**CDC** **States or local jurisdictions:** health agencies
Outbreaks attributed to ambient water contaminants *(core)*	1) Number of outbreaks by source (freshwater, marine, treated recreational water) and etiologic agent (biologic, toxic, other) *(core)*	**CDC** **States or local jurisdictions:** health agencies
Interventions		
Activity restrictions *(core)*	1) Number and type of health-based activity restrictions *(core)*	**EPA:** BEACH Program **FDA** **States or local jurisdictions:** shellfish and food safety programs in health, environmental protection, and natural resources agencies, especially those with indicator projects
Compliance with regulations and guidelines *(optional)*	1) Number of fines for noncompliance with CWA regulations or local guidelines *(optional)*	**EPA**
Public education *(optional)*	1) Public awareness campaigns about health hazards associated with on-lot wastewater treatment systems *(optional)*	**States or local jurisdictions:** health and environment agencies

(continues)

Water, Drinking

Indicators	Suggested Measures	Potential Data Sources
Hazards		
Monitored contaminants in drinking water *(core)*	1) Number and proportion of drinking water systems that fail to meet water quality regulations and guidelines (SDWA MCLs, CCLs, state lists) by type of water supply *(core)* 2) Measurements of SDWA MCLs, CCLs, and contaminants monitored under state regulations and guidelines by type of water supply *(core)* 3) Number of citations for noncompliance with local standards for free chlorine levels *(optional)*	**AWWA** **EPA:** SDWIS **States or local jurisdictions:** environmental protection agencies, especially those with indicator projects; Consumer Confidence Reports from local water utilities
Source water contamination *(optional)*	1) Number and type of point-source discharges into drinking water aquifers *(optional)* 2) Levels of naturally occurring toxicants *(optional)* 3) Levels and types of contamination of private water supplies *(developmental)*	**EPA** **USGS** **States or local jurisdictions:** environmental protection agencies, especially those with indicator projects
Exposures		
(None identified)		
Health Effects		
Methemoglobinemia *(core)*	1) Case of methemoglobinemia *(core)*	**States or local jurisdictions:** health agencies
Outbreaks attributed to drinking water *(core)*	1) Number by type of water supply (including bottled water) and etiologic agent (biologic, toxic, other) *(core)*	**CDC** **States or local jurisdictions:** health agencies

Water, Drinking Continued

Indicators	Suggested Measures	Potential Data Sources
Interventions		
Implementation of sanitary surveys *(core)*	1) Number and proportion of drinking water systems in which a sanitary survey has been conducted within past 5 years (by type of water supply) *(core)*	**EPA:** SDWIS **USGS:** sewage tracer program
Compliance with operation and maintenance standards *(core)*	1) Fines for noncompliance with SDWA regulations or local guidelines *(core)* 2) Citations for noncompliance with local water quality regulations or guidelines *(core)*	**AWWA** **EPA** **States or local jurisdictions:** health agencies; public water utilities
Boil-water advisories *(core)*	1) Number of boil-water advisories by type of water supply *(core)*	**States or local jurisdictions:** health agencies; public water utilities
Source water protection programs *(optional)*	1) Proportion of wellheads covered by protection programs *(optional)* 2) Proportion of surface-water supplies covered by watershed protection programs *(optional)*	**AWWA** **EPA** **States or local jurisdictions:** health agencies; public water utilities
Public education *(optional)*	1) Proportion of the population aware of availability and meaning of consumer confidence reports *(optional)*	**States or local jurisdictions:** health agencies; public water utilities

Lead

Indicator	Suggested Measure	Potential Data Source
Hazards		
Lead contamination in the environment *(optional)*	1) Proportion of housing stock built before 1950 *(optional)*	**CB** **HUD**

(continues)

Lead Continued

Indicator	Suggested Measure	Potential Data Source
Hazards Continued	2) Lead levels in sediment and in game or commercial fish *(optional)*	**States or local jurisdictions:** environmental protection agencies, especially those with indicator projects
Residence near metal processing industries *(developmental)*	1) Proportion of population residing near lead smelters *(developmental)*	**CB** **HUD**
Exposure		
Blood lead level (in children) *(core)*	1) Proportion of high-risk children with elevated blood lead level *(core)*	**CDC:** NHANES; Lead Surveillance Program **States or local jurisdictions:** prevalence surveys
Health Effect		
Lead poisoning (in children) *(core)*	1) Number of hospitalizations from lead poisoning in children *(core)*	**CDC:** NHAMCS; NHDS **States or local jurisdictions:** hospital discharge surveys
Intervention		
Lead elimination programs *(optional)*	1) Number of jurisdictions with lead training and certification programs *(optional)*	**CB** **CDC:** NHIS **EPA** **HUD** **States or local jurisdictions**
	2) Proportion of population living in pre-1950 housing that has been tested for the presence of lead-based paint *(optional)*	**Private sector:** industry monitoring systems
	3) Number of completed lead abatements *(developmental)*	

Pesticides

Indicator	Suggested Measure	Potential Data Source
Hazards		
Pesticide use and patterns of use *(core)*	1) Annual tons used *(core)* 2) Pounds applied *(core)* 3) Patterns of use in agriculture, home, and garden *(optional)*	**EPA (OPP, Health Effects Division)** **USDA (PDP)** **USGS (NAWQA, NASQAN)**

Pesticides Continued

Indicator	Suggested Measure	Potential Data Source
Hazards Continued	4) Number of worker and community complaints about possible pesticide exposure *(developmental)*	**States or local jurisdictions:** monitoring and reporting systems; environmental protection agencies, especially those with indicator projects; local USGS Offices
Residual pesticide in foods *(core)*	1) Proportion of foods with residual pesticide levels that fail to meet safe consumption regulations and guidelines *(core)*	**EPA** **USDA (FDA)**: Total Dietary Survey
Exposure Biologic markers of pesticides or pesticide metabolites in human tissue *(optional)*	1) 95th percentile blood and urine concentration levels for biomarkers of exposure to carbaryl (1-naphthol), methyl parathion and parathion (paranitrophenol), chlorpyrifos (3,5,6-trichloro-2-pyridinol), propoxur (isopropoxyphenol), 2,4-D, o-phenylphenol, permethrins, diazinon, chlordane, dieldrin, DDT, lindane *(optional)*	**CDC:** NHANES; NRHEEC **States or local jurisdictions:** survey data from human exposure capacity-building projects
	2) 95th percentile urine concentration level for six biomarkers of exposure to 28 pesticides: dimethyl phosphate, dimethyl thiophosphate, dimethyl dithiophosphate, diethyl phosphate, diethyl thiophosphate, diethyl dithiophosphate *(optional)*	
Health Effect Pesticide-related poisoning and illness *(core)*	1) Incidence of pesticide-related poisonings and illnesses in pesticide workers *(core)*	**AAPCC:** TESS **CDC:** NHDS; SENSOR/NIOSH surveillance systems; NVSS; terrorism surveillance

(*continues*)

Pesticides Continued

Indicator	Suggested Measure	Potential Data Source
Health effect Continued	2) Number of non-occupational pesticide-related poisoning and illness *(core)* 3) Number of pesticide-related poisoning and illness in children *(core)*	**States or local jurisdictions:** injury indicators surveillance; ME/Cs; pesticide poisoning surveillance programs; terrorism surveillance
Interventions		
Compliance with pesticide application standards *(core)*	1) Proportion of workers, handlers, and trainers in compliance with employee training standards *(core)* 2) Proportion of workers in compliance with recommendations for home and yard use *(developmental)*	**CDC:** NHIS **EPA** **OSHA** **USDA** **States or local jurisdictions:** pesticide programs within agriculture, environment, and health agencies
Public and professional education *(optional)*	1) Public awareness campaigns about pesticide hazards and safe application and use *(optional)* 2) Public and professional education about symptoms of low-level pesticide exposure *(optional)*	**EPA** **OSHA** **USDA** **States or local jurisdictions:** pesticide programs in agriculture, environment, and health agencies
Alternatives to pesticide use *(developmental)*	1) Number of jurisdictions in which "organic" foods are available *(developmental)* 2) Consumption patterns of "organically grown" foods *(developmental)*	**EPA** **OSHA** **USDA** **States or local jurisdictions:** pesticide programs in agriculture, health, and environmental agencies, especially those with indicator projects

Toxics and Waste

Indicator	Suggested Measure	Potential Data Source
Hazards		
Chemical spills *(core)*	1) Number of chemical spills by type and location *(core)*	**ASDR:** HSEES **DOT** **EPA** **States or local jurisdictions:** environment, transportation, and agriculture agencies
Toxic contaminants in foods *(core)*	1) Levels of toxic contaminants in foods *(core)*	**USDA (FDA):** Total Diet Survey
Hazardous waste sites *(optional)*	1) Proportion of leaking underground storage facilities that have not been remediated *(optional)* 2) Proportion of identified brownfield properties that have not been remediated *(optional)* 3) Tons of toxic substances and materials sold to general public *(optional)* 4) Proportion of population in close proximity to leaking underground storage facilities, brownfield properties, and sites on the National Priority List and RCRA lists *(optional)* 5) Number of worker and community complaints about possible toxic exposures *(developmental)*	**ATSDR** **CDC, NIOSH** **DOC** **EPA** **OSHA** **States or local jurisdictions:** agriculture and environmental protection agencies, especially those with indicator projects
Exposures		
Biologic markers of human exposure to heavy metals *(optional)*	1) Blood and urine concentration level (95th percentile) for lead, arsenic, cadmium, manganese, mercury *(optional)*	**CDC:** ABLES; NHANES; NRHEEC **States or local jurisdictions:** lead prevalence surveys

(continues)

Toxics and Waste Continued

Indicator	Suggested Measure	Potential Data Source
Exposures Continued		
Biologic markers of human exposure to persistent chemicals *(optional)*	1) Serum concentration level (95th percentile) for polychlorinated biphenyls (PCBs), dioxins, furans *(optional)*	**CDC:** ABLES; NHANES; NRHEEC
Health Effects		
Possible child poisoning *(core)*	1) Consultations for child poisoning *(core)* 2) Emergency department visit for child poisoning *(core)*	**AAPCC:** TESS **CDC:** NHAMCS; NHDS; NVSS **CPSC** **States or local jurisdictions:** injury indicators surveillance; ME/Cs; vital statistics
Morbidity and mortality associated with toxic substances *(optional)*	1) Number of non-occupational poisonings *(optional)* 2) Number of deaths from nonoccupational poisoning *(optional)* 3) Number of injuries resulting from chemical spills *(optional)*	**AAPCC:** TESS **CDC:** NHAMCS; NHDS; NVSS; NEISS; NIOSH **CPSC** **States or local jurisdictions:** CDI and injury indicators surveillance; health agencies, occupational health and safety divisions; ME/Cs; vital statistics
Interventions		
Use of surveillance and warning systems *(optional)*	1) Number of jurisdictions that have surveillance systems for detecting methemoglobinemia and acute poisoning from lead, arsenic, cadmium, mercury, pesticides, and other chemicals *(optional)* 2) Number of fish consumption advisories *(optional)*	**States or local jurisdictions:** health, environmental protection, and natural resources agencies
Waste and toxic substances reduction *(optional)*	1) Proportion of solid waste diverted from disposal *(optional)* 2) Identified sites with completed exposure pathways *(optional)*	**CDC:** NHIS **EPA** **States or local jurisdictions:** health, environmental protection, and natural resources agencies

Toxics and Waste Continued

Indicator	Suggested Measure	Potential Data Source
Interventions Continued		
Public education *(developmental)*	1) Public awareness campaigns about toxic and hazardous household products *(developmental)*	**Private sector:** marketing agencies; solid waste disposal companies
	2) Number of purchases of home safety and child-proofing devices (e.g., electrical outlet covers, cabinet locks, smoke detectors) *(developmental)*	

Sun and Ultraviolet Light

Indicator	Suggested Measure	Potential Data Source
Hazard		
Ultraviolet (UV) light *(core)*	1) Number of days in which the UV light index exceeds a safe threshold *(core)*	**EPA** **NOAA (NWS)** **States or local jurisdictions:** environmental protection agencies, especially those with indicator projects
Exposures		
(None identified)		
Health Effects		
Melanoma *(core)*	1) Incidence of melanoma *(core)*	**CDC:** NHDS, NVSS
	2) Melanoma mortality *(core)*	**States or local jurisdictions:** cancer registries; CDI surveillance hospital discharge surveys; vital statistics
Injuries attributed to UV light *(optional)*	1) Number of corneal burns *(optional)*	**CDC:** NHAMCS, NHDS
	2) Number of other eye injuries *(optional)*	
	3) Incidence of cataracts *(optional)*	

(continues)

Sun and Ultraviolet Light Continued

Indicator	Suggested Measure	Potential Data Source
Intervention		
Public education *(optional)*	1) Proportion of adults who follow protective measures to prevent melanoma and skin cancer *(optional)* 2) Proportion of adolescents who follow protective measures to prevent melanoma and skin cancer *(optional)* 3) Number and type of sun protection messages issued to the public *(optional)* 4) Number of purchases of sun-blocking products *(developmental)*	**CDC:** NHIS **NWS** **States or local jurisdictions:** health agencies **Private sector:** marketing agencies

Sentinel Events

Indicator	Suggested Measure	Potential Data Source
Hazard		
Unsafe or unhealthy environmental event or condition *(optional)*	1) Chemical spill *(core)* 2) Ambient ozone concentration that exceeds the safe level *(optional)* 3) Ambient temperature that exceeds safe threshold *(optional)* 4) Disaster (e.g., natural, sociopolitical) *(optional)*	**ATSDR** **DOT** **EPA** **NOAA, NWS** **States or local jurisdictions:** environmental protection agencies, especially those with indicator projects **USGS**
Exposures		
(None identified)		
Health Effects		
Illness or condition with suspected or confirmed environmental exposure *(core)*	1) Asthma-related death *(core)* 2) Case of methemoglobinemia *(core)*	**AAPCC:** TESS **CDC:** BRFSS; Food Net; Pulse Net; NHAMCS; NHDS; NHIS; NVSS

Sentinel Events Continued

Indicator	Suggested Measure	Potential Data Source
Health Effects Continued	3) Illness attributed to ambient or drinking water contaminants *(core)*	**CDC, ARC** **EPA:** NMMAPS **HCFA:** Medicare; Medicaid
	4) CO poisoning (not fire-related) *(core)*	**NOAA (NCDC; NWS; NSSL)**
	5) Hospitalization from lead poisoning in a child *(core)*	**States or local jurisdictions:** asthma, CDI and injury indicator surveillance; ambulatory care and hospital discharge data; ME/Cs; vital statistics
	6) Consultation or emergency department visit for possible poisoning in a child, including lead poisoning *(core)*	**Private sector:** HMOs, medical insurers
	7) Pesticide-related poisoning or illness *(core)*	
	8) Temperature-attributed death *(core)*	
	9) Foodborne illness *(optional)*	
Unusual pattern of illness or condition with suspected or confirmed environmental contribution *(core)*	1) Rates of acute asthma events *(core)*	**CDC:** MACDP; MADDSP; NBDPN; NVSS
	2) Rates of cardiovascular and respiratory events in persons with underlying disease on days when outdoor air standards are exceeded or when temperatures are at dangerous levels *(core)*	**HCFA:** Medicare; Medicaid **States or local jurisdictions:** asthma surveillance programs; cancer registries; CDI surveillance; hospital discharge surveys; ME/Cs; vital statistics
	3) Cancer incidence and mortality rates, specifically lung cancer in nonsmokers, mesothelioma, soft tissue sarcoma, and melanoma *(optional)*	**Private sector:** HMOs, medical insurance companies; health care databases, especially emergency department visits
	4) Incidence rates for adverse reproductive outcomes, specifically low and very low birth weight and pre-term and very pre-term births *(optional)*	

(continues)

Sentinel Events Continued

Indicator	Suggested Measure	Potential Data Source
Health Effects Continued	5) Incidence rates of developmental disabilities, specifically mental retardation and autism spectrum disorder *(optional)*	
	6) Incidence rates of birth defects, especially cerebral palsy *(optional)*	
	7) Syndromes with unknown etiologies that require emergency medical care or cause death *(developmental)*	
Intervention		
Use of surveillance and warning system *(optional)*	1) Number of surveillance systems for sentinel events, syndromes, and unusual patterns of disease that include environmental data *(optional)*	**CDC** **States or local jurisdictions:** health, environmental protection, and natural resources agencies
	2) Number of vector-control programs that use environmental data *(optional)*	

Noise

Indicator	Suggested Measure	Potential Data Source
Hazard		
Residence in noisy environments *(optional)*	1) Number of noise complaints *(optional)*	**States or local jurisdictions:** police, sheriff offices
	2) Level of noise monitored in a community *(optional)*	
Exposures		
(None identified)		
Health Effect		
Noise-induced hearing loss (nonoccupational) *(core)*	1) Proportion of noise-exposed adults with hearing loss *(core)*	**CDC:** BRFSS; NHANES; NHIS; YRBS **DOD (Recruiting Offices)**

Noise Continued

Indicator	Suggested Measure	Potential Data Source
Hazard		
Continued	2) Proportion of children and adolescents with hearing loss *(optional)*	**States or local jurisdictions:** prevalence surveys from health agencies, schools
Intervention		
Hearing protection practices *(optional)*	1) Proportion of population using appropriate ear protection devices and equipment *(optional)*	**CDC:** NHIS **OSHA**
	2) Number of jurisdictions with noise ordinances and prohibitions on specific activities *(optional)*	

Disasters

Indicator	Suggested Measure	Potential Data Source
Hazards		
Residence in a floodplain *(core)*	1) Proportion of resident population with homes in a floodplain *(core)*	**CB:** census data **FEMA** **USGS**
Geographic or climatic conditions that increase susceptibility to hazards *(optional)*	1) Number of days in which temperatures exceed safe thresholds *(optional)*	**FEMA** **NOAA** **USDA** **USGS**
	2) Amount of excessive rainfall *(optional)*	**States or local jurisdictions:** agriculture and environmental protection agencies, especially those with indicator projects
	3) Duration of drought conditions *(developmental)*	
	4) Number of days of flooding *(developmental)*	
	5) Number of floods in areas with high concentrations of pesticide through production, sales, or use *(developmental)*	
Residence in a temporary or unsafe structure *(optional)*	1) Proportion of population residing in damaged or destroyed home *(optional)*	**ARC** **CB:** census data **CDC**

(continues)

Disasters Continued

Indicator	Suggested Measure	Potential Data Source
Hazard		
Continued	2) Proportion of population residing in temporary shelter *(optional)*	**FEMA** **States or local jurisdictions**
Exposures		
(None identified)		
Health Effects		
Deaths attributed to extremes in ambient temperature *(core)*	1) Number of heat-attributed deaths *(core)* 2) Number of deaths from hypothermia *(optional)*	**ARC** **CDC:** NHAMCS; NHDS; NVSS **EPA:** NMMAPS **NOAA (NWS, NCDC, NSSL)** **States or local jurisdictions:** ME/Cs; vital statistics
Morbidity and mortality attributed to natural forces *(optional)*	1) Number of illnesses or injuries from natural disasters by type of disaster *(optional)* 2) Number of deaths from natural disasters by type of disaster *(optional)*	**ARC** **CDC:** NHAMCS; NHDS; NVSS **EPA:** NMMAPS **NOAA (NWS, NCDC, NSSL)** **States or local jurisdictions:** ME/Cs; vital statistics
Intervention		
Emergency prepared-ness, response, and mitigation training programs, plans, and protocols *(core)*	1) Proportion of jurisdic-tions for which multi-institutional exercises to prepare for disaster response are conducted annually *(core)* 2) Proportion of jurisdic-tions for which protocols exist for public education messages to elicit preventive behaviors among resident population *(optional)* 3) Proportion of jurisdic-tions for which early warning systems are in place *(optional)* 4) Proportion of jurisdic-tions for which sheltering programs exist *(optional)*	**CDC (NCEH)** **FEMA** **NOAA (NWS, NCDC, NSSL)** **States or local jurisdictions:** health and public safety agencies; local FEMA

Disasters Continued

Indicator	Suggested Measure	Potential Data Source
Intervention Continued	5) Proportion of jurisdictions for which safe building codes are enforced *(optional)*	

Potential Sources of Data and Information for Environmental Public Health Indicators

Source: Environmental Public Health Indicators Project; NCEH, EHHE; January 2006.

Federal Agencies

Agency for Toxic Substances and Disease Registry (ATSDR)

http://www.atsdr.cdc.gov/

Hazardous Substances Emergency Events Surveillance (HSEES) system: Provides information about releases of hazardous substances that need to be cleaned up or neutralized according to federal, state, or local law, as well as threatened releases that result in a public health action such as an evacuation.

http://www.atsdr.cdc.gov/HS/HSEES/

Centers for Disease Control and Prevention (CDC)

http://www.cdc.gov/

Behavioral Risk Factor Surveillance System (BRFSS): Tracks health risk through use of telephone surveys.

http://www.cdc.gov/brfss

FoodNet: Provides a network for active surveillance of foodborne diseases and related epidemiologic studies.

http://www.cdc.gov/foodnet/

Metropolitan Atlanta Congenital Defects Program (MACDP): Monitors all major birth defects in metropolitan Atlanta, Georgia, and serves as the model for many state-based programs and as a resource for the development of uniform methods and approaches to birth defects surveillance.

http://www.cdc.gov/ncbddd/bd

National Birth Defects Prevention Network (NBDPN): Maintains a national network of state and population-based programs for birth defects surveillance and research.

http://www.nbdpn.org/

National Program of Cancer Registries (NPCR): Establishes standards, model laws and regulations, computerized-reporting and data-processing systems; trains registry personnel; provides support for cancer prevention and control programs.

http://www.cdc.gov/cancer/npcr/

National Vital Statistics System (NVSS): Provides the nation's official vital statistics.

http://www.cdc.gov/nchs/nvss.htm

PulseNet: Provides a national network of public health laboratories that perform a DNA "fingerprinting" method on foodborne bacteria for disease surveillance.

http://www.cdc.gov/pulsenet/

Registry of Toxic Effects of Chemical Substances (RTECS®): Contains information about the toxic effects of chemical substances, including drugs, food additives, preservatives, ores, pesticides, dyes, detergents, lubricants, soaps, plastics, extracts from plant and animal sources, plants, or animals that are toxic by contact or ingestion, and industrial intermediates and waste products from production processes.

http://www.cdc.gov/niosh/rtecs.html

State Tobacco Activities Tracking and Evaluation (STATE): Summarizes data on tobacco use prevention and control.

http://apps.nccd.cdc.gov/statesystem/

Youth Risk Behavior Surveillance System (YRBSS): Tracks risky behaviors among youth.

http://www.cdc.gov/nccdphp/dash/yrbs/index.htm

Department of Commerce (DOC)

http://www.commerce.gov/

Census Bureau: Provides data about population, geography, and economics.

http://www.census.gov/

National Technical Information Service: Links to scientific and technical resources.

http://www.scitechresources.gov/

Department of Defense (DOD)

http://www.dod.gov/

Recruiting Offices: Links to the DOD recruiting sites.

http://www.dod.gov/sites/r.html

Department of Energy (DOE)

http://www.energy.gov

Energy Information Administration (EIA): Cites statistics by geography, sector, price, fuel, environment, forecast, and analyses.

http://www.eia.doe.gov/

Energy Data and Prices: Contains index of state, international, and national data on energy.

http://www.energy.gov/engine/content.do?BT_CODE=PRICESTRENDS

Department of Transportation (DOT), Federal Highway Administration (FHA)

http://www.fhwa.dot.gov/

Electronic Reading Room: Links to publications, reports, and statistics.

http://www.fhwa.dot.gov/pubstats.html

Nationwide Personal Transportation Survey (NPTS): Catalogs daily personal travel in the United States.

http://www.fhwa.dot.gov/ohim/nptspage.htm

Environmental Protection Agency (EPA)

http://www.epa.gov/

EPA—Air

Aerometric Information Retrieval System (AIRS): Contains information about ambient air pollution.

http://www.epa.gov/ttn/airs/

Air Data: Provides an index of air-related topics.

http://www.epa.gov/air/data/index.html

Air Facility System (AFS): Contains information about ambient air pollution.

http://www.epa.gov/Compliance/data/systems/air/afssystem.html

AIR NOW: Provides air-quality maps and ozone forecasts, publications, and consumer tips for reducing air pollution.

http://www.epa.gov/airnow/

Air Toxics: Contains information about air toxics regulations, assessments, programs, education, and partnerships.

http://www.epa.gov/ttn/atw/

Compliance Monitoring Data for Air: Provides information about three databases that contain compliance and permit data for regulated stationary sources; stores and tracks compliance information about owners and operators of asbestos demolition and renovation activities and memoranda issued by EPA on applicability and compliance issues associated with the New Source Performance Standards, National Emissions Standards for Hazardous Air Pollutants, and chlorofluorocarbons.

http://www.epa.gov/compliance/monitoring/index.html

Information Clearinghouse: Contains information about indoor air quality.

http://www.epa.gov/iaq/iaqinfo.html

National Air Quality and Emissions Trends Report: Contains information about criteria air pollutants.

http://www.epa.gov/ttn/chief/trends/

National Emissions Inventory (NEI): Characterizes emissions of criteria and hazardous air pollutants.

http://www.epa.gov/air/data/neidb.html

National Morbidity, Mortality, and Air Pollution Study (NMMAPS): Describes morbidity and mortality associated with air pollution in the United States based on a study conducted by the Health Effects Institute.

Office of Air and Radiation (OAR): Lists publications and reports about ambient air.

http://www.epa.gov/oar/oarpubs.html

Urban Air Toxics Program: Lists air toxics, source categories, and integrated strategies for reduction.

http://www.epa.gov/ttn/atw/urban/urbanpg.html

EPA—Miscellaneous

Compliance Monitoring Data: Provides access to data for air, hazardous waste, pesticides, toxics, and water.

http://www.epa.gov/compliance/monitoring/index.html

Databases and Software: Contains information about air, toxic substances, pesticides, solid waste, water, and "integrated media" (the relation between multiple environmental problems).

http://www.epa.gov/epahome/dmedia.htm

Environmental Monitoring for Public Access and Community Tracking (EMPACT): Indexes real-time environmental information for U.S. cities.

http://www.epa.gov/empact/index.htm

Global Warming: Provides information about global warming impacts by state.

http://www.epa.gov/globalwarming/index.html

Library Network: Provides access to agency decisions and environmental topics of interest through online publications and services for the public.

http://www.epa.gov/natlibra

EPA—Toxics

Compliance Monitoring Data for Toxics and Pesticides: Provides access to systems that track the amount of pesticides produced and compliance and enforcement activities.

http://www.epa.gov/compliance/monitoring/programs/fifra/index.html

Integrated Risk Information System (IRIS): Contains information about health hazards posed by approximately 5,000 substances.

http://www.epa.gov/iris/

Office of Pesticide Programs, Health Effects Division: Registers and reviews environmental and human health information about pesticides.

http://www.epa.gov/pesticides/about/aboutus.htm

Toxic Release Inventory/Emergency Planning and Community Right-To-Know Act (TRI/EPCRA): Lists approximately 600 designated chemicals that threaten human health and the environment. Authorized under EPCRA (1986), this system requires manufacturers to report releases of these chemicals to EPA and state governments.

http://www.epa.gov/tri/

EPA—Water

Beaches Environmental Assessment and Coastal Health (BEACH) Program: Focuses on improving public health and environmental protection programs for beachgoers and providing the public with information about the quality of beach water.

http://www.epa.gov/ost/beaches/2000/

Clean Water Act: Establishes the basic structure for regulating discharges of pollutants into U.S. waters.

http://www.epa.gov/r5water/cwa.htm

Compliance Monitoring Data for Water: Provides access to two information systems: the Permit Compliance System and the Safe Drinking Water Information System.

http://www.epa.gov/compliance/monitoring/programs/cwa/index.html

Environmental Information Management System: Provides access to the data used to develop national maps for watershed indicators.

http://oaspub.epa.gov/eims/eimsstart

National Drinking Water Contaminant Occurrence Database: Contains occurrence data from both Public Water Systems and other sources on physical, chemical, microbial and radiological contaminants.

http://www.epa.gov/ncod/

Office of Wetlands, Oceans, and Watersheds: Describes program information and introduces other relevant websites for statutes, publications, resource protection, maps, databases, and other topics.

http://www.epa.gov/owow/

Safe Drinking Water Act: Sets drinking water quality standards and oversees the states, localities, and water suppliers who implement those standards.

http://www.epa.gov/safewater/sdwa/sdwa.html

Safe Drinking Water Information System (SDWIS): Stores information needed to monitor U.S. public drinking water systems.

http://www.epa.gov/safewater/sdwisfed/sdwis.htm

Urban, Great Waters, and Regional Programs: Describes programs that characterize risks to human health and the environment from mercury, urban air toxics, and air pollution deposition in the Great Lakes.

http://www.epa.gov/ttn/atw/riskinit.html

Water Data and Maps: Includes information about data systems, databases, mapping, and water quality models.

http://www.epa.gov/owow/data.html

Water Science: Includes information about water quality criteria and standards, industrial water pollution controls, water quality tools, health advisories, training, guidance, and financial assistance.

http://www.epa.gov/OST/

Watershed Information Network: Catalogs geospatial displays and analyses of information important for watershed protection and restoration.

http://www.epa.gov/win/

Watershed Indicators Index: Provides a general overview of watershed indicators.

http://www.epa.gov/iwi/iwi-overview.pdf

Watershed Information Network: Provides national maps and fact sheets for all watershed indicators and candidate indicators through the Watershed Atlas.

http://www.epa.gov/win/

Food and Drug Administration (FDA)

http://www.fda.gov/

Total Diet Study (TDS): Measures dietary intake of food contaminants—such as pesticide residues, industrial chemicals, toxics, and radionuclides—and nutritional elements and vitamins.

http://www.cfsan.fda.gov/~comm/tds-toc.html

Federal Emergency Management Agency (FEMA)

http://www.fema.gov/

Environmental Program: Integrates resource considerations into disaster preparedness, mitigation, response, and recovery.

Flood Hazard Mapping: Outlines specifications and procedures.

http://www.floodmaps.fema.gov/fhm/tsdindex.shtm

Mapping Sources and Data: Provides information about flood hazards and mapping resources.

Miscellaneous Information: Links to sources for funding, related federal and state agencies, and legislation and laws.

Housing and Urban Development (HUD)

http://www.hud.gov/

Library: Contains an index of topics, including information about disaster relief, community environmental issues, and hazards from lead.

http://www.hud.gov/library/index.cfm

Data and Publications: Catalogs reports, publications, periodicals, and housing data.

http://www.hud.gov/library/bookshelf03/index.cfm

National Aeronautics and Space Administration (NASA)

http://www.nasa.gov/

Global Change Master Directory: Provides a directory of earth science data on agriculture, atmosphere, land surface, human dimensions, oceans, and other topics.

http://globalchange.nasa.gov/

National Institute of Environmental Health Sciences (NIEHS)

http://www.niehs.nih.gov/

National Toxicology Program: Links to information, fact sheets, and health and safety information.

http://ntp-server.niehs.nih.gov/

National Library of Medicine (NLM)

http://www.nlm.nih.gov/

TOXLINE: Contains a collection of online information about drugs and other chemicals.

http://toxnet.nlm.nih.gov/cgi-bin/sis/htmlgen?TOXLINE

National Oceanic and Atmospheric Administration (NOAA)

http://www.noaa.gov/

National Environmental Satellite, Data, and Information Service (NESDIS): Provides information services and access to global environmental data from satellites and other sources and conducts research to promote, protect, and enhance the nation's economy, security, environment, and quality of life.

http://www.nesdis.noaa.gov/

National Weather Service (NWS): Provides access to weather data, forecasts, and warnings.

http://www.nws.noaa.gov/

National Climatic Data Centers (NCDC): Maintains an active archive of weather data, responds to data requests, and produces climate publications.

http://lwf.ncdc.noaa.gov/oa/ncdc.html

National Severe Storms Laboratory (NSSL): Investigates all aspects of severe weather and conducts research to improve severe weather warnings and forecasts.

http://www.nssl.noaa.gov/

Occupational Safety and Health Administration (OSHA)

http://www.osha.gov/

Statistics and Data: Provides access to inspection data, federal statistics, and the Bureau of Labor's statistics on workplace injuries, illnesses, and fatalities.

http://www.osha.gov/oshstats/index.html

United States Department of Agriculture (USDA)

http://www.usda.gov/

Economics and Statistics System: Contains information about food, land, water, conservation, and other topics.

http://usda.mannlib.cornell.edu/

National Agricultural Statistics Service (NASS): Links to state and federal publications and data.

http://www.usda.gov/nass/

Pesticide Data Program (PDP): Collects data on pesticide residues in food.

http://www.ams.usda.gov/science/pdp/

United States Geological Survey (USGS)

http://www.usgs.gov/

Environment and Human Health: Links to reports, publications, data, and fact sheets.

http://www.usgs.gov/themes/environment_human_health.html

National Stream Quality Accounting Network (NASQAN): Contains monitoring data from large U.S. rivers.

http://water.usgs.gov/nasqan/

National Water Quality Assessment Program (NAWQA): Provides data about water chemistry, hydrology, land use, stream habitat, and aquatic life for major river basins and aquifers.

http://water.usgs.gov/nawqa/

NAWQA Pesticide National Synthesis Project: Produces a long-term assessment of the status of and trends in the quality of the nation's water resources.

http://water.wr.usgs.gov/pnsp/

Toxic Substances Hydrology Program: Provides bibliographies and publications about toxic substances in agriculture and mining.

http://toxics.usgs.gov/index.html

Water Resources Data: Links to water data, publications, technical resources, programs, and local information.

http://water.usgs.gov/

States and Local Jurisdictions

Note: States' data collection and reporting methods may differ, and some data may be collected but not reported.

Departments of Agriculture: Provides access to local services provided by the Farm Service Agency, Natural Resources Conservation Service, and Rural Development agencies and may provide information about land management practices, pesticides, pesticide alternatives, and water quality.

http://www.usda.gov/wps/portal/!ut/p/_s.7_0_A/7_0_1OB?navtype=MA&navid=AGENCIES_OFFICES

Environmental Protection and Natural Resources Agencies: Contains information about how state environmental agencies are organized and provides links to each state.

http://www.sso.org/ecos/states.htm

Medical Examiner and Coroner (ME/C) Offices: Provides contacts for each state and information about types of deaths investigated. Individual ME/C offices may provide information about specific deaths, including investigation, autopsy, and toxicology reports.

http://www.cdc.gov/epo/dphsi/mecisp/index.htm

Public Health Departments: Provides links to state health departments (scroll past birth data section).

http://www.cdc.gov/nchs/about/major/natality/sites.htm

Public Health Laboratories: Provides links to most state public health labs.

http://www.aphl.org/about_aphl/state_laboratory_listing.cfm

United States Geological Survey District Offices: Provides links to state offices.

http://www.usgs.gov/major_sites.html

Universities

Environment Databases: Provides access to a wide variety of online resources.

http://www.ulib.iupui.edu/subjectareas/gov/dbenviro.html

Environment, Health, and Other Government Statistical Documents: Provides a central reference and referral point for government information, political science, statistical data, and news.

http://www.lib.umich.edu/govdocs/stats.html

Nongovernment organizations

American Legacy Foundation: Provides data about tobacco use and information about tobacco control programs.

http://www.americanlegacy.org/

American Waterworks Association: Provides information about local drinking water issues.

http://www.awwa.org/

North American Association of Central Cancer Registries: Provides links to standards and technical assistance documents as well as to cancer incidence data.

http://www.naaccr.org/

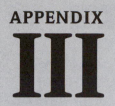
Selected Statistical Techniques and Tests

In this appendix, selected statistical techniques and tests are presented in Table A.1. These are only some of many approaches used in evaluating data. The choice of analysis and statistical test depends on the type of exposure and outcome variables. Discrete data are often treated statistically as a continuous variable. When the categories of the discrete variable are small, it may also be treated as a categorical variable.

A definition of the statistical techniques and tests shown in the table, along with corresponding Statistical Analysis System (SAS) procedure code (Institute Inc., Cary, NC, 2003), are also presented below. Because it is beyond the scope of this book to provide a thorough treatment of SAS programming, this code assumes that the reader has a basic understanding of SAS.

Briefly, SAS programs involve SAS statements. Each SAS statement ends with a semicolon; the semicolon completes the SAS statement. SAS statements are used to create SAS data sets and to run predefined statistical or other routines. A group of SAS statements used to define and create your SAS data set is called a Data Step. Data Step tells SAS programs about the data. For example,

```
DATA EXAMPLE;
INPUT SUBJECT $ AGE EXPOSED $ ILL $;
DATALINES;
 1 Male 44 Yes Yes
 2 Male 52 No No
 3 Female 39 Yes No
 .
 .
 .
 ;
```

The name of the data set is arbitrary and must begin with a letter. For categorical variables, follow the variable name on the INPUT line with "$". "DATALINES" comes prior to the data. Following the data set is a semicolon. It does not matter whether you choose to type words in upper or lower case.

PROC (meaning procedure) begins several predefined routines. Each PROC is followed by a specific option, like PRINT, SORT, MEAN, REG, ANOVA, FREQ, etc. We finish the procedure statements with "RUN". For example, to obtain the mean age for males and females separately, we first sort the data according to sex;

```
PROC SORT DATA=EXAMPLE;
Title 'Sorted Data by Sex';
  BY SEX;
RUN;
```

TABLE A.1 Classification of Statistical Techniques (and Tests) by Types of Variables

Exposure Variable	Outcome Variable			
	Continuous, normally distributed	**Continuous, not normally distributed, or Ordinal with > 2 categories**	**Nominal with > 2 categories (Multichotomous)**	**Nominal with 2 categories (Dichotomous)**
Continuous, normally distributed	Correlation coefficient Linear regression (t test, F test)	*Spearman rank correlation*	Analysis of variance (F test)	Logistic regression (likelihood ratio test)
Continuous, not normally distributed, or Ordinal with > 2 categories	*Spearman rank correlation*	*Spearman rank correlation*	*Kruskall-Wallis*	*Wilcoxon rank sum*
Nominal with > 2 categories (Multichotomous)	Analysis of variance (F test)	*Kruskal-Wallis*	Contingency table (Chi-square test)	Contingency table (Chi-square test)
Nominal with 2 categories (Dichotomous)	Comparison of means (t test)	*Wilcoxon rank sum* Polytomous Logistic regression (Likelihood ratio test)	Contingency table (Chi-square test)	Contingency table (Chi-square test or z statistic for one tail)

Note: Along the left column are types of exposure variables and along the top are types of outcome variables. The appropriate statistical analyses and tests for the different combination of exposure and outcome variables are presented in the table.

Nonparametric tests (shown in *italics*) are distribution free tests because they do not follow a specific distribution (e.g., normal).

Source: Adapted from Feigal D, Black D, Grady D, Hearst N, Fox C, Newman TB, et al. Planning for data management and analysis. *Hulley and Cummings, Designing Clinical Research: An Epidemiologic Approach.* Baltimore, MD: Williams & Wilkins; 1988.

Then run PROC MEANS, with the variable the means are to be computed for preceded by VAR and, because means is to be computed for males and females, add the line "BY SEX";

```
PROC MEANS DATA=EXAMPLE;
Title 'Mean Age by Sex';
  VAR AGE;
  BY SEX;
RUN;
```

SAS programs are typed into the SAS EDITOR. Once the DATA STEP and procedure(s) are entered into the SAS EDITOR, they are submitted. When the procedure is executed, it produces a SAS LOG and a SAS OUTPUT. The SAS LOG is an annotated copy of the original program, with the data excluded. Any procedure coding errors will be identified there, as well as information about the data set (e.g., number of observations and variables). The SAS OUTPUT provides the results computations and procures requested by the PROC statement.

- Parametric statistics involve techniques of statistical hypothesis testing based on the assumption that the distributions of variables being assessed belong to known probability distributions (e.g., the normal distribution).
- Nonparametric tests have less power than parametric tests when a distribution is known, but more power when the assumptions underlying the parametric test are not satisfied.
- Descriptive statistics describe variables: number of observations, mean, standard deviation, minimum, maximum, standard error, sum, first quartile, third quartile, interquartile range, coefficient of variation, skewness, kurtosis, and student's t testing the null hypothesis that the population mean is zero.

Example SAS code:

```
PROC MEANS DATA=EXAMPLE N MEAN STD MIN MAX STDERR
SUM Q1 Q3 QRANGE CV SKEWNESS KURTOSIS T;
Title 'Descriptive Statistics for the Variable X';
  VAR X;
RUN;
```

- Tests for normality and distribution plots are important for assessing the assumptions upon which we base our parametric tests.

Example SAS code:

```
PROC UNIVARIATE DATA=EXAMPLE NORMAL PLOT;
Title 'Tests and Plots for Assessing the Assumption
of Normality for the Variable X';
```

```
    VAR X;
RUN;
```

- Pearson's correlation coefficient quantifies the strength of the linear relationship between continuous or discrete exposure and outcome variables. It is sensitive to outlying values, particularly when the sample size is small. The estimated correlation coefficient should remain within the range of the data. PARAMETRIC

Example SAS code:

```
PROC CORR DATA=EXAMPLE PEARSON;
Title 'Correlation between X and Y Variables Using
Person's Correlation Coefficient';
    VAR X Y;
RUN;
```

- Spearman's rank correlation is a more robust measure of association than Pearson's correlation coefficient. This approach ranks the exposure and outcome data separately and calculates a coefficient of rank correlation. It is much less sensitive to outlying values. It can also be used if the exposure and outcome variables are ordinal. NONPARAMETRIC

Example SAS code:

```
PROC CORR DATA=EXAMPLE SPEARMAN;
Title 'Correlation between X and Y Variables Using
Spearman's Rank Correlation';
    VAR X Y;
RUN;
```

- Linear regression is a technique that explores the relationship between continuous random variables. If there is one independent variable, it is called simple linear regression and if there are two or more independent variables, then it is called multiple linear regression. It is distinct from simple correlation analysis in that a dependent variable (y) is specified as well as one or more independent variables (x's). The aim of regression analysis is to estimate the value(s) of the dependent variable that is associated with a fixed value of the independent variable(s). A linear relationship is assumed between the dependent and independent variable(s). PARAMETRIC

Example SAS code:
(Simple regression)

```
PROC REG DATA=EXAMPLE;
Title 'Simple Linear Regression';
  VAR Y=X;
RUN;
```

(Multiple regression)

```
PROC REG DATA=EXAMPLE;
Title 'Multiple Linear Regression';
  VAR Y=X1|X2;
RUN;
```

The "|" between the variables will cause Y to be regressed on X1, X2, and X1*X2.

- T-test for assessing the difference between two independent means.

  Example SAS code:
  (Two levels of exposure: yes vs. no)

```
PROC TTEST DATA=EXAMPLE;
Title 'Test for Difference in Mean Birth Weight for
Exposed and Unexposed';
  CLASS EXPOSED;
  VAR BIRTHWEIGHT;
RUN;
```

- T-test for assessing the difference between two dependent means.

  Example SAS code:

```
PROC TTEST DATA=EXAMPLE;
Title 'Test for Change in Means from Baseline to
Follow-up';
  PAIRED TIME1*TIME2;
RUN;
```

- Wilcoxon rank-sum test for assessing the difference in medians between two independent groups. NONPARAMETRIC
  Example SAS code:

```
PROC NPAR1WAY DATA=EXAMPLE WILCOXON;
CLASS EXPOSED;
  VAR BIRTHWEIGHT;
  EXACT WILCOXON;
RUN;
```

- The Kruskal-Wallis test is a generalization of the two-sample Wilcoxon rank-sum test to three or more groups. If EXPOSED in the previous SAS example was three or more levels (e.g., none, low, medium, high) that code would have automatically produced the Kruskal-Wallis test.

- Analysis of variance (ANOVA) is a collection of statistical models and their associated procedures that compare means by splitting the overall observed variance into different parts. One-way ANOVA is used to tests for differences among three or more independent groups; One-way ANOVA for repeated measures is used when the subjects are dependent groups; 2×2 ANOVA is a common type of factorial analysis of variance used when the experimenter wants to simultaneously study the effects of two treatment variables. ANCOVA is used instead of ANOVA if there is a covariate or covariates present. Covariates are typically used as control variables.

Example SAS code:
(Three or more categories of exposure; e.g., low, medium, high)

```
PROC ANOVA DATA=EXAMPLE;
  CLASS EXPOSED SEX;
  MODEL BIRTHWEIGHT=EXPOSED|SEX;
  MEANS EXPOSED|SEX / SNK;
RUN;
```

(Repeated measures)

```
PROC ANOVA DATA=EXAMPLE;
  CLASS GROUP;
  MODEL PREEXPOSURE POSTEXPOSURE=GROUP/NOUNI;
  REPEATED TIME 2 (0 1);
  MEANS GROUP;
RUN;
```

For unbalanced data PROC GLM is required.

- Contingency tables are counts arranged in tabular format and involve nominal data grouped into categories. A contingency table has r rows and c columns with (r-1)(c-1) degrees of freedom. The association between variables in contingency tables can be assessed using the chi-square test.

Example SAS code:

```
PROC FREQ DATA=EXAMPLE ORDER=DATA;
  TABLE X*Y/CHISQ;
RUN;
```

Suppose we are interested in assessing the relationship between X and Y, controlling for Z. Then the code is modified as follows:

```
PROC FREQ DATA=EXAMPLE ORDER=DATA;
  TABLE Z*X*Y/CMH NOPRINT;
RUN;
```

The NOPRINT option supresses the combination of contingency tables. The output provides summary statistics for x and y controlling (or adjusting) for z. The odds ratio (OR) and relative risk (RR) estimates are also presented. We can obtain the RR using PROC GENMOD.

Suppose we wanted to calculate the RR of illness (yes vs. no) according to exposure status (yes vs. no), adjusted for age. The following will calculate the adjusted RR.

```
PROC GENMOD DATA=EXAMPLE;
  CLASS=EXPOSED;
  MODEL Ill=EXPOSED AGE/DIST = BIONOMIAL LINK = LOG;
  ESTIMATE 'BETA' EXPOSED 1 -1/EXP;
RUN;
```

Suppose we wanted to determine the effect of a worksite safety program on people's behaviors. We can compare safety compliance before and after the intervention. This experimental design is called a paired or matched design because the subjects are observed before and after the intervention. McNemar's chi-square test is appropriate here and can be obtained using the SAS procedure code

```
PROC FREQ DATA=EXAMPLE ORDER=DATA;
Title 'McNemar's Test for Paired Samples';
  TABLE BEFORE*AFTER/AGREE;
RUN;
```

McNemar's chi-square test is also appropriate for matched case–control data.
- Logistic regression is a technique used to measure the association between a dependent and independent variable, where the dependent variable is dichotomous (has two levels) rather than continuous. Multiple logistic regression is an extension of logistic regression of two or more independent variables. NONPARAMETRIC

Example SAS code:

```
PROC LOGISTIC DATA=EXAMPLE DESCENDING;
  CLASS X;
  MODEL Y=X;
  RISKLIMITS;
RUN;
```

(Multiple logistic regression)

```
PROC LOGISTIC DATA=EXAMPLE DESCENDING;
  CLASS X SEX;
  MODEL Y=X SEX AGE;
  RISKLIMITS;
RUN;
```

- Polytomous logistic regression involves an extension of logistic regression where the response is dichotomous to a multichotomous response (e.g., no pain, slight pain, substantial pain). The response may be nominal or ordinal. For details on this method and accompanying SAS code, the reader may wish to refer to Stokes ME, Davis CS, Koch GG. Categorical data analysis using the SAS system. SAS Institute Inc., SAS Campus Drive, Cary, NC 27513.

The procedure statements in SAS may include the WHERE option, prior to MODEL, to subset the sample for analysis; the BY option, which performs the analysis on the levels of sorted variables; and the CLASS statement to create dummy variables. In addition to these commonly used options, there is an extensive array of possible options available with the different procedures, and the interested reader should refer to the SAS manuals for a list of and information about these options.

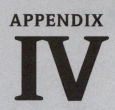

Exposure History Questionnaire

The following is an example of an exposure history questionnaire developed in 1992 by the Agency for Toxic Substances and Disease Registry (ATSDR) in co-operation with the National Institute for Occupational Safety and Health.

Part 1. Exposure Survey

Name: _____ Date: _____

Birth date: _____ Sex (circle one): Male   Female

Please circle the appropriate answer.

1. Are you currently exposed to any of the following?   no   yes
    dust or fibers   no   yes
    chemicals   no   yes
    fumes   no   yes
    radiation   no   yes
    biologic agents   no   yes
    loud noise, vibration, extreme heat or cold   no   yes
2. Have you been exposed to any of the above in the past?   no   yes
3. Do any household members have contact with metals,
    dust, fibers, chemicals, fumes, radiation, or biologic agents? no   yes

If you answered yes to any of the items above, describe your exposure in detail—how you were exposed, to what you were exposed. If you need more space, please use a separate sheet of paper.

4. Do you know the names of the metals, dusts, fibers,
    chemicals, fumes, or radiation that you are/were
    exposed to?   no   yes

If yes to question 4, list them below.

5. Do you get the material on your skin or clothing?   no   yes
6. Are your work clothes laundered at home?   no   yes
7. Do you shower at work?   no   yes
8. Can you smell the chemical or material you are working
    with?   no   yes

9. Do you use protective equipment such as gloves, masks, respirator, or hearing protectors?   no   yes

If yes to question 9, list the protective equipment used.

10. Have you been advised to use protective equipment?   no   yes
11. Have you been instructed in the use of protective equipment?   no   yes
12. Do you wash your hands with solvents?   no   yes
13. Do you smoke at the workplace?   no   yes
    At home?   no   yes
14. Are you exposed to secondhand tobacco smoke at the workplace?   no   yes
    At home?   no   yes
15. Do you eat at the workplace?   no   yes
16. Do you know of any co-workers experiencing similar or unusual symptoms?   no   yes
17. Are family members experiencing similar or unusual symptoms?   no   yes
18. Has there been a change in the health or behavior of family pets?   no   yes
19. Do your symptoms seem to be aggravated by a specific activity?   no   yes
20. Do your symptoms get either worse or better at work?   no   yes
    at home?   no   yes
    on weekends?   no   yes
    on vacation?   no   yes
21. Has anything about your job changed in recent months (such as duties, procedures, overtime)?   no   yes
22. Do you use any traditional or alternative medicines?   no   yes

If you answered *yes* to any of the questions, please explain.

Part 2. Work History
A. Occupational Profile

The following questions refer to your current or most recent job:

Job title: _____

Description: _____

Type of industry: _____

Name of employer: _____

Date job began: _____

Are you still working in this job?   yes   no

If *no*, when did this job end?

Fill in the table below listing all jobs you have worked including short-term, seasonal, part-time employment, and military service. Begin with your most recent job. Use additional paper if necessary.

Dates of Employment	Job Title and Description of Work	Exposures*	Protective Equipment

*List the chemicals, dusts, fibers, fumes, radiation, biologic agents (i.e., molds or viruses) and physical agents (i.e., extreme heat, cold, vibration, or noise) that you were exposed to at this job.

Have you ever worked at a job or hobby in which you came in contact with any of the following by breathing, touching, or ingesting (swallowing)? If *yes*, please check the circle beside the name.

_ Acids	_ Ammonia	_ Pesticides	_ X-rays
_ Chloroprene	_ Dichlorobenzene	_ Trinitrotoluene	_ Carbon
_ Methylene	_ PCBs	_ Benzene	tetrachloride
chloride	_ TDI or MDI	_ Fiberglass	_ Ketones
_ Styrene	_ Arsenic	_ Phenol	_ Rock dust
_ Alcohols	_ Ethylene	_ Vinyl chloride	_ Other (specify)
(industrial)	dibromide	_ Beryllium	_ Chlorinated
_ Chromates	_ Perchloroeth-	_ Halothane	naphthalenes
_ Nickel	ylene	_ Phosgene	_ Lead
_ Talc	_ Trichloroeth-	_ Welding fumes	_ Silica powder
_ Alkalies	ylene	_ Cadmium	_ Chloroform
_ Coal dust	_ Asbestos	_ Isocyanates	_ Mercury
_ PBBs	_ Ethylene	_ Radiation	_ Solvents
_ Toluene	dichloride		

B. Occupational Exposure Inventory

Please circle the appropriate answer.

1. Have you ever been off work for more than 1 day because of an illness related to work?   no   yes
2. Have you ever been advised to change jobs or work assignments because of any health problems or injuries?   no   yes
3. Has your work routine changed recently?   no   yes
4. Is there poor ventilation in your workplace?   no   yes

Part 3. Environmental History

Please circle the appropriate answer.

1. Do you live next to or near an industrial plant, commercial business, dump site, or nonresidential property?   no   yes
2. Which of the following do you have in your home?

    Please circle those that apply.

    Air conditioner   Air purifier   Central heating (gas or oil?)   Gas stove
    Electric stove   Fireplace   Wood   Humidifier

3. Have you recently acquired new furniture or carpet, refinished furniture, or remodeled your home?   no   yes

4. Have you weatherized your home recently?   no   yes

5. Are pesticides or herbicides (bug or weed killers; flea and tick sprays, collars, powders, or shampoos) used in your home or garden, or on pets?   no   yes

6. Do you (or any household member) have a hobby or craft?   no   yes

7. Do you work on your car?   no   yes

8. Have you ever changed your residence because of a health problem?   no   yes

9. Does your drinking water come from a private well, city water supply, or grocery store?   no   yes

10. Approximately what year was your home built?   _____

If you answered *yes* to any of the questions, please explain.

Answers to Odd-Numbered
Chapter Questions

Chapter 1

1. Environmental epidemiology is the study of distribution and determinants of health-related states or events in specified human populations that are influenced by physical, chemical, biological, and psychosocial factors in the environment.

3. Environmental epidemiology originally focused on pathogens, water quality and supply, waste control, and food quality. This focus shifted toward chemical and physical agents that affect chronic illness and injury, and that disrupt social conditions.

5. Humans are often exposed to contaminants through soil, food, water, and air. Soil can be contaminated when hazardous materials (chemicals, pathogens, etc.) either become attached to soil particles or are trapped in spaces between soil particles. Contaminates can be mixed into the soil by falling from the air or from water that flows through or over it. Exposure through food occurs when food contaminated by biological agents (pathogens such as salmonella) or harmful chemicals are consumed. Water-borne transmission occurs when poisonous chemicals or pathogens are carried into drinking water, pools, or lakes. Airborne transmission occurs when hazardous chemicals (carbon monoxide, ozone, anthrax) or harmful biological agents (viruses, bacteria, fungi) are carried through the air and inhaled.

7. A comprehensive and accurate evaluation of how humans interact with their environment is referred to as a "systems approach." In this situation, the entirety of the environmental problem is considered; in other words, the source and nature of all environmental pollutants in a region are determined; assessment is made on how and in what form people come in contact with the pollutants; studies are conducted to identify the effects the pollutants have on human health; and appropriate control measures are applied.

9. Refer to Table 1.2.

Chapter 2

1. A research problem should be specific. It should define the population of interest and variables that will be used. Finally, it should be written before conducting the study to focus the research investigation.

3. A variable is a characteristic that differs from one observation to the next and can be measured or categorized. The distinction between a dependent and independent variable relates to the research purpose. The researcher chooses how to view the variables, basing the decision on the research problem. A change in a dependent variable is measured in response to an imposed change in the independent variable. For example, how does the risk of lung cancer in uranium miners vary according to level of exposure to airborne radon and its decay products?

5. Exposure data measure the intensity and duration of potential risk factors in an epidemiological study. Exposures can be specific events or divided into durations or doses. Continuous data are often the most informative, allowing us to compute dose–response relationships. However, noncontinuous data can also be useful. Outcome data measure the occurrence or quality of the health condition of interest. While they are typically dichotomous data, they can be ordinal or continuous data as well. Standard case definitions are vital for accurate outcome data.

7. Fate and transport refers to the determination of the transport speed and synergistic effects of chemicals in their environments (groundwater, soil, gas, and atmosphere) in an effort to effectively manage ecological and human exposures to selected chemicals.

Chapter 3

1. Physical conditions and substances in the human environment that influence health.

3. Chemical contaminants monitoring programs can involve:
   a. Identifying the source
   b. Measuring the discharge at the source
   c. Determining the route of transmission
   d. Identifying transfer among the specific media
   e. Determining any transformation in the environment

5. Biomarkers are traditionally used to measure the actual level of absorption of an agent or the bioaccumulation of metabolite within the body.

7. The Centers for Disease Control and Prevention.

9. Identifying at-risk populations and limited data.

11. Meta-analysis combines studies with the same conceptual hypothesis, whereas reviews summarize and describe results from many studies.

13. Environmental injustice refers to current and future inequalities that lead to disproportionate environmental impacts on the poor and people of color. Because these groups are more likely to be exposed to environmental risks at home and at work, environmental justice is concerned with protecting people where they live, work, and recreate. Beginning in the early 1960s, the environmental justice movement, a grassroots effort, has sought to combat the distributional inequities of environmental risks through protests and dissemination of studies showing the presence of environmental injustice. Efforts such as these led the Environmental Protection Agency (EPA) to form the Office of Environmental Equity in November 1992. In addition, certain regional offices adopted specific policies to address the issue of environmental justice; in 1993, EPA New England issued a policy to ensure "the fair treatment and meaningful involvement of all people, regardless of race, color, national origin, or income, with respect to the development, implementation, and enforcement of environmental laws, regulations and policies."

Chapter 4

1. A study design is the method used to collect, analyze, and interpret observations. It allows for statistical inference between exposures and health outcomes and defines the population to which the results can be generalized. Some study designs used in environmental epidemiology are cross-sectional studies, cohort studies, and experimental studies.

3. Observational studies are studies in which health events of the subjects are observed without altering them. They are susceptible to confounding and bias and cannot establish causation as easily as experiments. Experiments are studies that analyze the effects of intervention on a health outcome. They are the best way to establish causality, but can be infeasible due to ethical concerns, rarity of outcome, time, and cost.

5. Because a case–crossover design measures exposure levels of a potential risk factor long before and immediately before its corresponding outcome occurs, dangers due to multiple exposures within a short time period can be assessed. This is useful for air pollution research especially.

7. The six primary methods or activities within meta-analysis are:
   a. Assessing evidence that a relationship or law exists and that it is relatively nonartificial

b. Examining the form of a relationship
c. Analyzing the causal or key conceptual components of the independent and dependant variables
d. Assessing the scope of a relationship
e. Analyzing the mediating process that underlies a relationship
f. Developing a model that accounts for the variance among study outcomes

Chapter 5

1. (1) Final step of editing; (2) characterize study participants; (3) provide support and rationale for the study hypothesis; and (4) provide guidance on the appropriate analytic statistical techniques to use.

3. Statistical inference is the process of using probability to make conclusions about a population based on information taken from a sample. Hypothesis testing is the method by which the ability to statistically infer a result is realized. Statistical inference also uses probability to establish a level of reliability in the rejection or lack of rejection of the study hypothesis.

5. While the numerator is the same for both types of incidence (i.e., number of cases), the denominator in the probability calculation is the number of at-risk participants at the beginning of the study for cumulative incidence. For incidence density the denominator in the rate calculation is the sum of the person-time at-risk for participants in the study.

7. e, a, c, b, d.

9. Pearson's correlation coefficient and linear regression. Both measures assume a linear association between exposure and outcome variables. Simple regression means only one independent variable, whereas multiple regression means more than one independent variable. The latter method is useful for adjusting for potential confounding factors.

The correlation coefficient merely tells us whether a linear relationship exists between two variables; it does not specify whether the relationship is cause-and-effect. This statistic is limited to linear relationships and can be misleading if outliers exist. In such cases, Spearman's rank correlation coefficient would be more appropriate.

Simple linear regression measures the association between two continuous variables, with fixed values of the explanatory variable. The method of least squares is used to estimate the regression coefficients. Statistical inference is made on the regression coefficients. Plots of the data should be considered prior to fitting a regression line to the data to identify outlying observations, if they exist, and evaluate model assumptions (e.g., linearity and constant variance).

11. Nonparametric methods are called distribution-free methods (i.e., they make fewer assumptions). Examples of nonparametric statistical tests are the Wilcoxon signed-rank test (for paired data) and the Wilcoxon rank sum test for comparing independent groups. Advantages of nonparametric methods are that the underlying populations are not required to be normally distributed, these methods can be performed relatively quickly for small samples, they are less sensitive to measurement error, and they permit the use of ordinal rather than continuous data. The disadvantage of nonparametric methods is that if the assumptions underlying a parametric test are satisfied, the nonparametric test has less power. Because nonparametric tests rely on ranks rather than on the actual values of the observations, nonparametric tests do not use everything that is known about a distribution. In addition, if a large number of observations are tied, a correction term must be added to the calculations.

Chapter 6

1. Causal inference is a conclusion about the association between the presence of a disease and reasons for its existence. It is based on connections between health and factors that can affect health (such as genetics, environment, or presence of pathogens). It provides the scientific justification for medical and public health action.

3. Consistency: Consistency exists when multiple studies using different methods, settings, and researchers all result in the same association. For example, many different studies found a link between smoking and lung cancer. In another example, multiple studies have shown that exercise reduces heart disease.

    Strength of Association: The stronger the association between the exposure and the disease, the more likely there is a causal relationship. This strength is measured by statistical methods.

    Temporality: The exposure must temporally precede the disease for a reasonable amount of time to have causal inference. This time period is called the incubation period for acute diseases and the latency period for chronic diseases.

Biologic coherence: Causal inference also requires an association between the exposure and the disease that is supported by basic human biology.

Specificity: When an exposure is associated only with one disease or a disease is associated with only one exposure, there is strong specificity. As more exposures and diseases are added, specificity decreases.

5. Predisposing factors are conditions already present that create a susceptibility to a health problem without actually causing it. Examples of predisposing factors are having AIDS with any infectious disease or skin with little pigmentation with susceptibility to ultraviolet radiation. Enabling factors assist the health problem in beginning and continuing its course. For example, prolonged exposures to high levels of ultraviolet radiation enable skin aging. Also, malnourishment enables a number of diseases, such as tuberculosis, malaria, and HIV. Precipitating factors are essential to the development of health problems. For example, failures in the genes that regulate cell growth can precipitate cancer, or the blockage of a heart valve can be a precipitating factor in a heart attack. Reinforcing factors can either support the production and transmission of health problems or support and improve a population's health status. An example of a negative reinforcing factor is the social stigma against AIDS in some countries that causes infected persons to avoid testing and treatment. An example of a positive reinforcing factor is education about clean water to those that do not know about the effects of drinking contaminated water.

7. Causal inference is built upon the appropriate use of epidemiologic study designs, statistical methods, and theory to provide a basis for making informed and effective individual and public health decisions to prevent and control adverse health outcomes.

Chapter 7

1. a) **Sentinel Event** Because the extreme heat is unexpected, so also is the number of cases of heat stroke during June. The number of cases exceeded the number of cases expected, but the cause was clearly known: exposure to increased temperatures is directly responsible for heat stroke.

   b) **Cluster** Here you may think it likely to be a sentinel event because the storm is likely responsible for the disease. However, we do not know if the storm did in fact cause the disease, and if it did we do not know what it was about the storm that brought on the disease; either contaminants got into the drinking water supply, an infectious bacteria contaminated the food sources, people's immune systems were suppressed by the weather conditions, or some other factor could have contributed to the sickness in question.

c) **Cluster** The facts that cases are continually increasing over the period of time and that factories are nearby suggest that pollutants in the air are likely contributing to respiratory problems. However, unlike lead poisoning where only one cause can be responsible, many contributors influence respiratory infection, and further investigation would be necessary to establish a significant causal relationship.

d) **Neither** The problem here is the researchers' methodology; to verify a cluster, boundaries need to be clearly defined, and should the researcher "seek out" those with the condition, he or she lays the potential for bias in his study by way of boundary shrinkage. A better way would be to collect information by way of random sample.

e) **Neither** This may look like a sentinel event because the cause is known, but the allergies during spring are not unexpected; if more people than usual experienced allergic reactions during a given season, then this would be grounds for a cluster that would require further investigation to determine the reason(s) for the rise.

3. Attack rates are calculated at the assessment stage of the investigation.

5. First, when a cluster is in search of a cause, post hoc hypotheses are involved. Hypotheses of this type are problematic because the conventional P value is interpretable only with a priori hypotheses, that is, those hypotheses established without prior knowledge of the level of the health events in a specified population. Second, with cluster investigations, disease rates have the danger of being overestimated due to "boundary shrinkage" of the population where the cluster is assumed to exist.

7.

Age	Population in Cluster Area	Expected Rate per 100,000	Expected Counts
< 40	1,612,003	4	64
40–49	299,056	4	11
50–59	224,625	10	23
60–69	135,299	34	46
70–79	93,967	41	39
80+	55,758	78	43
Total			

9. Yes.

$$z = 2(\sqrt{304} - \sqrt{226}) = 4.8$$

The P value corresponding to this z score is $p < 0.0001$, indicating that the observed number of leukemia cases is significantly higher than the expected, with almost zero probability that the result is due to chance.

11. These questions may include the following:
    1) Have only males/females or elderly/young been affected?
    2) How long have the affected individuals lived in the given area?
    3) Has there been a recent influx of people into the area (e.g., new military base, company, etc.)?
    4) Has all useful information been provided, that is, information on potential confounding factors?
    5) Is the health problem rare?
    6) Might the health problem be explained by chance?
    7) Have any new diagnostic procedures related to the health problem been recently adopted in practice?
    8) Have any new reporting procedures been put into practice?
    9) Do diagnosed cases represent reporting from a single physician?
    10) Do people have any reason, due to media or other, to now be more aware of the health problem under investigation?

Chapter 8

1. Hidden patterns and relationships are often more apparent using spatial analysis than with other methods.
3. There are two primary types of data used in GIS: geologic data and attribute data. Geologic data reference location on the earth using some coordinate system. Attribute data refer to characteristics or properties that can then be connected with the spatial data.
5. The population density can influence the distribution of cases. Perhaps a cluster of disease in a given area is merely because that area was more densely populated than in other areas. For this reason rates are preferred to counts. Rates can be compared among the affected areas or with neighboring areas, particularly rates that adjust for age, race, and gender differences among populations.

7. Vector data use x and y coordinates to construct lines, polygons, or individual points and can be used to mark roads, boundaries, or other important lines. Raster data divide an image into individual pixels where the quality of each pixel is the smallest unit of data, such as in a scanned image of a photo. As you might have guessed, raster files are much larger than vector files, and do in fact have some advantages, because they can spatially associate dramatically different factors, such as topography and health data.

9. Mapping may be used to create a visual aid in describing the health state according to place. This is a fundamental application of descriptive epidemiology. Mapping is also beneficial when investigating disease etiology because its spread and origin can be visually diagrammed. Mapping may also lead to clues about a health-state based on attribute data, which, through techniques such as multiple regression, can reveal an association of some attribute in a geographic area that is a risk factor for the event.

Chapter 9

1. If the dependent variable (y) is displayed as real data, then a change in x corresponds to a *direct* change in y. If the dependent variable is displayed as the natural log of the data, then a change in x corresponds to a *percent* change in y.

3. a) The shape of this curve shows a seasonal effect. Therefore, two cohorts of people, one living in this city and one living in a different city of similar **environment**, might be followed over time to see if there is a difference in rate for respiratory disease between people in the two cities. Other variables, such as pollution levels or pollen levels, can be included to help identify causal relationships that are believed to be biologically related to respiratory illness. You should consider autocorrelation, which can be done using lagged variables ($t - 1$, $t - 2$, etc.), and thus control the effect of the previous month's occurrence on this month's occurrence.

   b) Dependence is another way of naming autocorrelation. Differencing can control for dependence and reestablish stationarity in the model.

   c) An age effect is not likely here. However, both a period effect and a cohort effect may exist.

5. Although longitudinal data are less susceptible to confounding as ecologic studies, time-varying environmental factors (e.g., secular trend; carryover

effect–residual influence of the intervention on the outcome) can result in confounding.

Chapter 10

1. Air pollution is a broad term applied to chemical, physical (e.g., particulate matter), or biological agents that modify the natural characteristics of the atmosphere. The six common ambient air pollutants regulated by the EPA are ozone, particulate matter, carbon monoxide, nitrogen dioxide, sulfur dioxide, and lead.

3. Ground-level ozone is formed from nitrous oxides (NO_x) and volatile organic compounds (VOC) in the presence of sunlight. Sources of NO_x and VOC include motor vehicle exhaust, industrial emissions, gasoline vapors, and chemical solvents. Therefore, high levels of ozone occur in industrialized and urban areas. In addition, because sunlight is a catalyst for the reaction of NO_x and VOC to form ozone, ozone levels are typically higher during the summer than during other seasons of the year. The chemical reaction for ozone can be summarized as:

$$VOC + NO_x + Sunlight = Ozone$$

5. Two epidemiologic methods for studying air pollution are time series and geographical studies. Time–series studies are designed to compare the same population over short periods of time. Their findings relate to short-term (e.g., day-to-day) changes in a contaminant such as air pollution on health events (morbidity or mortality counts). Limitations to time–series studies include measurement errors that result from assuming that every person in a group has the same exposure level; uncontrolled confounding factors that may bias the results; recall bias or differential that are present if a group knows it is in a high-exposure category; lack of standardization of equipment for monitoring air pollutants may result in biased results; and difficulty identifying the overall health effect of air pollution from time–series studies may result from a harvesting effect (mortality displacement), which is when very ill people die only a few days earlier because of the environmental pollution. In addition, time–series analysis is not effective at identifying chronic health effects of air pollution. Geographical studies involving air pollution compare the health events of populations that have had various long-term exposure levels to ambient air pollution. It is also

possible to compare the health effects of air pollution in the same population, only at different time periods over an extended length of time with geographic studies.

7. To monitor carbon dioxide and mold, individuals can purchase carbon monoxide detectors as well as humidity monitors. Individuals can also control mold by closely monitoring pipes for leaks, isolating any leaks, and cleaning mold spots with bleach. If mold problems are substantial, individuals can hire professionals to remove mold. Professionals can also be hired to test for asbestos and radon gas.

Chapter 11

1. The two broad groups of food contaminants are chemicals such as lead, cadmium, mercury, sodium, phosphates, nitrites, nitrates, and organic compounds and biologic agents such as bacteria, viruses, parasites, and mold.

3. Fertilizers are beneficial in that they add nutrients, such as nitrogen, phosphorus, and potassium, to soil to enhance the quantity and quality of crop production. Some fertilizers also contain micronutrients, such as iron, zinc, and other metals, known to enhance plant growth. However, fertilizers can be harmful when they are not used properly or in excess. For example, nitrogen fertilizers containing nitrates and nitrites cause adverse health conditions such as methoglobinemia if used in excesses.

5. Food additives are substances that are intentionally and unintentionally added to a food product during its processing or production.

7. Acid deposition occurs when acidic pollutants in the air are deposited on the ground. Acid deposition has two parts, wet and dry. Wet deposition occurs when mild acids mix with rain, fog, snow, or hail and fall to the earth where they deposit sulfuric and nitric acids. Dry deposition refers to particles that form an acid when they mix with water in lakes and rivers. Acid deposition can alter the composition of soil, limiting important nutrients to plants and damage fish and other living organisms, materials, and human health.

Chapter 12

1. Waterborne diseases are infectious diseases that are spread primarily through contaminated water. Hepatitis, cholera, typhoid, and intestinal worms are the more common waterborne diseases. Poor sanitary conditions are prin-

cipal factors in the occurrence and propagation of water contamination. Health outcomes associated with contaminated water include diarrhea; cardiac defects; spontaneous abortions; various cancers; damage to neurological, hepatic, and immunologic function; and congenital malformations. Table 10.1 summarizes additional waterborne diseases and health outcomes.

3. Although freshwater for agriculture represents about 69% of total annual use of freshwater worldwide, followed by industry (23%) and then domestic (8%), developed countries tend to use a smaller percentage of their freshwater for agriculture and more for industry and for personal use (e.g, showers and toilets) compared with developing countries. However, developed countries suffer more from chemical discharges into water, mainly groundwater, than developing countries. Water pollution in developing countries is mainly attributed to agricultural runoff in water sources. Individuals in the developed world typically have better access to clean water than individuals in the developing world. An estimated 1.1 billion people do not have access to an adequate supply of drinking water, and 2.6 billion fail to have access to basic sanitation. Over half live in China and India.

Chapter 13

1. Natural
   - Radioactive elements in the earth's crust (radon gas, uranium, etc.)
   - Solar radiation in sunlight

   Human-made
   - Industrial: power plants, nuclear reactors, nuclear weapons, etc.
   - Radioactive wastes from industrial processes
   - Medical uses: radiation therapy, X-rays, etc.
   - Consumer products: luminous clocks and watches, glazes, tobacco, etc.

3. UVC is the most dangerous, but generally doesn't reach earth because of protection from the stratospheric ozone layer.

   UVB can cause DNA damage, leading to health hazards. It can pass through weakened areas of the ozone layer, exposing humans, and it is found in sun-tanning lamps.

   UVA is the most common form on earth, passing freely through the ozone layer. It is not generally harmful.

5. Inhalation: breathing radiation into the lungs.

   Ingestion: swallowing radioactively contaminated material into the digestive system.

   Direct or external: being in close proximity to radioactive materials.

7. Children's bodies are growing and developing, so their cells are dividing more quickly than adults. If they receive DNA damage from radiation, the cells containing damaged DNA will continue to replicate, spreading the damage over a larger portion of their bodies. This could lead to substantial future health problems.

9. Radiation-monitoring agencies and institutions are necessary because radiation poses a real health threat. Monitoring institutions seek to limit harmful forms of radiation exposure. Some of the duties of the EPA, NRC, and OSHA in monitoring and regulating radiation exposure include:
   - The EPA is the federal government agency responsible for monitoring levels of radiation and developing guidelines and regulations for safe levels of exposure.
   - The NRC regulates nuclear power plants, reactors, and wastes to ensure that they are safely handled and comply with regulations.
   - OSHA seeks to ensure safety in the workplace. It sets regulations for the hazardous jobs that may require employees to handle radioactive materials.

Chapter 14

1. Weather is a short-term event (e.g., a rainstorm, a windy day), whereas climate is the average weather conditions of an area over a long period of time (e.g., a dry, humid climate). Weather conditions are discrete events that can be linked to related health events. The relationship between climate and health has many confounding factors involved, making the research much more complex.

3. Natural
   - Melting glaciers, hurricanes, and evaporation of oceans cause a higher concentration of water vapor in the atmosphere, trapping in heat and solar radiation.
   - Increased cloud cover traps heat in the lower atmosphere.
   - Solar rays/flares increase the amount of solar energy the earth receives.
   - Volcanic eruptions fill the atmosphere with dust, gases, and aerosols that can increase the greenhouse effect.

   Human
   - Industrial processes such as burning fossil fuels, producing cement, refining oil and metals, etc. can produce and release large amounts of CO_2, which can contribute to the greenhouse effect.
   - Production of halocarbon gases deletes the ozone layer, allowing excess UV light to enter the earth's atmosphere.

5. The stratosphere contains the ozone layer—the atmosphere's key filter to keep out harmful UV light. The depletion of the ozone layer leads to global warming.

 The troposphere is where clouds and surface weather occur. Increased cloud coverage (a product of increased water vapor and temperature) can also lead to an increased greenhouse effect.

7. Decreased arctic sea ice; increased ocean levels; increased atmospheric water vapor.

9. The humidity and standing water could allow mosquitoes to populate the area. If certain species of mosquitoes moved into the area, it could bring in new diseases that previously weren't present in the area. As the mosquito population increased, the likelihood of human infection would also increase. Mosquitoes are a primary vector linked to many diseases, including yellow fever, malaria, West Nile virus, dengue fever, and viral encephalitis. Mosquito-borne diseases such as malaria cause as many as 2 million deaths each year.

11. Decrease in medicinal plants and species; ecological imbalances that lead to the emergence and spread of infectious diseases; loss of habitat leading to disappearance of predators and increase in disease-carrying prey.

13. Humans
   - Skin cancer (melanoma, basal or squamous cell carcinoma)
   - Actinic keratoses
   - Cataracts
   - Immune suppression

   Plants
   - Disrupted physiological process
   - Altered competitive balance
   - Increased plant diseases
   - Reduced survival of phytoplankton

   Animals
   - Damaged early developmental stages for several animals
   - Disruption of the food chain

Glossary

A priori hypothesis Formulation of the hypothesis before observation of an event such as an excess of cancer; that is, the hypothesis is established without prior knowledge of the level of the health events in a specified population.

Absolute risk (or just risk) The probability of disease at a given time period. It is measured by the cumulative incidence rate.

Acid Having a pH of less than 7. Any of a class of substances whose aqueous solutions are characterized by a sour taste, the ability to turn blue litmus red, and the ability to react with bases and certain metals to form salts.

Acid deposition Acidic pollutants in the air that are deposited on the ground. Wet deposition falls to earth by mixing with rain or fog, forming mild acids, or by mixing with snow or hail, forming sulfuric and nitric acids as they melt. Sunlight tends to increase the rate of these reactions. Dry deposition refers to particles that form an acid as they mix with water in lakes and rivers and as dry deposition of gases and particles.

Acid precipitation (rain) Air pollution produced when acids that form in the atmosphere because of industrial gas emissions (primarily sulfur dioxide, nitrogen oxides, burning coal and other fuels from certain industrial processes) are incorporated into rain, snow, fog, or mist.

Accuracy Measure indicating the degree to which something is correct. The accuracy of an epidemiologic finding is the extent that it is free from error.

Actinic keratoses (also called **keratosis**) A scaly or crusty bump that forms on the skin surface; the most common precancer, resulting from prolonged exposure to ultraviolet light such as sunlight.

Acute exposure   Exposure characterized by a large, single dose or series of doses of a substance in a short time period, with adverse health outcomes manifesting themselves relatively quickly.

Adjusted rate   A summary rate that through statistical modification removes the confounding effect due to factors such as age, sex, or race/ethnicity.

Age effect   The primary change in risk for a given health condition is age.

Age-adjusted rate   A statistical procedure that adjusts for differences in age distributions within a group over time or among groups at a specific time. It is calculated by taking the weighted average of the age-specific rates, where the weights are the proportions of persons in the corresponding age groups of a standard population. These rates are often preferred over crude rates because they can be compared between groups or over time without the differences influenced by the confounding effect of differences or changes in the age-distribution.

Age-standardized rates   A synonym of age-adjusted rates.

Aggregate measures   Summaries of observations based on individuals within a group.

Air pollution   A broad term applied to chemical, physical (e.g., particulate matter), or biological agents that modify the natural characteristics of the atmosphere.

Alpha level (α)   The chance of committing a Type I error that a researcher is willing to take when testing a hypothesis. The standard alpha level is 0.05, but 0.1 and 0.01 are commonly used.

Alpha particles   A tiny mass of material composed of two protons and two neutrons. They do not travel far from their radioactive source and cannot penetrate human skin. Hence, they are not considered to be an external exposure hazard. However, alpha particle sources within the human body may pose an internal health hazard if they are present in sufficiently large quantities.

Analytic study designs   A type of epidemiologic study that tests one or more predetermined hypotheses about associations between exposure and outcome variables. These designs involve a comparison group.

Analytic time–trend analysis   The ecologic association between average exposure change and disease rate change is made for a population in a single geographic area.

Atmosphere Layer of gases surrounding the earth. It is retained by the earth's gravity. The earth's atmosphere consists of 78% nitrogen, 21% oxygen, and 1% other gases.

Attack rate A cumulative incidence rate involving a specific population during a limited time period, such as during a disease outbreak.

Attribute data Generally defined as additional information on the characteristics of the object under investigation.

Attributes Demographic characteristics of those affected, such as socioeconomic status, education, and other personal variables, or features of a suspected source of disease.

Becquerel (Bq) The international standard for radioactivity (i.e., rate radioactive materials decay). One Bq refers to the amount of radioactive material required for disintegration in one second.

Beta particles A high-speed electron or positron, especially one emitted in radioactive decay. They can penetrate the dead skin layer, resulting in burns. They may cause a serious direct or external radiation threat, depending on the amount received. They may also pose a serious internal radiation threat if ingested or inhaled.

Bias A factor to consider when trying to establish the validity of a statistical association. Nonrandom (systematic) error in a study that causes a deviation of the results from the truth. In epidemiologic studies bias may result in an overestimation or underestimation of a measure of association. Common types of bias in case control studies are selection bias and measurement (recall, interviewer) bias. A common type of bias in cohort studies is loss to follow-up bias, which is a type of selection bias.

Biological coherence A criterion for judging if an association is causal. It indicates whether the association between an exposure and disease outcome is supported in terms of basic human biology.

Biological contaminants Living organisms or their associated toxins. These contaminants include bacteria, viruses, fungi, molds, and house dust. Biological contaminants can be found in water, soil, plants, and animals. They are also common in various occupational settings. Biologic agents may affect food in several ways and affect human health by producing allergic reactions, serious medical conditions, or even death.

Biologic plausibility A criterion for judging if an association is causal. It has a similar meaning to biologic coherence; however, it is broader in the sense that laboratory proof is not necessary.

Biomarkers Anatomic, physiologic, biochemical, or molecular substances that are associated with the presence and severity of specific disease states and are detectable and measurable by a variety of methods including physical examination, laboratory assays, and medical imaging.

Biomonitoring The approach of measuring pollutant levels in tissue or fluid samples.

Biosphere Part of the earth where life occurs (air, land, surface rocks, and water) and where biotic processes in turn alter or transform.

Blinding The process by which the investigator and/or the subjects are not aware of treatment assignments in experimental studies.

Boundary shrinkage The boundary where a possible disease cluster exists is ill-defined, accentuating the apparent risk by focusing the investigation tightly on the cases making up the cluster.

Carbon cycle The biogeochemical cycle in which carbon is exchanged between the biosphere, geosphere, hydrosphere, and atmosphere in the earth. The four major reservoirs (atmosphere, terrestrial biosphere, oceans, and sediments) of carbon are interconnected by pathways of exchange.

Carbon monoxide Carbon monoxide (CO) is a colorless, practically odorless, and tasteless gas or liquid. It results from incomplete oxidation of carbon in combustion.

Case definition A set of standard clinical criteria to establish if a person has a particular disease.

Case evaluation The second of three phases of the assessment stage in a cluster investigation. It involves an attempt to ensure that a biological basis is present. Diagnostic verification may involve examination of the patient's record, access to pathology and medical examiner's reports, if possible, and histological reevaluation may be warranted. However, obtaining confirmation and reevaluation may not be possible. Some conditions, injuries, or behaviorally caused occurrences have no laboratory tests that are applicable, and occupational or environmental disorders or conditions are often difficult to diagnose. Also, case evaluation is one of the phases of assessment in a cluster investigation.

Case–control study   An observation epidemiologic study where the presence of a potential risk factor or factors is compared between those with and those without the health outcome of interest. The study begins by identifying cases and controls and then investigating whether the cases were more or less likely to have been exposed than the controls. Case–control studies are best suited for chronic conditions where the latency period from exposure to disease is years or decades.

Case–crossover design   This is an observational epidemiologic study that involves comparing the exposure status of a case immediately before its occurrence with that of the same case at a prior time. Individuals serve as their own controls, with the analytic unit being time—where the time just before the acute event is the "case" time compared with some other time, referred to as the "control" time. The rationale for this study design is that if precipitating events exist, they should occur more frequently immediately prior to the onset of disease rather than during a period more distant from the disease onset. The case–crossover study design is especially appropriate where individual exposures are intermittent, the disease occurs abruptly, the incubation period for detection is short, and the induction period is short.

Case study   A snapshot description of a problem or situation for an individual or group. A case study involves a qualitative description of the facts in chronological order.

Cause   A factor that produces a change in another factor.

Causal criteria   Standards or expectations determined as necessary for there to be a causal association, such as a valid statistical association, an established time sequence of events, biologic plausibility, consistency among studies, specificity, and experimental evidence.

Causal inference   A conclusion about the presence of a disease and reasons for its existence.

Chance   A factor to consider when trying to establish the validity of a statistical association. Chance may explain a relationship between an exposure and disease outcome when the measured association is based on a sample of the population of interest. If everyone in the population is considered, then chance does not play a role. An association may exist merely because of the luck of the draw—chance. As the sample size increases, the sample becomes more like the population and the role of chance decreases. The degree to which chance variability occurs may be monitored by the P value.

Chemical contaminants   Chemicals that pose an unacceptable threat to human health and/or the environment.

Chemical poisoning   Chemical foodborne illness. Metals associated with environmental contamination and cause chemical poisonings include arsenic, antimony, cadmium, lead, and mercury.

Chi-square test of independence   A statistical test of significance that is commonly used to evaluate whether two nominal variables are associated by comparing the observed with the expected cell frequencies in a contingency table.

Chronic exposure   Long-term continuous or frequent recurrent exposure at low doses over an extended period of time.

Clean Water Act   Standards for regulating discharges of pollution in ambient water. Under the Clean Water Act, the Environmental Protection Agency (EPA) has the authority to set standards on the types and amounts of pollutants introduced into water and the task of overseeing efforts to monitor water and ensure these standards are kept. Although the Clean Water Act has historically focused on chemical pollutants and point sources of contamination, today the act addresses physical and biological pollutants, as well as watershed-based approaches to tracking contamination.

Climate   The average weather conditions of an area over a long period of time (e.g., a dry, humid climate).

Climate forcing power   A measure of imposed perturbation to the earth's energy balance.

Cluster   An unusual aggregation, real or perceived, of health events that are grouped together in time and space and that are reported to a health agency.

Cluster investigation   A review of an unusual number, real or perceived, of health events (for example, reports of cancer) grouped together in time and location.

Cohort effect   The change in the rate of a condition according to birth year.

Cohort study   An observation epidemiologic study where individuals are followed over time in order to describe the incidence or the natural history of a condition. Several outcome variables may be associated with a single exposure. This study design may be retrospective or prospective and is best suited for assessing exposure-disease relationships with a short latency period.

Common source outbreak   An outbreak traced to an exposure at a point in time, an intermittent exposure, or a continuous exposure over days, weeks, or years.

Completely ecologic analysis   The units of analysis on all variables are ecologic measures, such as the proportion exposed, the rate of injury, or the rate of disease.

Computer cartography   Computer-generated maps.

Condensation   When water vapor cools, forming clouds and sometimes rain.

Confidence interval   The probability range where a population parameter lies based on a random sample of the population. The most common reported confidence interval represents the range of values where one can be 95% confident that the population parameter lies. Confidence intervals are typically calculated for rates and measures of association in epidemiology.

Confounding   A factor to consider when trying to establish the validity of a statistical association. Confounding occurs when the relationship between a risk factor and outcome is influenced by an extrinsic factor. A confounding factor is associated with the outcome variable and independent of that association; it is also associated with the exposure.

Contingency table   A table of counts. The combination of row and column categories are called cells. One variable determines the row categories and the other variable defines the column categories.

Continuous data   Measurable values on a continuum.

Continuous source   In the context of an epidemic, it denotes the cause resulting from persons being continually exposed to a substance over a given time period, but at relatively low levels.

Criteria pollutants   Six common air pollutants dangerous to human health and environmental conditions: carbon monoxide, lead, nitrogen dioxide, ozone, particulate matter, and sulfur dioxide.

Cross-sectional study   An observational epidemiologic study where the exposure and outcome status are assessed simultaneously. They are generally descriptive but may be analytic if the hypothesis is determined prior to evaluating the data.

Cumulative incidence   The proportion of incident cases to the at-risk population at the beginning of the observation period. The denominator is the number of individuals at risk. It indicates the probability that a disease will occur in a given time period.

Cyclic pattern   Periodic, usually predictable, increases and decreases in the frequency of a selected cause of morbidity or mortality in a given population.

Data   Numerical information from selected variables; observations or measurements of a phenomenon of interest such as exposure to environmental contaminants or disease information collected about a patient, family, or community.

Dependence   In a time series, dependence refers to the correlation of observations of a variable at one point in time with observations of the same variable at prior points in time.

Dependent variable   The outcome, response, or effect that is influenced or predicted by other independent variables in a study. In environmental epidemiology, the dependent variable is typically the outcome status, based on one's exposure status, the independent variable.

Descriptive statistics   Numerical summaries from a sample that characterize the sample without any attempt to test a particular hypothesis.

Discrete data   Data that represent quantities (integer values), not just labels. A natural order exists among the data. Because it is meaningful to measure the distance between levels of discrete observations, application of arithmetic computations is appropriate, such as the mean, median, and mode.

Descriptive study design   An observational epidemiologic study that has no predetermined hypotheses. This study design simply describes what exits in a population according to person, place, and time. There are four common types of descriptive studies—case report, case series, cross-sectional, and exploratory ecologic. These studies are useful for generating hypotheses.

Differencing   A time–series concept that involves a step taken to de-trend data to control autocorrelation and achieve stationarity.

Disease investigation   An effort to enable researchers to identify possible links between environmental exposures and injury or disease. Disease investigations are a response to public concerns about disease outbreaks or clusters.

Dose–response relationship   The relationship between the amount of exposure (dose) to a substance and the resulting changes in the body function or health (response).

Ecologic study   An observational epidemiologic study where the units of analysis are groups of people rather than individuals. Generally descriptive but can be analytic if the hypothesis is formulated before analyzing the data.

Electromagnetic radiation   A stream of photons (particles with zero mass) traveling in a wave-like pattern at the speed of light. Each photon contains a certain amount of energy: those with the highest energy have the shortest wavelengths. Electromagnetic radiation can ionize an atom (remove an electron from its orbit) if the energy per photon is high enough (i.e., wavelength short enough).

Electromagnetic spectrum   A kind of radiation where electric and magnetic fields vary simultaneously, from power lines to visible light to gamma rays.

El Niño   A warming of the ocean surface off the western coast of South America. It occurs every 4 to 12 years when upwelling of cold, nutrient-rich water does not occur. El Niño affects Pacific jet stream winds, alters storm tracks, and creates unusual weather patterns throughout the world.

Endemic   In biology and ecology, endemic means that something is unique to its own place or region. In epidemiology, endemic refers to the constant presence or usual frequency of a specific disease in a particular population.

Environment (natural environment)   That which includes all living and non-living things that occur naturally on earth.

Environmental epidemiology   The study of distribution and determinants of health-related states or events in specified populations that are influenced by physical, chemical, biological, and psychosocial factors in the environment. It also involves the application of this study to prevent and control health problems. Its population focus and emphasis on identifying causal relations distinguishes it from environmental health, which is more comprehensive. It seeks to clarify the relation between environmental factors and human health by focusing on specified populations or communities. It is based on the observation that most diseases are not random occurrences, but rather are related to environmental factors that vary according to subgroups of population, place, and time.

Environmental health The theory and practice of assessing, correcting, controlling, and preventing those environmental factors that have a potentially harmful effect on human populations.

Environmental justice A process primarily concerned with combating current inequalities and preventing future inequalities that lead to disproportionate environmental impacts on the poor and people of color, who are more likely to be exposed to environmental risks at home and at work. Environmental justice is concerned with protecting people where they live, work, and recreate.

Environmental measures Physical characteristics of a place such as a home or work site for members of a group.

Environmental Public Health Indicators Project A project sponsored by the Centers for Disease Control and Prevention's Division of Environmental Hazard and Health Effects and the National Center for Environmental Health, which has compiled a summary of core indicators related to adverse health outcomes, a comprehensive list of suggested measures for these environmental health indicators, and potential data sources.

Environmental tobacco smoke (also called secondhand smoke or passive smoke) Smoke generated from the burning end of a cigarette, pipe, or cigar and the exhaled mainstream smoke that is puffed by the smokers of cigarettes, pipes, and cigars.

Epidemic A condition where an increase in the number of cases of disease occurs above what is normally expected for a given time and place.

Epidemic curve A graphic representation (histogram) of the distribution of disease cases by time of onset.

Epidemiology The study of the distribution and determinants of health-related states or events in specified populations, and the application of this study to control for health problems.

Estimated annual percent change A common measure used to describe change in trend data. It is calculated by fitting a regression line to the natural logarithm of the rates (r) using calendar year as a regressor variable.

Experimental study   An epidemiologic study where the participants in the study are deliberately manipulated for the purpose of studying an intervention effect. An intervention is assigned to selected participants to determine its effect on a given outcome. Two common types of planned experimental studies in epidemiology are randomized controlled trials and community trials. With the exception of the experimental study, all study designs are observational.

Exploratory time–trend analysis   In an exploratory time trend (or time series) a comparison of injury/disease rates over time is made for a population in a single geographic area. Age-period-cohort analysis is a special type of exploratory time–trend analysis.

Exposure   May involve an actual exposure to a substance (e.g., toxic chemical or microorganism, a behavior (e.g., where one works or socializes), or an individual attribute (e.g., age, sex, race).

External validity   The extent the results of a study are relevant to people who are not part of the study (representativeness).

Fate and transport   An important issue in managing hazardous pollutants. Fate and transport involves the determination of the transport speed and synergistic effects of groundwater, soil, gas, and chemicals in their environments.

Fertilizers   Synthetic (chemical) sources of nutrients (usually nitrogen, phosphorous, and potassium) that assist plant growth.

Fisher's exact test   A statistical test used to determine if there are nonrandom associations between two categorical variables where sample sizes are small.

Food additives   Substances that become part of a food product, by intention or not, during the processing or production of that food. Food additives can maintain product consistency, improve or preserve the nutrient value, maintain the wholesomeness of the food, control acidity and alkalinity, and enhance flavor and color.

Food contaminants   Metals or chemicals (e.g., mercury, pesticides, herbicides, aflatoxins) that make food dangerous for humans if consumed.

Gamma ray   Electromagnetic radiation emitted by radioactive decay with energies ranging from 10 thousand to 10 million electrons.

Geocoding   A geographic information system process for converting implicit information (e.g., street addresses) into explicit map images (i.e., displayed features on a map).

Geographic information system   A computer system used to store, view, edit, and analyze geographical information.

Geographic reference   May be explicit or implicit. Explicit refers to geographic information absolutely tied to the earth; it is described in terms of geographic coordinates (latitude and longitude or some national grid coordinates). On the other hand, implicit geographic reference refers to geographic information being described as a street address, census track, postal code, or forest stand identifier.

Geographical studies   The investigation of an area of the earth's surface (region) by specific underlying characteristics. The investigation may involve assessment of the interrelationships of phenomena (especially of the relationship between human society and the land, as in ecology), with regionalization, and with ties among areas.

Geosphere   The solid earth that includes continental and oceanic crust and various layers of the earth's interior.

Global measures   Attributes of groups for which no analogue at the individual level exists, such as population density, number of private medical clinics, or laws.

Global positioning system   A system of satellites, computers, and receivers that can determine the latitude and longitude of a receiver on earth by calculating the time difference for signals from different satellites to reach the receiver.

Global warming   An average increase in the earth's temperature, which in turn causes climate change as a result of both natural causes and human activities, including greenhouse gases, ozone depletion, deforestation, and volcanoes, to name a few.

Greenhouse effect   The "trapping" of infrared radiation from the earth by greenhouse gases in the atmosphere.

Greenhouse gases   Any gas that absorbs infrared radiation in the atmosphere, including water vapor, carbon dioxide, methane, nitrous oxide, chlorofluorocarbons, ozone, phosphofluorocarbons, hydrofluorocarbons, and hydrochlorofluorocarbons.

Gray   An international unit measure of absorbed dose of radiation, with 1 gray equivalent to 100 rad.

Ground-level ozone   Ozone near the earth's surface. It is a secondary pollutant formed by the action of sunlight on primary pollutants (nitrogen oxides from vehicle emissions and industry and volatile organic compounds from vehicles, solvents, and industry).

Halocarbon substances   Greenhouse gases that contain carbon and one or more halogens (i.e., chlorine, fluorine, or bromine), such as fluorocarbon, and are known to degrade ozone.

Hazard rate   An instantaneous probability of the event at a small time interval (close to zero). It is conditional in the sense that the person was at risk at time t. The hazard rate may be calculated at each specific point in time during the follow-up.

Health   The World Health Organization's definition of health is a state of complete physical, mental, and social well-being and not merely the absence of disease or infirmity.

Health-related states or events   A term used in the definition of epidemiology to capture the fact that epidemiology involves more than just the study of disease states (e.g., respiratory illness), but also includes the study of events (e.g., injury) and behaviors and conditions associated with health (e.g., hand washing).

Heavy metals   A group name for metals and semimetals (metalloids) that have been associated with contamination and potential toxicity or ecotoxicity.

Hydrological cycle   (See **Water Cycle**.)

Hydrosphere   The collective mass of water found on earth in oceans, seas, lakes, ponds, rivers, streams, underground water, ice, and atmospheric water vapor (clouds).

Hypothesis   A tentative suggestion that certain associations exist in certain activities or a chain of events. The initial hypothesis is generally based on observation, which refers primarily to empirical findings from data systematically collected.

H_2O   The chemical symbol for water. It is an odorless, tasteless, colorless liquid made up of a combination of hydrogen and oxygen. It is the most abundant molecule on the earth's surface.

Incidence   The frequency of a health-related state or event within a particular population or area. This measure captures the magnitude of a public health problem (burden).

Incidence density   Measure of the proportion of incident cases to the population at risk in the course of a given time period. The denominator is the sum of the time periods contributed by the individuals at risk of the event in the numerator.

Incidence proportion   Synonym for cumulative incidence rate or attack rate.

Incubation period   The time between exposure to an infectious agent and the development of the first signs or symptoms of a disease.

Independent variable   That which is expected to influence or predict the dependent (outcome) variable. In environmental epidemiology, the independent variable is typically exposure status, which predicts the outcome status, the dependent variable.

Internal validity   The extent that the results of a study are not attributable to bias or confounding.

Ionization   The physical process of converting an atom or molecule into an ion. This occurs by changing the difference between the number of protons and electrons.

Ionizing radiation   Radiation with shorter wavelengths and higher frequency. Ionizing radiation has enough energy to remove electrons from atoms or molecules (groups of atoms), with the high potential of damaging living tissue.

Koch's postulates   Three postulates or guidelines, published in 1880, applied by Koch to establish the etiology of anthrax and tuberculosis, although they can be generalized to other diseases. The parasite occurs in every case of the disease in question and under circumstances that can account for the pathologic changes and clinical courses of the disease. These postulates are (1) the parasite occurs in every case of the disease in question and under circumstances that can account for the pathologic changes and clinical courses of the disease; (2) it occurs in no other disease as a fortuitous and nonpathogenic parasite; and (3) after being fully isolated from the body and repeatedly grown in pure culture, it can induce the disease anew.

Kyoto Protocol   Named after the location where the conference was held, Kyoto, Japan; on December 11, 1997, delegates from the United Nations created an agreement to strengthen United Nations Framework Convention on Climate Change by setting standards for greenhouse gas emissions among countries that ratified the protocol.

Latency period   The time it takes for a disease to develop once the causes are in place. A term used with chronic diseases.

Lead   A metal found in natural deposits that is commonly used in household plumbing materials and water service lines. The long-term health effects of lead can be severe, including decreased growth, hyperactivity, impaired hearing, and brain damage.

Level of significance (also called **significance level**)   The probability value in statistics used to reject the null hypothesis.

Linear regression   A mathematical technique where a straight line is fitted to a set of data points to measure the effect of a single independent variable on the dependent variable. The slope of the line indicates the average change in the dependent variable that occurs for a unit change in the independent variable.

Lithosphere   The crust of the uppermost mantle of the earth.

Logistic regression   A form of regression in which the dependent variable is dichotomous (coded into variables of 0 and 1) and the independent variable is any type.

Longitudinal data   The same sample of respondents are observed in subsequent time periods.

Longitudinal study   An observation epidemiologic study where the same people are studied over time.

Mantel-Haenszel chi-square   A test for evaluating overall trend that is commonly used in evaluating dose–response relationships in epidemiologic studies.

Mapping   The act or process of making a map. In epidemiology, mapping of disease counts or rates is a useful approach for identifying patterns of disease according to geographic location. Disease patterns can also be shown in relation to the potential source of the disease.

Matched-paired analysis   Used to analyze matched case–control studies. The odds ratio in a matched-paired study is interpreted the same as in an unmatched case–control study, but is calculated as b/c.

McNemar's chi-square   Used to test associations between variables where paired matching was employed in a case–control study.

Meta-analysis   The process or technique of synthesizing research results by using various statistical methods to retrieve, select, and combine results from previous separate but related studies.

Moderator variable   An independent variable that moderates the association between an exposure and disease outcome; that is, the association depends on the level of the moderating variable. For example, the relationship between exercise and heart disease may be moderated by sex. If the relationship between exercise and heart disease was two times stronger for males than females, for example, then the relationship is dependent on one's sex.

Monitoring programs   A plan to measure and estimate physical conditions and substances in the human environment that influence health.

Montreal Protocol   The protocol, signed in 1987, is an international treaty to protect stratospheric ozone by stopping the emission of halocarbon gases and other substances.

Morbidity   A nonfatal condition; a disease or injury; any departure from good health.

Multilevel analysis   A modeling technique that combines information at two or more levels. For example, an individual-level analysis within each group could be performed. Then, using the results from the individual-level analysis, ecologic analysis of all groups could be performed.

Multiple logistic regression   Analogous to multiple linear regression methods when the dependent variable is dichotomous.

Multiple regression   A straightforward generalization of simple regression where there are two or more independent variables.

Nitrogen cycle   The biogeochemical cycle that describes the transformations of nitrogen and nitrogen-containing compounds in nature.

Nitrogen oxides   Gases that contain nitrogen and oxygen in varying amounts. They may be colorless and odorless. However, nitrogen dioxide (NO_2) is a common pollutant that combines with particles in the air to produce a reddish-brown appearance.

Nominal data   Data that fall into unordered categories. They are sometimes called qualitative data because they describe the quality of a thing or a person. Distinct levels differ in quality, not quantity. The categories are often represented by numbers.

Nonattainment areas Those areas where monitored concentrations of air pollution exceed the EPA standards a given number of times over a 3-year period. Regulatory consequences occur for nonattainment areas.

Nonionizing radiation Any type of electromagnetic radiation that does not carry enough energy per quantum to ionize atoms or molecules.

Nonparametric test Such tests are called distribution-free tests. They do not make assumptions about the distribution of data being considered. Examples of nonparametric statistical tests are the Wilcoxon signed-rank test (for paired data) and the Wilcoxon rank sum test for comparing independent groups.

Nonpoint-source pollution Pollution that comes from many sources rather than a single source.

Normal distribution The term is synonymous with the standard normal distribution. The normal distribution is a bell-shaped symmetric curve with scores concentrated near the mean and decrease in frequency as the distance from the mean increases. The probability density function of the standard normal distribution has mean 0 and variance 1.

Observational study Epidemiologic studies where the investigators have no control over the exposure status of the persons being assessed. Observational studies may be descriptive or analytic.

Occurrence evaluation The third of three phases of the assessment stage in a cluster investigation that involves defining the step the characteristics of the cluster.

Ocean The principal component of the hydrosphere composed of saline water. About 70% of the earth's surface is covered by ocean.

Ordinal data The ordering among categories provides additional information beyond the information provided by nominal data.

Outbreak This term carries the same definition as "epidemic," but is typically used when the event is confined to a more limited geographic area. It also may be less threatening to the public than the word "epidemic."

Outcome The health-related state or event that is being investigated in the study.

Ozone A molecule made up of three atoms of oxygen. Ozone occurs naturally in the stratosphere, providing a protective layer shielding the earth from harmful ultraviolet radiation.

Ozone depletion   Destruction of the stratospheric ozone layer that shields the earth from ultraviolet radiation harmful to life. It is caused by certain chlorine- and/or bromine-containing compounds that break down when they reach the stratosphere and then destroy ozone molecules.

Pandemic   An epidemic that is extensive, involving large regions, countries, or continents.

Panel study   A series of cross-sectional studies conducted on the same subjects (the panel) over successive time intervals.

Parameter   A measure from the population.

Partially ecologic analysis   A combination of individual- and group-level data in the analysis. For example, infant birth weight may be associated with environmental exposure to biogas from a landfill.

Particulate matter   A criteria air pollutant. Particulate matter includes dust, soot, and other tiny bits of solid materials that are released into and move around in the air.

Pathogens   An agent that causes disease, especially a living microorganism such as a virus, bacterium, parasite, or fungus.

Period effect   A change in the rate of a condition affecting an entire population at a given point in time.

Person-time rate   The rate that new cases are occurring in a population. The rate is calculated by dividing the new cases occurring during a specified time period by the total person–time units at risk of becoming a case. This measure allows each subject's contribution to the denominator of the rate calculation to be only as much time as observed in the at-risk population.

Pesticides   The descriptor applied to chemicals that are used to kill pests in order to minimize their impact on agriculture and human health. Pesticides are typically classified according to the organisms they control for, such as fungicides, herbicides, insecticides, molluscicides, rodenticides, and so on.

pH scale   A scale from 0 to 14 that reflects the concentration of hydrogen ions in solution. The lower numbers represent acidic conditions. The higher numbers represent basic, or alkaline, conditions.

Phosphorous cycle   The biogeochemical cycle that describes phosphorus as it moves through the lithosphere, hydrosphere, and biosphere.

Point prevalence   A proportion, typically expressed per 100 people, that is a measure of the magnitude of the health problem (burden).

Point source   In the context of an epidemic, it denotes the cause resulting from persons being exposed to the same exposure over a limited time period.

Poisson regression   A regression method that is appropriate when the dependent events occur infrequently, the events occur independently, and the events occur over some continuous medium such as time or area. The probability of a single event occurring is influenced by the length of the time interval. Counts or rates of rare diseases are well suited for modeling with Poisson regression.

Polycyclic aromatic hydrocarbons   A group of over 100 different chemicals that are formed during the incomplete burning of coal, oil and gas, garbage, or other organic substances such as tobacco or charbroiled meat.

Population attributable-risk   The amount of absolute risk of a disease in a population that can be attributed to the exposure. It assumes that a causal association exists between the exposure and outcome variables. It may also be thought of as the measure of excess risk due to the exposure.

Population attributable-risk percent   The percent of the absolute risk of a disease in a population that is attributed to a specific exposure.

Post-hoc hypothesis   Formulation of the hypothesis after observation of an event, such as an excess of cancer.

Precipitation   Water falling to the earth's surface in any form, such as rain, snow, sleet, or hail.

Precision   That part of accuracy concerned with the consistency or stability of the results. For example, the results of studies involving large samples are more likely to produce precise results because of the smaller chance of sampling error.

Preliminary evaluation   The first of three phases of the assessment stage in a cluster investigation. Its purpose is to quickly estimate whether an excess of the health event has occurred and to provide a description of the characteristics of the cluster.

Prevalence The number of cases of a given health-related state or event that exists in a defined population at a specified time. Prevalence is a measure that combines incidence and duration (survival, recovery).

Prevalence ratio The ratio of the prevalence rate in the exposed group to the prevalence rate in the unexposed group. This measure of association is occasionally used in cross-sectional studies.

Propagated outbreak A progressive outbreak that is transmitted from person-to-person or in some cases from indirect transmission through a vector.

Proportional hazards A useful model for analyzing time-to-event (or survival) data. The model indicates the probability that a person will experience an event (e.g., death) in the next interval of time, given that they have survived until the beginning of the interval. The model assumes an underlying hazard function, which describes how hazard (or risk) changes over time for a baseline or reference group (e.g., risk among the unexposed).

P **value** The probability that a given result is due to sampling error. The higher the *P* value, the more likely sampling error accounts for an observed association. An association is typically considered to be statistically significant when the corresponding *P* value is equal to or less than 0.05. In exploratory studies, the *P* value may be higher (such as 0.1). If the researcher wants to be more conservative, the *P* value may be lower (such as 0.01).

Rad (radiation absorbed dose) Measures the amount of radiation energy transferred to some mass of material, typically humans. One roentgen of gamma radiation exposure results in about one rad of absorbed dose. For gamma rays and beta particles, 1 rad of exposure results in 1 rem of dose.

Radionuclide Radioactive elements, naturally occurring or synthetic, that emit various types of energetic radiation (e.g., alpha and beta particles and gamma radiation). Their half-lives may be as little as a minute fraction of a second or as much as many thousands of years.

Random error A nonsystematic type of error that occurs by chance. Sampling error is an example of random error.

Raster data An abstraction of the real world, where the raster is a form of spatial data stored as a matrix of cells or pixels. Raster data are represented by a grid of rectangular cells covering a given area.

Rate base A unit of measure commonly used in expressing rates. It is used to avoid fractional rates and allows the rate to be expressed per 10^m, where m is typically between 2 and 5. For example, an incidence rate of female breast cancer for women ages 50 years and older of 0.0035 may be expressed as 350 per 100,000, using 100,000 as the rate base.

Rate ratio Ratio of the person–time incidence rate in the exposed group to the person–time incidence rate in the unexposed group. It measures the strength of association between the exposure and outcome variables.

Regression A statistical analysis for assessing the association between two variables.

Relative risk (also called **risk ratio**) The ratio of the absolute risk of a health-related state or event among the exposed group to the absolute risk of the disease among the unexposed group. It is a measure of the strength of association between exposure and outcome variables.

Rem (roentgen equivalent man) A unit that relates the dose of any radiation to the biological effect of that dose.

Research problem Formulation of the interrelationship among a susceptible host, agent of disease or injury, and permissive environment that produces disease or injury according to person, place, and time.

Research question Specific inquiry about the association between an exposure and health outcome.

Risk The probability of an event occurring in a given time period.

Risk assessment A process in which information is analyzed to determine if an environmental hazard might cause harm to exposed persons and ecosystems.

Risk factor A factor that is associated with the increased probability of a human health problem.

Risk management The integration of recognized risk, risk assessment, development of strategies to manage risk, and mitigation of risk through managerial resources.

Risk ratio (See **Relative risk**.)

Safe Drinking Water Act Established in 1974 to protect the quality of drinking water in the United States. The law covers all waters that may be used for drinking use, whether above or below ground. The act authorizes the EPA to set safe quality standards for drinking water.

Seasonal trend   Periodic increases and decreases in the occurrence, interval, or frequency of disease. These patterns tend to be predictable.

Secular trend   A long-term change in the rate of a given disease, injury, or death in a specified population.

Semi-ecologic cohort   Combination of ecologic and individual-level data.

Sensitivity   The proportion of patients with a given outcome who have a positive test.

Sentinel event   Occurrences of unexpected health-related states or events that occur from specific, recognized causes that are known to be associated with the health event.

Sievert   A radiation-related definition that is a unit used to derive a quantity called equivalent dose. It is intended to reflect the biological effects of radiation, not the physical effects, which are characterized by the absorbed dose, measured in grays.

Skewed distribution   Asymmetry in the distribution of the sample data values; that is, values on one side of the distribution are farther from the middle than values on the other side. For positive (or right) skewness, the usual measures of location will be different values (mode < median < mean). For negative (or left) skewness, the measures of location will also be different values (mode > median > mean).

Small-particle pollution   Fine particles of soot produced by power plants or diesel engines.

Smog   Air pollution that is a mixture of smoke and fog.

Spatial data   Data that pertain to spatial elements, such as location, and may contain information about the shape and size and relationship to other entities.

Specification   A time–series concept that involves testing for linear versus nonlinear dependence, followed by specification of the model (e.g., autoregressive moving average, threshold autoregressive, exponential autoregressive, etc.).

Specificity   The proportion of individuals without a given outcome who have a negative test.

Standardized mortality ratio   The ratio of the number of observed deaths in the comparison population to the number of expected deaths based on the specific rates in the standard population.

Standardized registration ratio   The ratio of the number of observed incident events in the comparison population to the number of expected incident events based on the specific rates in the standard population.

Stationarity   In a time series, results when the mean value of the series remains constant over time (i.e., there is no trend).

Statistic   A measure from the sample. Statistics are used to characterize data from a sample and measure associations between variables.

Statistical Analysis System   A software programming language for performing selected analyses.

Statistical inference   Inference about a population from a sample taken from the population; that is, the use of statistics to make inferences about some unknown aspect of the population.

Strength of association   A criterion used for judging if an association is a causal association. A strong direct association between an exposure and disease outcome increases the likelihood of there being a causal association. In general, weak associations provide little support of causal association. Stronger associations are less likely explained by chance, bias, or confounding.

Study design   The program that directs the researcher along the path of systematically collecting, analyzing, and interpreting results; it is a formal approach of scientific or scholarly investigation.

Study hypothesis   Suggested explanation for the presence of a certain pattern or association between elements of a system, such as a chemical exposure and adverse health outcome.

Study subjects   Persons that are the object of scientific investigation.

Sulfur cycle   Compounds such as sulfur dioxide, elemental sulfur, sulfuric acid, salts of sulfate, or organic sulfur, which are transported by physical processes like wind or erosion by water, by geological events like volcanic eruptions, or by biological activity. They are also transformed by chemical reactions.

Sulfur dioxide   The chemical compound with the formula SO_2; that is, a compound composed of one sulfur and two oxygen molecules. It is a toxic gas that comes from volcanoes and industrial emissions.

Systems approach   Viewing a health problem in its entirety by determining the source and nature of each environmental contaminant or stress; assessing how and in what form it comes into contact with people; measuring the health effect; and applying controls when and where appropriate.

Target population   The population for which the results are intended to be generalized.

Temporality   A criterion used for judging if an association is a causal association. For an exposure to cause a disease it must temporally precede the disease at a reasonable interval.

Teratogenic   Capable of disturbing the growth of an embryo or fetus. Many different chemicals and environmental factors are teratogenic in humans, including ionization, radiation, certain infections (e.g., herpes virus, rubella virus, syphilis), metabolic imbalance (e.g., alcoholism, diabetes, folic acid deficiency), drugs and environmental chemicals (e.g., chlorobiphenyls, Dioxin, ethanol, teteracyclines, uranium).

The inner versus outer environment   From the perspective of the human body, there are two environments, the inside and the outside. Three barriers separate these environments: the skin, the gastrointestinal tract, and the lungs.

The personal versus ambient environment   The personal environment refers to that in which people have control (e.g., hygiene, diet, sexual practices, exercise) compared with the ambient environment in which they have virtually no control.

The physical, chemical, biological, and psychosocial environments   These are four avenues or mechanisms by which selected factors may affect human health. Physical factors include workplace injuries, traffic accidents, excessive noise, heat, and cold, and radiation exposure; chemical factors include toxic waste, pesticides, and preservatives; biological factors include organisms that may contaminate food and water, organisms transmitted by fomites or vectors, and those transmitted from person to person; and psychosocial factors include education, income, nutrition, medical care, and other factors that affect one's psychological development.

The solid, liquid, and gaseous environments   Each of these environments is subject to pollution. What occurs in one environment often affects another environment. People interact with each of these environments.

Time–series designs   A sequence of measurements of some numerical quantity made at or during successive periods of time.

Time–series studies   Studies designed to compare the same population over short periods of time. Their findings relate to short-term (e.g., day-to-day) changes in a contaminant such as air pollution on health events (morbidity or mortality counts).

Toxicokinetics   An area of study of how a substance enters the body and the course it takes while in the body.

Ultraviolet radiation   Electromagnetic radiation with a wavelength shorter than that of visible light. For radiation in the ultraviolet region of the spectrum, wavelengths are measured in nanometers (nm), with 1 nm = one millionth of a millimeter.

Unit of analysis   That which is being studied; that is, the object of a study. The unit of analysis may be a person or a population (as in an ecologic study).

United Nations Framework Convention on Climate Change   An international body that has taken steps to reduce greenhouse gas emissions and respond to the impacts of climate change.

United Nations Global Environment Monitoring System (GEMS)   Established in 1978, it is the primary source for global water-quality data. Key activities include monitoring, assessment, and capacity-building throughout the world. The state and trends of regional and global water quality are provided through GEMS.

U.S. Clean Air Act   A comprehensive federal law that regulates all sources of air pollutants emissions. In 1970, the Clean Air Act (CAA) authorized the Environmental Protection Agency to establish National Ambient Air Quality Standards (NAAQS) to protect the environment and the public health. In 1977, the CAA was amended to set new goals and dates for achieving NAAQS. Regulations were also established to prevent any deterioration in air quality above an established baseline level. In 1990, the CAA was further amended to meet problems such as acid rain, ground-level ozone, stratospheric ozone depletion, and air toxics.

UVA radiation   Band of ultraviolet radiation that has wavelengths just shorter than visible violet light (wavelengths 320–400 nanometers). It is not absorbed by stratospheric ozone.

UVB radiation   Band of ultraviolet radiation that is mostly absorbed by stratospheric ozone (wavelengths 280–320 nanometers). UVB that does contact earth (or received from sun lamps) can damage DNA, crops, and marine organisms. In humans it is a risk factor for melanoma of the skin and other types of skin cancer.

UVC radiation   Band of ultraviolet radiation entirely absorbed by stratospheric ozone and normal oxygen (wavelengths shorter than 280 nanometers). It is responsible for generating ozone. UVC rays have the highest energy and the most dangerous type of ultraviolet light.

Validity   That component of accuracy reflecting the level of systematic error in the study.

Variable   A characteristic that differs from one observation to the next and can be measured or categorized.

Vector   An invertebrate animal (e.g., tick, mite, mosquito, bloodsucking fly) capable of transmitting an infectious agent among vertebrates.

Water   A common chemical substance that is essential to all known forms of life.

Water cycle   Movement of water around, over, and through the earth: water storage in ice and snow, water storage in the atmosphere, groundwater storage, precipitation, groundwater discharge, stream flow, snowmelt runoff, surface runoff, freshwater storage, water storage in oceans, and evaporation.

Water pollution   Adverse effects upon bodies of water (lakes, rivers, oceans, groundwater) produced by human activities, making them unsafe for drinking, fishing, swimming, and other activities.

Weather   A short-term event (e.g., a rainstorm, windy day), whereas climate is the average weather conditions of an area over a long period of time (e.g. a dry, humid climate). Weather conditions are discrete events that can be linked to related health events.

Webs of causation   Graphical, pictorial, or paradigm representations of the complex conditions or events caused by an array of activities connected to a common core (the disease or injury).

Wilcoxon rank sum test   A nonparametric statistic used to compare the locations of two populations, to identify if one population is shifted compared with the other. The sum of ranks is compared with this method.

Index

Page numbers followed by *f* denote figures; those followed by *t* denote tables